THE THYROID DEBACLE

ERIC BALCAVAGE AND KELLY HALDERMAN

BALBOA.PRESS
A DIVISION OF HAY HOUSE

Copyright © 2022 Eric Balcavage and Kelly Halderman.

All rights reserved. No part of this book may be used or reproduced by any means, graphic, electronic, or mechanical, including photocopying, recording, taping or by any information storage retrieval system without the written permission of the author except in the case of brief quotations embodied in critical articles and reviews.

Balboa Press books may be ordered through booksellers or by contacting:

Balboa Press
A Division of Hay House
1663 Liberty Drive
Bloomington, IN 47403
www.balboapress.com
844-682-1282

Because of the dynamic nature of the Internet, any web addresses or links contained in this book may have changed since publication and may no longer be valid. The views expressed in this work are solely those of the author and do not necessarily reflect the views of the publisher, and the publisher hereby disclaims any responsibility for them.

The author of this book does not dispense medical advice or prescribe the use of any technique as a form of treatment for physical, emotional, or medical problems without the advice of a physician, either directly or indirectly. The intent of the author is only to offer information of a general nature to help you in your quest for emotional and spiritual well-being. In the event you use any of the information in this book for yourself, which is your constitutional right, the author and the publisher assume no responsibility for your actions.

Any people depicted in stock imagery provided by Getty Images are models, and such images are being used for illustrative purposes only. Certain stock imagery © Getty Images.

Print information available on the last page.

ISBN: 979-8-7652-2799-2 (sc)
ISBN: 979-8-7652-2797-8 (hc)
ISBN: 979-8-7652-2798-5 (e)

Library of Congress Control Number: 2022907838

Balboa Press rev. date: 06/01/2022

This book is dedicated to the millions of people struggling with hypothyroidism and other chronic health problems. It is dedicated to those feeling lost, frustrated, and ignored. It is dedicated to those stuck on the medical merry-go-round with no idea how to get off the hellish ride.

We know what you are experiencing is real. We know there is a better way to improve your health and quality of life than what you have been offered.

You have inspired us to write this book. It is our hope that you will use the information in this book to find your path to a higher state of health and vitality.

DISCLAIMER

Though every effort has been made to ensure the accuracy of information presented herein, the authors are not engaged in providing any type of professional advice or other services to the individual reader. The material contained in the book is not intended to be, and cannot be taken as, a substitute for the advice and counsel of one's physician or other professional licensed health-care providers. The authors shall not be liable for any loss, injury, or damage allegedly arising from any information or suggestions in this book.

No part of this publication may be reproduced or distributed in any form or by any means, electronic or mechanical, or stored in a database or retrieval system, without prior written permission from the publisher and authors.

ACKNOWLEDGMENTS

First and foremost, we would like to thank our families. Writing this book has been a long, arduous, time-consuming road, and we know we would not have been able to cross the finish line without your patience and support for our passion.

To our teachers, mentors, and friends who have contributed immeasurably to our knowledge and skill, we thank you. To our current and past patients, thank you for challenging us, trusting us, and teaching us through your healing journeys. We are honored to be able to help you and are committed to the advancement of care.

CONTENTS

Foreword xiii
Introduction xvii

PART 1: CONFESSIONS OF AN ALLOPATHIC DOCTOR

Chapter 1:   The Journey from Physician to Patient 1
Chapter 2:   Thyroid Anatomy and Physiology 14
Chapter 3:   Pathologies of Thyroid Physiology 21
Chapter 4:   Thyroid Evaluation and Treatment 39
Chapter 5:   Challenges with the Current Thyroid Model 64

PART 2: HYPOTHYROIDISM SEEN THROUGH A NEW LENS

Chapter 6:   A Paradigm Past Its Prime 83
Chapter 7:   A New Perspective 97
Chapter 8:   Looking Beyond TSH 107
Chapter 9:   The Evolution of a Hypothyroid Condition 137
Chapter 10: Hypothyroidism Is a Spectrum Disorder 152
Chapter 11: The Impact of Cellular Hypothyroidism 168
Chapter 12: Interpreting Thyroid Lab Tests 191

PART 3: THE STRATEGIC THYROID SOLUTION

Chapter 13: The Dichotomy of Health 219

Chapter 14: Dietary Fitness 226

Chapter 15: Sleep Fitness 245

Chapter 16: Respiratory Fitness 261

Chapter 17: Emotional Fitness 277

Chapter 18: Physical Fitness 292

Chapter 19: Habitual Fitness 308

Chapter 20: Environmental Fitness 318

Chapter 21: Metabolic Fitness 333

Chapter 22: Genetic Fitness 343

Chapter 23: Epilogue 355

Endnotes 361

FOREWORD

As a medical student, you want to think your medical school and supervising physicians are doing the right thing. You want to believe that you're getting the best possible training from the best in the business. In time, the realization sets in, and you find out this is not the case.

I didn't enroll in just any medical school. I enrolled in the top naturopathic medical school in the nation, Bastyr University. It was here that I was going to learn how the body functions, how it breaks, and how to restore it naturally. Yes, naturally. I wasn't interested in big pharma. I wasn't interested in surgery. I was fascinated by how the body has an inherent ability to heal. Our job as naturopathic physicians is to assist patients in healing using nutrition, mindset, sleep, and a clean environment.

Patient after patient, shift after shift, I saw patients diagnosed with hypothyroidism. Instead of herbal tinctures, supplements, or lifestyle changes, I found myself being told to prescribe thyroid medications of various types. At first I was okay with that because I was writing prescriptions, and I saw some patients getting better. Over time, though, I questioned why we were doing it. I recall a conversation in which this statement stood out: "It's the standard of care, and it's very economical."

I wasn't interested in what was standard. I already knew what was standard, which is why I had decided to become a naturopathic physician instead.

Over and over, I tried using naturopathic principles versus following the standard of care when I had a patient diagnosed with hypothyroidism. I didn't come here to prescribe meds to people. My supervising doctors shot me down. So out came the script pad, and down went the usual prescription of Synthroid, sometimes Armour, and, when we were being really fancy, a combination of Synthroid and Cytomel.

Thankfully, I ended up getting called into the dean's office, where I was informed that I had caused quite a stir among students who felt the same way I did regarding the treatment of our hypothyroid patients. I listened to the dean explain why we did things the way we did and how we had to follow the guidelines. I nodded without smiling and shared my honest feelings about why I was displeased.

After my talking-to, a few of the supervising physicians approached me personally. They told me they would make more of an effort to use the naturopathic principles around treatment. Some did change their ways, but others decided not to.

It's easy to fall into the habit of prescribing thyroid meds. It is indeed inexpensive, fast, and, at times, effective. Results can come quickly, and patients are happy. But that happiness is short-lived, as the underlying cause of hypothyroidism continues to fester.

Some patients got worse. They felt anxious, couldn't sleep, and still struggled with symptoms of hypothyroidism: hair falling out, dry skin, brain fog. They were confused, and so were the supervising doctors.

After I graduated, I continued not treating people with thyroid disorders in the way I was taught. In fact, I learned from a fantastic naturopathic physician, a couple of them, who treated lots of patients with hypothyroidism without even addressing the thyroid. Instead they focused on other things. It worked, and it worked very well.

I never treated the thyroid directly when it came to thyroid disorders. I still don't.

You'll learn in this book why it makes sense. You'll also learn why oftentimes you and countless others actually feel much worse than you otherwise would when taking thyroid meds to treat your hypothyroidism.

Look, my wife struggles off and on with Hashimoto's thyroiditis. There is no cure for her. There is no cure for anyone. The cure doesn't exist. The job of patients with this disease is to keep the body in homeostasis, and that isn't easy.

My wife feels worse when taking thyroid meds. She feels worse when stressed out, when she doesn't sleep well, when routine sets in, and when she doesn't get to do her hot yoga or spend time in her sauna. There are times when she decides to take a nibble of dairy or taste something with gluten in it. I know what's going to happen, and so does she.

Years of running labs and seeing her patterns allow me to understand when she's going to have antibodies against her thyroid and when her thyroid parameters will be off. In fact, I've basically told her there is no point in ordering thyroid labs anymore because we know when they're going to be off and what has to be done about it. These are basic fundamentals.

Dig into this book. Learn how your thyroid works, what dirties it, and how you can clean it up. If you're taking thyroid medications and they are helping you, perhaps you can dig deep in the preceding pages and learn how to taper off your meds with your doctor and get off of them completely. On the other hand, if you're on thyroid medications and they are not helping you, you, too, will benefit from diving in deeply and learning why you're struggling.

Some of you have no thyroid gland and need thyroid meds to survive. Keep taking them, but do follow the guidelines in this book so you can help your meds work better. In time, you'll feel better than ever.

This is not your usual thyroid book—thank goodness. It brings in two great minds.

Dr. Kelly was trained in the traditional medical management of hypothyroidism in medical school. She brings in the perspective of what she learned in medical school and residency on treating hypothyroidism. She is able to add the perspective of how your doctor may currently be managing your hypothyroidism based on medical guidelines. Because of her own diagnosis of hypothyroidism and her frustration with having symptoms despite being on medication to normalize her thyroid-stimulating hormone (TSH), she sought to learn from doctors like Dr. Eric how to really recover. And she did.

Dr. Eric, whom I've known for a long time, digs and digs. He doesn't stop until he understands all the nuances of something. He is a go-to for me when it comes to thyroid stuff, and now you're holding the work of a book.

Get after it and enjoy finally learning what you really need to know about thyroid physiology.

—Dr. Ben Lynch, author of the best-selling book *Dirty Genes*

INTRODUCTION

I'm Dr. Eric Balcavage, and I have spent two decades helping my patients recover from chronic hypothyroid symptoms. I've lectured to doctors, explaining how the current medical model of thyroid care, including the tests used to evaluate thyroid physiology, is outdated. Many times it's ineffective at improving symptoms and, in my opinion, potentially detrimental to long-term health.

When most people, doctors included, think about thyroid conditions, they are referring to the thyroid gland, the butterfly-shaped gland positioned just about in the middle of your neck. This gland produces several hormones; the most significant are thyroxine, or T4, and triiodothyronine, or T3.

What is often missed is that thyroid physiology includes the whole cycle from the production of thyroid hormones to their use by cells and tissues, which extends well beyond the thyroid gland. I believe that the most critical aspect of thyroid physiology is not what occurs within the thyroid gland but what is happening away from the gland, especially in the individual cells of the body.

Why would I say that? Because hypothyroid symptoms are caused by reduced amounts of thyroid hormone reaching the receptors inside the cells. Ultimately, as you will learn through this book, thyroid physiology is influenced by so much more than how much thyroid hormone is produced by the thyroid gland. The gland is important, but if the thyroid gland is damaged, destroyed, or removed, and all the downstream complexity of thyroid physiology is working optimally, treatment with thyroid hormone replacement will keep thyroid physiology in the cells functioning properly. The treatment should eliminate the signs and symptoms of hypothyroidism. A person's metabolism and health can return to normal. However, when the thyroid physiology away from the thyroid gland and away from thyroid hormone production is compromised, no amount or type of thyroid hormone, whether made by the gland or provided as medication, will restore optimal thyroid physiology.

It is my opinion that traditional or allopathic medicine has a myopic view of thyroid physiology. Its focus has always been on the thyroid gland and the overproduction or underproduction of T4. Allopathic medicine has forgotten or disregarded the fact that thyroid hormones primarily function within our cells and tissues.

I don't make these claims lightly. I've read hundreds of published papers. I've been in the trenches with patients. I've seen firsthand the frustration that so many people struggle with when they know something is wrong with their health, and often specifically with their thyroid physiology. Most people don't use that term, but they just know that something is wrong, regardless of their thyroid hormone levels or what their medical doctors say. I have seen the exasperation of people who waited months to see endocrinologists only to be told that nothing was wrong with their thyroid gland because one or two of their lab test results were normal.

An antiquated view of thyroid physiology has ruined people's health, their relationships, and even their lives. That seems harsh, but it's true. When you feel chronically unwell and doctors tell you that nothing is wrong, your unrelenting sense that something is wrong wears on you, your relationships, and your quality of life. I have patients who cry in frustration during the initial consultation as they explain the impact that their chronic symptoms have had on their lives. They tell me about how their family and friends start to think of them as hypochondriacs since their doctors can't find anything wrong with them.

My aim in writing this book is not to blame anyone for what I call the "the thyroid debacle." Instead I want to provide people like you, who are struggling under the current medical model of thyroid care, with answers. I also want to give health-care practitioners a different lens through which to look at thyroid physiology. I know many patients and doctors are frustrated with the current medical model of thyroid care. By offering a different view and explanation of thyroid physiology, I hope to help doctors and patients grasp why thyroid physiology extends beyond the thyroid gland and TSH. Ultimately this understanding will change diagnoses and treatments, and provide relief for those with chronic symptoms.

When doctors and patients look at thyroid physiology through this new lens and address the root causes of its alterations, the struggle with chronic thyroid symptoms can fade away. Whether you have a specific thyroid diagnosis or not, whether you are taking thyroid hormone replacement therapy or not, this new approach can restore your health and quality of life.

MY STORY

I never intended to focus on thyroid challenges. However, I was pulled into thyroid physiology because I wanted to help a family member diagnosed with hypothyroidism. It didn't take me long to realize there were problems with the current medical model of thyroid care.

Allopathic doctors (a.k.a. medical doctors) are taught to consider just two lab values when evaluating thyroid physiology: thyroid-stimulating hormone (TSH) and free T4 (fT4). (T4 in the blood is bound to a protein or is free. Free thyroid hormone can enter the cells.) Those who have been through the grinder of thyroid care may be familiar with these two hormones and the blood tests that measure them. For those that haven't, it's okay. We will get to what these lab tests are and what they represent in the following chapters.

It is assumed that these two values, the amount of these hormones in the blood, can determine the state of thyroid physiology throughout the whole body. Even if you have symptoms commonly associated with hypothyroidism, the medical guidelines say that you don't have hypothyroidism if your TSH and fT4 values are within a normal range. However, as soon as your lab test results are abnormal, even by a tenth of a point, your doctor is likely to say you have a thyroid condition and will treat you with thyroid hormone replacement therapy. This model did not make sense to me.

Laboratory testing was not new to me. Before I became a doctor of chiropractic, I was a medical technologist. My job was to administer and process laboratory tests, including thyroid panels, which measure a group of thyroid hormone levels in the blood. Throughout my training, I was taught that these tests were carried out to confirm a diagnosis and that only tests that could provide evidence supporting the suspected thyroid problem should be performed. My problem with this approach is the same problem I have with most of the tests doctors typically order today: They aren't thorough enough.

Limited testing looks only for what the doctor already assumes is most likely to be causing the problem, disorder, or disease. It works well if the doctor's thought process and diagnosis are accurate. It works well if the culprit is a disease. It works well if you are looking to change only one variable with drug treatment. It may work well in crisis care. And it works really well if the goal is to contain costs, at least initially.

This model breaks down because when a thyroid panel of blood tests is limited to TSH (and maybe fT4), it's impossible to get a complete picture of what is happening in a person. One lab value can be influenced by many factors, making it appear normal or abnormal. Without an extensive panel of blood tests, a doctor can't determine whether one particular test result is significant or not.

Throughout this book, you will find that one test result by itself often has little value. Why? Because when we look at lab values, we must consider what is happening with the person. We must consider *why* a value is out of range. Lab test results should tell us something about our patients. They are signposts of problems but not *the* problem.

The current medical model for many situations is focused on normalizing lab values. Of course, we also try to normalize them with appropriate treatment in functional medicine, but the approach is different. For instance, if your cholesterol level is elevated, the traditional medical approach is to prescribe a statin to lower it into the normal range. The idea is that a high value is bad, and if a medication can inhibit cholesterol production and reduce the cholesterol level, then your health is improved.

In functional medicine, we look at that high cholesterol value differently. We ask what would cause cholesterol levels to be elevated. There are many reasons cholesterol could become elevated, but one of the primary reasons is reduced thyroid hormone in the cells of the liver. Without sufficient thyroid hormone (T3) reaching the thyroid receptors inside liver cells, cholesterol can't be cleared from the body, causing it to build up in the blood. Sure, we could suppress cholesterol with medication, but that does not address the cause. It doesn't address the hypothyroid state in the liver or the cause of the hypothyroid state in the liver.

The medical solution for high cholesterol requires lifetime treatment with a statin medication to keep the value suppressed and never addresses the root cause. Instead it allows the real issue to fester on, contributing to a downward spiral of health, more symptoms, and more medications.

When we run a broader array of tests, we see a more comprehensive picture of what is going on and the clues as to why a lab value is out of range. For example, beyond cellular hypothyroidism in the liver, a few other possibilities may cause cholesterol levels to rise. So the way to narrow the field of possibilities is to look at the clues provided by a comprehensive set of lab tests. We can decipher clues within more complex lab panels and find answers to why a person has high cholesterol. If only a few targeted tests are done, a doctor will miss those clues entirely.

Allopathic medicine focuses on treatment with pharmaceuticals and surgery. The tools in the traditional toolbox are directed toward normalizing the lab values, often without consideration as to the impact that the forced normalization will have on the rest of a patient's physiology. Many medications used to push a lab value into a normal lab reference range have significant side effects.

Also, if you read the label of medication or look up its mechanism of action—that is, how it works in the body—you'll often find that it's unknown. For example, in the case of an elevated cholesterol level, a statin may lower a patient's cholesterol, but at what cost to the rest of his or her physiology? Lowering cholesterol with a drug does not address the compromised physiology causing it to rise in the first place. It is not the medical doctors' fault; this is the model they were taught.

You might think of it this way: If the oil light came on in your car, wouldn't you want to know why? Is your vehicle low on oil, or is there a problem with the oil sensor? Does putting a piece of tape over the oil light so you can't see it change the fact that it came on in the first place? Wouldn't fixing the cause be a better long-term solution?

Lab values are meant to be interpreted, not just read as high or low and then forced back into a normal range. They provide information that helps your doctor understand how the body is working. Your doctor should be determining why the test value is out of range and what the abnormal value indicates, not just hammer it back into a normal range artificially.

Limited testing is a significant problem throughout health care, especially in thyroid physiology. When doctors run only narrow thyroid panels, they can't see what is really happening with thyroid physiology. The thyroid gland and the specific hormones it produces have a significant impact on metabolism. Measuring only the levels of TSH and maybe fT4 in the blood cannot provide a doctor with a proper understanding of your thyroid physiology. It doesn't reveal what is happening in your peripheral cells, the cells located away from your thyroid gland. Without the rest of a comprehensive thyroid and metabolic panel, there is no context to help determine whether the TSH value is appropriate or inappropriate.

By the way, the term "comprehensive" means different things to different practitioners. An endocrinologist considers a comprehensive thyroid panel of blood tests to be a test for TSH and fT4. A functional medicine practitioner includes an additional eight thyroid blood tests. Our comprehensive metabolic panels measure sixty-five different components plus urinalysis. An allopathic physician might consider a comprehensive metabolic panel to be eighteen tests or less.

Looking only at TSH and deciding whether thyroid physiology is functioning appropriately is like taking one word out of a novel and thinking you know what the whole book is about. It's crazy! But let me get back to my own story.

I started attending functional medicine conferences to learn more about thyroid physiology. The education and training helped me understand that the medical model is too simplistic and basic to fully evaluate the gland and the action of its hormones. I quickly realized that the medical model is directed toward diagnosing, treating, and managing the disease of the thyroid gland while giving little attention to understanding why the thyroid gland stopped working properly. In the medical model, the cause of hypothyroidism doesn't matter, because the only treatment is the normalization of TSH with thyroid medication. The only solution, the only tool in the toolbox, is a lifetime of taking medicine.

I love the concept of functional medicine, which focuses on finding the root cause of hypothyroidism and reduced health. In the United States, hypothyroidism's primary cause is Hashimoto's thyroiditis, which is an autoimmune condition. Functional medicine trains doctors to look for the cause of Hashimoto's thyroiditis and not merely treat its symptoms pharmaceutically or manipulate TSH back into range. I was taught Hashimoto's thyroiditis is the result of an out-of-control immune system. If we find what is triggering the autoimmune attack—an organism, toxin, or food—and remove it, we can reduce the attack on the gland and improve the health of the person with hypothyroidism.

The functional medicine philosophy works well, but it didn't answer all the questions swirling around in my head, such as, 'Why does the immune system start attacking the thyroid gland in so many people?' and, 'Why is the immune system out of control?'

In my functional medicine training, I was told that among the reasons why the immune system loses control and attacks the body is a phenomenon known as molecular mimicry. The theory is that sometimes foreign antigens and self-peptides (self-tissue) look so similar to the immune system that not only do our bodies attack the foreign antigen, but they attack our own tissue as well. I continued to study functional medicine and asked many questions of my mentors. Some of the answers didn't make sense to me, but I was busy with my practice, my family, coaching, and training, and I decided to accept their answers for the time being.

MY HYPOTHYROIDISM

Throughout most of my life, I have been an endurance athlete. I love running, biking, and adventure racing. In my early forties, I decided to start training for triathlons. So, on top of everything else on my plate, I started spending even more time training, which meant less sleep to fit everything into my daily schedule.

I decided to have some blood tests just as a routine checkup. My bloodwork had always been pristine. I was shocked when I saw my results. They indicated that I was struggling with insulin resistance and had positive antibodies associated with Hashimoto's thyroiditis. How could this be? I had followed a strict gluten-free diet for years. I also followed a low-carb, moderate-fat, moderate-protein diet. I had not been ill, and my GI tract was working great. Now I felt just like one of my patients: frustrated, angry, and confused.

I had to ask myself how I really felt. Was I sick? Was I struggling with chronic symptoms? I was tired and sore, and my muscles and joints ached, but I chalked those issues up to training. If I was honest with myself, I had put on a bit of fat around my midsection. I think people call this a muffin top. But I was in my forties. And come to think of it, my bowels were a bit slower than in the past.

I decided to have a few blood tests to identify whether some organism in my body was triggering the autoimmunity. My tests showed yeast and bacteria overgrowth, so I started the same gastrointestinal and detoxification support protocols that I often prescribed to my patients. I also began to eat a strict anti-inflammatory diet. These steps seemed to work initially, but the insulin resistance didn't change; nor did my thyroid test results. I did not want to end up on thyroid medication. There had to be something I was missing.

A friend and colleague, Ben Lynch, ND, introduced me to a paper by Robert K. Naviaux, MD, titled "Metabolic Features of the Cell Danger Response."[1] This paper changed everything for me. Dr. Naviaux explains that humans are hardwired to adapt to stress. Our cells perceive the stress, which ultimately determines how our tissues, organs, and body systems respond to the stress. Naviaux explains that the triggers of cellular stress don't matter so much to the cell. But if the stress created by the trigger is excessive, it can initiate a cell danger response (CDR). The CDR then sets off a cascade of changes in the stressed and surrounding cells to prompt defensive and protective strategies. Many of the signs and symptoms we perceive as illness result from the CDR. In other words, they are often the body's normal response to danger. This danger response can be initiated at the cellular level regardless of whether the stress trigger is physical, chemical, emotional, or microbial.

This was a massive aha moment for me. Dr. Naviaux discusses how the cell's danger response to stress sets a cascade of events into action that can alter hormone levels, induce inflammation, trigger autoimmunity, potentially resulting in depression, anxiety, inflammation, and a multitude of changes in hormone levels in the blood.

What I read in that paper also helped me understand why supplements taken with good intentions often have unintended results. For example, taking B6 supports growth and development. But in times of cell stress and CDR, that supplementary B6 might be headed in a totally different direction. Since the nutrient helps cell defense, it enhances the production of inflammatory and toxic substances already being generated to kill the cellular threat. Now it was all starting to make sense.

I was humbled by the concept that what the body's cells do with the supplements and nutrients we provide is beyond our control. I was frustrated by my naivete. To assume that the nutrients I gave my patients would follow the particular cellular path I wanted was just ignorance. Sure, this is what we were taught: give a person vitamin B6 to support one specific pathway—simple. But life and cellular physiology just aren't that simple. The metabolism of our cells, tissues, and systems is incredibly complex. The cells and tissues do what they want with the nutrients we give them. Dr. Naviaux explains that cells use micronutrients (vitamins and minerals) to best support their needs, given their circumstances at the time.

> ### The Good News about Inflammation
>
> Many people assume that inflammation is a bad thing that always needs to be suppressed or eliminated. This, however, is not the case. Inflammation is a vital part of the immune system's response to injury and infection. It is the body's way of signaling the immune system to heal and repair damaged tissue and defend itself against organisms and toxins.

Dr. Naviaux doesn't spend much time in his paper explaining the role that thyroid hormone plays in the CDR in terms of both how the hormone functions within the cells and how the direct impact of the CDR affects the thyroid gland. I needed to know more. I needed to connect the dots.

Eager to find answers to my questions, I voraciously dug into scientific research. As I read paper after paper, I started to pull concepts together. Eventually I came across the work of a group of medical researchers in Germany who were writing some fascinating papers refuting the TSH-fT4 model of thyroid physiology, which I explain in part 2. The work of this group of brilliant minds allowed me to tie some of the loose ends together and inspired me to write this book with my friend Kelly Halderman, MD.

I ultimately learned that thyroid physiology is less about the gland and more about what is happening within the cells. I learned, for instance, that the cellular stress Dr. Naviaux discusses changes thyroid physiology within the cells to adapt to the perceived stress or danger.[2] The German researchers present this explanation in an article published in the medical journal *Frontiers in Endocrinology*. This paper's authors do a fantastic job explaining the adaptive role of thyroid hormones and how thyroid physiology changes when cells are in a nonstressed state versus a stressed state.

This means that peripheral cells play a massive and active role in thyroid physiology. The cells themselves determine whether to increase or decrease their metabolism by increasing or decreasing cellular *triiodothyronine* (T3). Cells in stress work to slow their metabolism as a protective measure, and they do this by deactivating the thyroid hormone that reaches the cells. The deactivation of thyroid hormone induces a state of cellular hypothyroidism, which causes symptoms.

The peripheral cells' ability to self-regulate independently of serum thyroid hormone levels is why you may have normal blood levels of TSH and fT4 and yet still have hypothyroid symptoms. The cells themselves can activate or deactivate thyroid hormone entering the cell to adapt to their stress response.

If stress occurred in a few cells of one tissue and was a local phenomenon, you might not even know it was happening. But what if it happened in hundreds, thousands, or millions of cells at the same time, in one tissue or multiple tissues? You would experience the signs and symptoms of hypothyroidism, which initially may be totally unrelated to the health of your thyroid gland. In other words, your signs and symptoms occur because of what is happening in your body's peripheral cells and tissues.

How does this relate to me and you and thousands of other people? For me, heavy athletic training was a stressor. Lack of sleep was a stressor. Disordered breathing—such as mouth-breathing during long runs and sleeping—was a stressor. The bacterial imbalance in my GI tract was a stressor. The chemical stress from the treated water I was drinking and swimming in was a stressor. All these stressors were stimulating a CDR throughout my body. Even though much of what I was doing was well-intended and considered healthy, my cells were overwhelmed, stressed, and sensing danger. My thyroid physiology was being altered in response to what my cells and tissues perceived as excessive stress and a threat.

You may be in a similar situation. The impact of all the stressors in your life may be more than your cells and tissues can adapt to, triggering a cell danger response. Disrupted sleep, subclinical infections, toxicity from your environment, emotional stress, unhealthy food choices, life stress, and trauma may be pushing your body's cells into an unhealthy state. As a result, the CDR is causing your cells to favor the deactivation of thyroid hormone, instigating chronic hypothyroid symptoms and, for some people, all-out thyroid gland disease.

For many men and women, there isn't a defining moment when thyroid physiology noticeably stopped working optimally. Instead it is often a slow, insidious progression. As the stress in your life becomes chronic and progressive, the scale can tip, triggering CDR and cellular hypothyroidism. Therefore, people can experience chronic hypothyroid symptoms, including weight gain, fatigue, thinning hair, brain fog, and constipation for weeks, months, or years before being diagnosed with primary hypothyroidism. Their hypothyroidism didn't start when their TSH and fT4 blood levels were out of the standard lab reference range. Instead, that's the end stage. Hashimoto's thyroiditis doesn't happen by accident or because of an out-of-control immune system. Typically it occurs as part of a protective response to globally slow down metabolism as a result of chronic, long-term excessive cellular stress.

Allopathic medicine has been looking at thyroid physiology from a perspective that the thyroid gland—and thyroid physiology, for that matter—is broken. Allopathic physicians approach it as if it's something that can't be fixed, but only managed with medication. Allopathic medicine believes thyroid physiology can simply be addressed by adding sufficient thyroid hormone to normalize TSH and fT4 blood levels. It's as if the only thing that matters is having adequate thyroid hormone in the blood. However, thyroid physiology is far more complicated than two lab values can represent.

Allopathic medicine aims to use thyroid medication to return the lab values of TSH and fT4 to the lab reference range. It is assumed that by doing this, what is termed "biochemical euthyroidism," optimal thyroid physiology in the body, will be restored. But unfortunately, while the lab values may be back within the reference range, this often doesn't come close to making the patient feel well or restoring his or her health.

The current allopathic thyroid care model is a debacle, and it's illogical. The allopathic model never addresses the root cause or causes of hypothyroidism. It prioritizes two lab tests over what the patient is actually experiencing. It ignores what's really going on. It discounts the research of the last two decades showing the complexity of thyroid physiology and why two tests just aren't good enough to evaluate thyroid physiology. In the allopathic model, hypothyroidism doesn't occur until 90 percent of the thyroid gland has been destroyed. That's far too late!

WHERE WE ARE HEADED

Through this book, Dr. Kelly and I hope to help you understand thyroid physiology. First, we discuss this physiology from a cellular perspective, including cellular thyroid allostasis, which is how the body responds to stressors to regain homeostasis. Next we discuss hypothyroidism as a spectrum disorder, meaning that there are many phases of hypothyroidism. And in part 3, Dr. Kelly and I describe strategies you can use for improving your thyroid physiology.

If you picked up *The Thyroid Debacle* to find a supplement formula to fix your thyroid or the best supplements to treat your GI tract or libido, this isn't that book. Nor is it a diet book. It's not a supplement protocol book, either. Instead, *The Thyroid Debacle* explains the factors that cause hypothyroidism, the condition, and its symptoms. You will learn what may be contributing to your cellular stress, deactivating your thyroid hormone, and causing hypothyroidism in all its forms.

We decided to take this approach for several reasons. The first is based on a wise proverb: "Give a man a fish, and you feed him for a day; teach a man to fish, and you feed him for a lifetime." We want you to know what is causing your reduced health and why. When you have a better understanding of what those things are, you have control.

The second reason is that most people gravitate toward taking a pill or supplement over changing their diet or lifestyle. Why? Let's be honest; it's easier. As you read this book, you will find out that things you can control, such as modifying how you eat and changing aspects of your day-to-day lifestyle, can significantly impact your hypothyroid symptoms. And many of the things you can do don't necessarily require a health-care professional's help. They don't require you to buy a device or supplement.

Nutritional supplements can be great tools to help you recover, but they are not *the* tool to fix what ails you. Likewise, medications can be a valuable tool, but they are not *the* tool. Supplements cannot correct a poor diet, bad habits, or a compromised lifestyle; they just can't. Unfortunately, too many functional medicine professionals blast allopathic medicine for prescribing lots of medications but then put their patients on fifteen or twenty supplements. We call this "medical greenwashing." Make no mistake; we use supplements as a tool, but they are not *the* tool.

Yes, there are foundational principles, and we present them in the upcoming chapters. But the solution does not come in a bottle. There is no magic supplement or device that fixes thyroid physiology or any of the chronic symptoms caused by thyroid-related issues. Instead the solutions lie in uncovering your cellular stressors, reducing or removing them to the best of your ability, and then supporting cell, thyroid, and full-body recovery.

Supplement use must be strategic. It should not be a shotgun approach. In most cases, supplements should not be a forever therapy. Similarly, this is why medicine doesn't fix thyroid physiology; it only manages your TSH and fT4 blood levels as your health often continues to decline.

> ### Know Your Stressors
>
> There is no one protocol to improve cellular hypothyroidism, Hashimoto's thyroiditis, primary hypothyroidism, or hyperthyroidism, because everyone's cellular stressors are a bit different. Your diet, lifestyle, relationships, and sleep quality will not be the same as those of your friend or a family member with hypothyroidism. Therefore, the solution can't possibly be the same for everyone.

Many of the people who pick up this book are struggling with Graves' disease or hyperthyroidism. You may even have been treated for hyperthyroidism and are now hypothyroid. While this book focuses on hypothyroidism, it is essential to understand that the same concepts hold true for hyperthyroidism. In a hyperthyroid state, something triggers the immune response to produce antibodies called thyroid-stimulating hormone receptor antibodies (TSHr Ab). Just as occurs with hypothyroidism, in hyperthyroidism physical, chemical, emotional, or microbial factors trigger an autoimmune response. So while this book is focused on hypothyroidism, the foundational principles still apply to the cause of, and recovery from, hyperthyroidism.

If you've picked up this book, you are likely one of the many who are frustrated, fatigued, and failing under the current thyroid care paradigm. We feel your pain. What Dr. Kelly and I want you to get from this book is a clear and comprehensive understanding of what causes hypothyroid symptoms and thyroid gland dysfunction, why allopathic medicine is failing you, and how to overcome chronic hypothyroid symptoms.

Make no mistake, recovering from chronic hypothyroid symptoms is not solved with medication or the latest miracle vitamin. Addressing the root cause of your hypothyroid symptoms will take work—and there may be more than one cause. In addition, it will take time for your body to undo the effects of months, if not years, of altered physiology.

When you understand how thyroid physiology works, why people become hypothyroid, and how to address the causes of hypothyroidism, your effort will be well worth it. You will have significantly improved control over your own health and well-being, and you will see your chronic hypothyroid symptoms dissipate. Your energy will be restored. Your hair will stop falling out. Your bowel function will improve. You'll stop struggling with weight problems. Your sex life will be better. Most importantly, your outlook on life will become one of hope versus one of despair.

You might be asking how two doctors could be right and so many others could be wrong. This is not about being right or wrong; this is about following the science. Most doctors and endocrinologists are following an outdated model of thyroid physiology. It's what they were taught in medical school, by pharmaceutical reps, and in largely biased research papers. We are not the only two doctors bringing the current thyroid debacle to light. There are many, and the ranks are growing in both functional and allopathic medicine.

In the process of questioning whether what I'd been taught all this time was, in fact, inaccurate, I began digging into the literature. Looking for answers, I found that my thoughts about thyroid physiology were not crazy but were closer to reality than the allopathic model.

The science I was uncovering in the published literature helped explain why my patients were getting better under my treatment model. In addition, the science was validating my beliefs that the hypothyroid symptoms my patients were experiencing were caused by cellular events and were not always reflected in their TSH and fT4 blood levels.

The science also validated my belief that hypothyroid symptoms and hypothyroidism are not caused by mistakes or random dysfunction of the thyroid gland. Instead, I believe that hypothyroidism, in most cases, is a protective mechanism. As you will discover in this book, the body's cells make deliberate changes to adapt to cellular threats. Alteration of thyroid physiology within the cells, the tissues, and the thyroid gland itself are part of the adaptive response to cell danger.

I'm confident that I will hear plenty of opposition to what I write in this book from some in allopathic medicine and possibly some in functional and integrative medicine as well, and that's okay. I'm not writing this book for them. I'm writing the book for you, for the hundreds of thousands of men and women struggling with chronic hypothyroid symptoms, and for the frustrated doctors working in a model where they realize that normalizing lab values does not always correlate with the restoration of health in their patients.

You need to know that what you are experiencing is real. You are not lazy. You are not crazy. You are unhealthy, and it's time someone provided you with the answers you need to turn your health around. It's time we stop managing lab numbers and help patients regain their health and vitality.

The Thyroid Debacle needed to be written to help lay people like you and doctors understand why

- you have chronic hypothyroid symptoms,
- you feel lousy although your lab test results are normal,
- you can have normal TSH and fT4 blood levels when you have many symptoms associated with hypothyroidism,
- thyroid hormone prescriptions can normalize TSH and fT4 blood levels yet allow symptoms to persist,
- your doctor may blame you for your symptoms, and why
- your doctor may blame your symptoms on other conditions.

You might ask why doctors are using an outdated model of thyroid physiology when new research indicates that the current treatment model is not working effectively. This would be a great question to ask your doctor, but you are not likely to get a satisfying response. I've been asking the same question for fifteen years.

To shed some light on why doctors continue to use this outdated model, my coauthor, Dr. Kelly, describes in part 1 why the medical model of thyroid care, including thyroid physiology, is still in common practice. She discusses how that model is used to evaluate, screen, diagnose, and treat hypothyroidism in detail. In part 2, I explain the new understanding of thyroid physiology. Finally, in part 3, we team up to help you address the root causes of your hypothyroid symptoms.

We hope you find the information in this book enlightening and beneficial. And we hope that it helps you improve your thyroid physiology, your overall health, and your quality of life as it has for us, our families, and our patients.

PART 1

CONFESSIONS OF AN ALLOPATHIC DOCTOR

I'm Dr. Kelly Halderman, and I have written part 1 of *The Thyroid Debacle* from my perspective—that is, one of a traditional family practice medical doctor. I will cover details of my allopathic medical journey as well as my personal health struggles. I will also describe basic medical knowledge about thyroid physiology and the diagnosis, treatment, and management of hypothyroidism, or underactive thyroid function, from an allopathic perspective. It is important to note that although I learned how to manage hypothyroidism as a resident from physicians who follow American Association of Clinical Endocrinologists (AACE) guidelines for treating various thyroid conditions, I do not.

In fact, I do not "treat" hypothyroidism at all; nor do I "treat" any other disease. And let me be clear when I say I no longer practice medicine because I found a better way to help myself and others. My strategy goes much more in-depth and relies on uncovering the root causes of why the body creates states such as hypothyroidism. This may sound crazy, but trust me; this strategy is why I am still alive despite having been diagnosed with not one, not two, but three serious medical conditions from which I have fully recovered. One diagnosis was Hashimoto's thyroiditis, a common type of hypothyroidism. I am living proof that a new model of thyroid care works. I use the strategies you will learn about in part 3 not only on the people in my care but also on me and my family.

Nevertheless, before you read about these new ways of addressing health issues, specifically hypothyroidism, it is important to understand why your traditional medical doctor treats your hypothyroidism the way he or she does. When you understand how your doctor was taught and the guidelines he or she has been told to follow, you will better understand why your concerns may fall on deaf ears. For instance, you'll know why your physician ignores or dismisses your symptoms because your "thyroid numbers look good."

Part 1 reviews the basics of what I refer to as the "the rules of the game," the AACE clinical practice guidelines for hypothyroidism in adults. It also discusses the traditional standard-of-care approach to hypothyroidism: when to diagnose, what to treat, when and how to treat, and how to monitor treatment. In part 2, Dr. Eric Balcavage will dazzle you with the science behind our new model of thyroid care, which we have been using successfully for over five years!

CHAPTER 1

THE JOURNEY FROM PHYSICIAN TO PATIENT

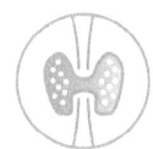

You may be asking why a person trained in allopathic medicine like me would coauthor a book like this, calling the widely accepted medical model for managing thyroid problems a "debacle." My honest answer to that question is that I never wanted to challenge that model. I loved allopathic medicine. I loved my white coat. I loved my colleagues. I loved being part of the club. Granted, the journey of learning and practicing allopathic medicine was arduous and completely exhausting, not to mention costly, but, as my teenager would say, it was "my jam."

I did not love the fact that I would sometimes lie in bed at night and wonder why no one was really getting better by taking the medication I prescribed; that concern needed to remain unspoken at the time. Even today, if doctors ask those kinds of questions, they risk ruffling feathers and hurting egos, and it may even get them kicked out of the club. So instead of speaking up about my concerns, I remained silent. This silence meant dismissing patients' valid symptoms when their thyroid lab test results were normal. It meant ordering studies for the elderly that harmed them more than they helped. It entailed writing prescriptions for antipsychotics for adolescents and for toenail fungus drugs that tragically destroyed a young father's kidney function and life. (He passed away after two unsuccessful kidney transplants.)

I still wade in remorse when thinking about these cases, yet all of my clinical decisions were determined by guidelines I had to follow, not by what I thought was the right thing to do. I was taught and encouraged not to think independently but to do what I was instructed. On top of that, I didn't even know that these decisions were bad ones. I saw poor outcomes on a daily basis, but I was locked into the standard protocol. I honestly believed that I was doing the right thing, despite the opposing evidence. Sadly, since the introduction of managed care, more and more doctors have been stripped of their ability to make their own decisions and forced to adhere to the same standard guidelines across the board. People continue to suffer significantly from this broken system.

In medical school and during residency, no one ever taught me how to read medical journals—I mean "read" as in reading them closely, digging into the science and taking the time to carefully consider what was valid information and what was manipulated or paid for by a pharmaceutical company. I was taught to use a standard set of guidelines to treat the patients in my care and never to dare question those guidelines. I was given hundreds of free lunches sponsored by pharmaceutical companies whose jobs were supposedly to update doctors on current science. (Riiiiiiiight!)

These so-called "updates" felt a lot more like sales pitches. And yet I still bought into what they were selling despite my misgivings. I continued to go along with the club and its rules for far too long. But, as the saying goes, hindsight is twenty-twenty. Looking back, I firmly believe that the structure of allopathy and the methods by which we allopathic doctors are trained allow, and even encourage, perfectly intelligent people to perform in perfectly illogical ways, thinking they are following sound principles backed by science. It boggles my mind just thinking about it.

I did some things in the past, prescribed some things, and said some things that I now find to be asinine and am ashamed of. How did this happen? How was I blinded, duped, manipulated, and used by the system? Perhaps it had to do with money. Or maybe it had to do with money's best friend, power. All I know is that it cost me a lot—and I mean *a lot*—not just in terms of the monetary impact but also from a physical, emotional, and profoundly personal standpoint. This still pains me daily.

It was quite an unexpected shock when the tables turned and I was the one given a grave medical diagnosis. This life-altering moment changed everything for me. With great courage, I faced the facts and began asking the tough questions. This is my personal story about how my long-held belief and trust in the standard medical guidelines came to a screeching halt when I was suddenly the one with the diagnosis, the one sitting in the patient's seat instead of the doctor's. This experience would forever shift the entire paradigm of what I believe health and healing should be.

THE PARADIGM SHIFT

Nothing is as powerful in having the capacity to change one's thought process and beliefs as raw experience. Until you've experienced something firsthand, you're not equipped to respond as optimally as someone who has firsthand knowledge. It is akin to writing a PhD dissertation on honey when you've never even tasted it or writing love poems without ever having been in love. I really wouldn't trust or care what you had to say about either of these topics if you hadn't truly experienced either of them in your body.

When the raw experience is lacking, there is a disconnect—perhaps better stated as an "incomplete knowing." When firsthand experience has been gained, an undeniable clarity and connection between the objective and subjective can blossom. When my body started to fail me in 2009, I went from having book knowledge about disease to actually living in a diseased body. This incredibly intimate experience was my biggest struggle and, in the same breath, my most influential teacher.

I now understand why it is commonly said that the best healers are the "once wounded," or those who have cultivated high levels of empathy through experiencing their own travails or the struggles of loved ones. These are the people I now trust the most with my health, because their knowledge comes from a more profound and more personal place than just a textbook. Before diving further into my eventual diagnosis and personal health story, let's start where my journey began, with my training.

Before I ever started medical school, I had heard a friend who just finished the grueling four years of her medical education say, "Medical school is like trying to drink water from a fire hose." Or maybe I heard Dr. McDreamy from *Grey's Anatomy* say that? Nonetheless, I thought it was just an amusing metaphor until I was actually living it during my first year of medical school. I was genuinely drowning in information. The knowledge we had to absorb, process, and regurgitate felt like mental torture at times. Yet I loved it. Hundreds of hours were spent in lecture halls and the laboratory learning the ins and outs of the human body and its beautiful and complex biochemistry and physiology. The training was vigorous, exams were challenging, sleep was minimized, and caffeine was maximized. Still, I knew without a doubt that I was exactly where I needed to be.

By the second year of medical school, doctors-in-training move on from learning such basics as anatomy, biochemistry, and physiology to more advanced topics, such as clinical medicine. This was where they use the basic knowledge they previously learned about how the body works and apply it to symptom patterns in real human beings.

For example, we were taught that when a person has hair loss, hoarseness, and weight gain, these signs and symptoms typically correlate with a thyroid gland that is not functioning properly. We were instructed to run a series of blood tests, other studies, or both, depending on the current guidelines, to confirm or dismiss the suspicion. It was a relatively simple model to follow: Take a person's history, perform a physical exam, and decide what his or her dysfunction is likely to be. In most cases, the next step is to order tests to prove or disprove the "disease" diagnosis. Actually, very few diagnoses in traditional medicine are "clinical," meaning that the diagnosis is made based on symptoms alone, without supporting test results. The overwhelming majority of diagnoses are based on what doctors see on a piece of paper—lab values and CT scan reports, for example—and not people's symptoms.

Since I am a type A, left-brained, follow-the-rules-to-a-T kind of person, I thrived in using this formulaic model. A blood test showing a high thyroid-stimulating hormone (TSH) level and a low level of T4, a type of thyroid hormone, equals a diagnosis of hypothyroidism. Normal TSH and T4 levels equal no hypothyroidism. I was so good at knowing this and other diagnostic formulas that I scored in the ninety-ninth percentile on my medical boards. I didn't miss anything when it came to using my allopathic medical tools correctly.

Did I actually help anyone by stringing together symptoms, correlating them with lab test results, and then ordering the appropriate medication? Maybe sometimes at best, but probably not as much as I thought. Honestly, I didn't think to question anything at the time, and it felt so good to be patted on the back by my peers for such work. I'm not saying it didn't cross my mind quite often that this system of matching symptoms with pills may not be working, but we, as traditional doctors, are not taught to adequately address the root cause of a person's illness. We are not trained to ask why. In fact, in retrospect, I think "why" was excised from my vernacular during medical school. Not until I suddenly became the one with a diagnosis and the one being put on medications without an ounce of information from my colleagues did it really matter enough to me to finally dare ask, "Why? Why is my body killing itself?"

In 2009, I suddenly started having strange neurological symptoms, such as problems walking, migraines, and urinary incontinence. At that time in my life, I was practicing medicine, was married to an extremely busy anesthesiologist, had two very young children, and lived in Northern Minnesota (a.k.a. the tundra). Not to mention that I had a pile of other unfortunate epigenetic stressors, such as being a junk-food vegan, a caffeine and sugar addict, and a couch potato to boot. By the time I finished work, cooked dinner for everyone, and took care of my kids, I was too exhausted and had no time to spare for regular exercise.

> Epigenetic stressors are factors that influence how your genes function.

I reported these strange symptoms to my colleagues and was quickly shuffled to "the best neurologist in town." He looked at me, holding my MRI in his hands, and said, "It looks like you have multiple sclerosis."

What? Me? Wait, I am a doctor, not a patient. Let me check the name on that report, because doctors do not get sick, I thought to myself. The next couple of weeks passed in a blur. I do remember thinking at the time, *Well, thank God I am a doctor, so I'll get the best care for this crippling, incurable disease!* Ha! The "best care" was nothing more than a prescription and a measly pat on the back to imply my doctor's condolences.

As I have always done throughout my entire life, I pulled myself up by my bootstraps and decided that I needed to take charge. The tools I had spent years in school learning and hundreds of thousands of dollars in tuition to achieve were worthless. However, I refused to give up. My parents taught me that hard work and determination are not optional life skills but are essential in every situation. Therefore, I knew I needed to be the one to help myself now, because I had come to realize that my "club" was not in the business of getting me out of the mess that I was in.

And so the path of my career and life completely changed. I honestly thank God that it did; if it hadn't, I'd probably be dead. This shift in perspective and my personal health experience are the reasons I understand how people feel if they've been diagnosed with a medical condition or if they've not been diagnosed but still believe there's something wrong. Whether you are a struggling patient or a silently frustrated physician, I've been in your shoes.

I was able to recover from multiple chronic illnesses, including multiple sclerosis and Hashimoto's thyroiditis, because I stopped using the current medical guidelines to treat myself, started asking the difficult questions, and got answers to my whys. I learned through my own very personal experience that true healing lies in addressing the root causes of signs and symptoms and not just in foolishly covering them up with prescription drugs.

How's that for a paradigm shift? When we know better, we do better. For those who provide medical care and do not know better yet, I am sorry if you are struggling. Here, in *The Thyroid Debacle*, you will find answers to help your suffering patients beyond the outdated "rule-following" protocol. If you are struggling with hypothyroidism, a plethora of hope awaits in these pages.

FOLLOWING THE RULES, NOT THE SCIENCE

It is an unfortunate truth that the majority of physicians do not regularly read medical journals in which the latest and most relevant scientific information is found. Most doctors claim that they routinely read them, but the current research statistics on this topic suggest that they don't.

This isn't exactly breaking news. Almost two decades ago, Claude Lenfant, MD, director of the National Heart, Lung, and Blood Institute, published an article in the *New England Journal of Medicine* titled "Clinical Research to Clinical Practice—Lost in Translation?"

In this article, he discusses "... the lack of success we [physicians] have had in translating research findings into medical practice ...". He cites *Harrison's Principles of Internal Medicine,* in which the editors "express their view that 'the practice of medicine combines both science and art. The role of science in medicine is clear.' What may be less clear," Dr. Lenfant notes, "is the 'art' part of medicine, [which] to the editors of Harrison's is the combination of medical knowledge, intuition, and judgment.'"

Today everyone recognizes that a great deal of the "knowledge" element of this combination is there for the taking. Libraries cannot be built fast enough to keep up with the number of scientific journals being published. Also, moving this knowledge off the shelves and into practice by making it relevant and accessible to practitioners and achieving a true marriage of knowledge with intuition and judgment requires the art of translation. And this translation is, indeed, a delicate and elusive art. Luckily, Dr. Eric and I are fluent in the language of current scientific research in all matters of the thyroid. Our translation of this science in part 2 will explain how it can be applied in practice. Once this knowledge is put into action, as we explain in part 3, you will be equipped with the power to dramatically improve your health.

Another issue with the current system—apart from the lack of application of research—can be attributed to "pharmaceutical education." It is commonplace for scientific updates, which are often disguised as "medical education," to be provided by pharmaceutical companies whose cherry-picked research findings somehow always seem to substantiate the use of more and more of their brands of medication. Follow the money on this problem.

Yet a third problem facing the system is that even if the scientific research results are valid and haven't been manipulated, doctors often still have difficulty putting these findings into practice. In other words, even when good, solid science says that a particular therapy or drug is valid and efforts are made to make doctors aware of these findings, doctors may choose not to use the more current research in practice.

Take, for example, the results of the Beta-Blocker Heart Attack Trial in 1981. The results of this clinical trial were so impressive that an alert was published in the *Journal of the American Medical Association* stating that there is a clearly established benefit in using beta-blockers for patients recovering from heart attacks. Yet in 1996, nearly fifteen years after the results of the trial were made known, beta-blockers were being prescribed for only 62.5 percent of patients who had suffered a myocardial infarction.

This oversight cannot be chalked up to the intervention being too complicated or potentially cost-prohibitive, because writing a prescription for a relatively cheap drug is a fairly simple task. It begs the question, Where is the disconnect? Why can't simple, scientifically-backed interventions be used in clinical practice? I could postulate until the cows come home, but I am all for utilizing new strategies and not continuing to use outdated methods or overlooking new ones that work.

To recap, these issues present a multifaceted conundrum. The practice of allopathic medicine seems to have trouble translating current, relevant research results into practice. Allopathic physicians also seem to have difficulty following the best and most reliable science and making appropriate recommendations based on randomized control trials. And wait, it gets better: the guidelines that are most used in clinical allopathic practice today are largely based on so-called "expert opinion" and consensus statements, which the World Health Organization reports are the worst level of evidence to support clinical practice. (Randomized control trials and meta-analyses are the best.)

> *The World Health Organization and other large entities have ranked the strength and accuracy of various types of evidence used in the medical decision process. In all scoring systems, the highest strength of evidence is randomized control trials and meta-analyses, with lower scores for other types of evidence. All grading systems place consensus statements and expert opinion by respected authorities (societies) as the poorest level*

of evidence because historically they have failed to adopt new concepts and treatments based on new knowledge or new-found understanding demonstrated in the medical literature.

—Kent Holtorf, MD

How are we expected to be anything but sick if allopathic doctors

- are too busy and overworked to read the latest and greatest science,
- are not encouraged to stay up to date with the newest science,
- are not experienced in translating relevant science into regular practice,
- often receive "education" by the pharmaceutical companies, and
- follow outdated guidelines?

These oversights and omissions are why millions of us may be receiving antiquated and ineffective care and suffering because of it. You may be familiar with the saying "The definition of insanity is doing the same thing over and over again and expecting different results." Perhaps no sentiment could better apply here. The rules and model of medicine need a scientifically backed and much-needed upgrade. It's not hard to understand why so many people are still suffering and being forced to wait to see whether they are listened to and whether the true art of translation ever happens.

The *New England Journal of Medicine* reported that, at best, it could take up to seventeen years for new best practice guidelines to reach the average physician. Seventeen years? How can this be? And who has that kind of time when he or she doesn't feel well and can't enjoy his or her life? When I read about how much time it takes to get new science into doctors' offices, I was both in total agreement and infuriated—so infuriated that I have committed my life to changing these circumstances. Check out my website for more information: www.drkellyhalderman.com.

I review the standard practice guidelines in depth throughout part 1 so you can be informed about how your allopathic doctor is likely to treat you. The information you read here will help you understand why your doctor may dismiss your symptoms when your TSH and T4 levels are normal, why physicians rely so heavily on the TSH test, and why they believe that normalizing lab test results means they are treating you appropriately. I think you'll agree with Dr. Eric and me when we say that it's time for a change.

TIME FOR A CHANGE

Before I became ill, I could claim ignorance. I now think that most doctors are just ignorant—not bad people purposely providing inadequate care. They are good people. I didn't know that there were flaws in the system. I didn't realize that the rules of the game were wholly inadequate for some conditions. The shift to becoming an unwell patient receiving standard medical care allowed me to experience the allopathic model firsthand. When I was given a diagnosis of multiple sclerosis (a.k.a. a death sentence) and handed those prescriptions and told to "get my affairs in order," I had the most significant "WTH" moment of my life. But this dramatic reversal of roles was what finally changed my thinking and made me take a deeper look into what exactly I was practicing.

Looking back, I don't think I fully realized that prescribing medications to cover up symptoms was missing the mark. Your current doctor may be toeing the line of allegiance to the club, much as I was before I got sick. Or your doctor may see that the current model of thyroid care isn't working but feels helpless because there's no time to figure out why following the current medical guidelines aren't working or how to fix them. Or perhaps your doctor sees that the long-accepted treatments aren't working and is trying his or her best to provide you with better care.

Whatever the case may be, this book outlines a science-based strategy for change—a new paradigm for thyroid care. As I stated, Dr. Eric, my friend, colleague, and coauthor, has devoted countless hours of research and clinical application of this new approach to providing us with the facts on why the current model of thyroid care is the problem and offers a comprehensive method for fixing it. I am forever indebted to him, as the information I've learned from his research and experience has changed my life.

In part 2, Dr. Eric covers the science behind a new model of thyroid care. This progressive model supplants the old one and gets straight to the causes of thyroid problems and other related conditions, such as insulin resistance, depression, and lipid abnormalities. After you read part 2, you will see why the time has come for us to unite and upgrade how we manage hypothyroidism.

I know change isn't easy. It's not in our human nature to want to change what has already been established. However, we've arrived at the dire point where we *must* speak up, because people are suffering. We must call a spade a spade. The current model of thyroid care is broken. The new model will revolutionize thyroid care and your health.

THE FIRST STEP IS THE MOST IMPORTANT

So where do we begin? A good starting point comes from a story told by Brendon Burchard, one of the world's top experts on human performance, about an Olympic sprinter he coached. The sprinter had won a couple of world championships but never a gold medal. "I was working with her after she [finally] won a gold, and I said, 'What happened? You had these years, two Olympics where you didn't medal, and then you did. What changed?' She said, 'I finally decided to start asking and telling people that I wanted a gold medal. I'd never verbalized it. I'd never asked for it. I'd never pushed for it. I learned that when you shout from the rooftops what you really want in life, will the village idiots come out and scream at you? Yes, but the village leaders will also come out.'"

Within these pages, Dr. Eric and I explain where the standard model of thyroid care isn't working and advocate for a new model based on current, relevant, and solid science. Whether or not you are a doctor, you can be a village leader and raise your voice to help effect change. We can unite and shout from the rooftops together so that millions of people suffering will be helped, including you. Once the science backing this needed change is elucidated in part 2, I honestly do not know how it will not revolutionize the prevailing paradigm.

Well, actually, I do, and you can probably guess why this is the case. Just check out how many drug advertisements dominate TV and computer screens and magazine pages, reminding us to "ask your doctor," followed by a rapidly delivered overview of numerous possible and probable side effects that are debilitating at best and potentially lethal at worst. In spite of this, we hope that this book lands in the hands of patients who will share this information with their doctors and also in the hands of health-care practitioners who have the ability to implement these strategies. Yet, as the brilliant German philosopher Arthur Schopenhauer once said, "All truth passes through three stages. First, it is ridiculed. Second, it is violently opposed. Third, it is accepted as being self-evident."

Dr. Eric and I hope we can defy the odds of processing truth by jumping to the third phase, where this revolution in thyroid care helps allopathic practitioners and people with hypothyroidism alike. We are all in this together.

CHAPTER 2

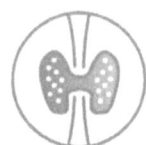

THYROID ANATOMY AND PHYSIOLOGY

Medical students begin their education on the thyroid by studying its anatomy and physiology. Anatomy is the study of bodily structures. Physiology is the study of how these anatomical structures function in a healthy person. In medicine, it is said that structure determines function, so it is vital for students to examine various body parts of cadavers before they put their hands on their patients. It is also important for doctors-in-training to look at thyroid tissue under a microscope to fully understand its complex biological processes, otherwise known as its physiology.

The thyroid gland lies in the center of the neck in front of, or anterior to, the trachea, or windpipe. It consists of a middle region, or isthmus, and two wing-shaped left and right lobes. Each of these lobes has parathyroid glands embedded on its bottom surface. The tissue of the thyroid gland is composed mainly of thyroid follicles. The follicles have a central cavity filled with a sticky fluid called colloid, which is the center of thyroid hormone production and is dependent on having a sufficient supply of the mineral iodine.

Figure 2.1: Thyroid gland and local anatomy.

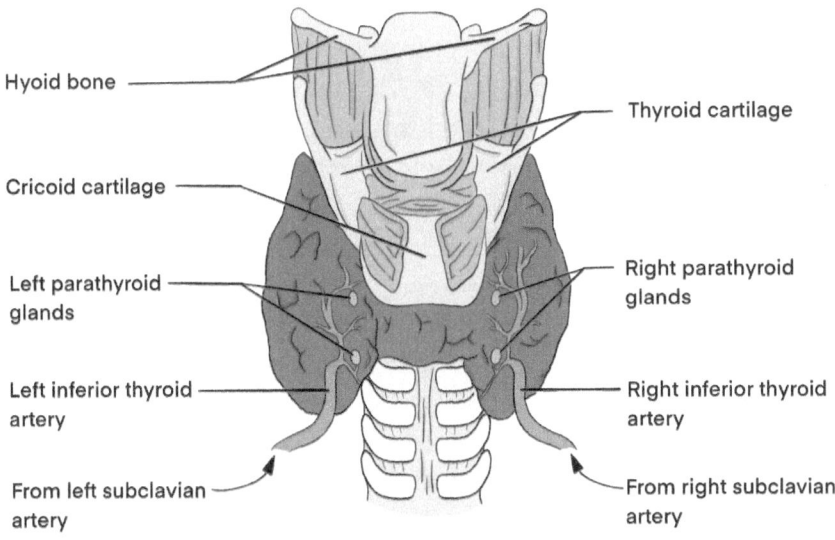

The gland itself is relatively small, weighing less than an ounce. Despite its size, it plays a significant role in maintaining the health of the entire human body.

Doctors-to-be learn early that the thyroid gland's main job is to produce thyroid hormones, which have far-reaching, critical effects, such as regulating metabolism, maintaining body heat, and assisting protein synthesis. Therefore, thyroid disorders can have severe and widespread negative consequences. Medical school professors teach that thyroid physiology problems begin in the thyroid gland.

You will find that Dr. Eric and I have a different perspective on thyroid physiology. Our belief and recent research are yielding evidence that many times, problems with thyroid physiology begin in the peripheral tissues far away from the gland. This is one reason a person can have hypothyroid symptoms despite having a properly functioning thyroid gland and normal thyroid hormone levels in the blood. In many cases of thyroid dysfunction, we believe that damage to the gland is the long-term effect of altered thyroid physiology, not the beginning.

HORMONES AS MESSENGERS

Thyroid hormones assert their control by binding to receptors on cells, similar to how a key opens a lock. The target cell has receptors for thyroid hormone (the locks), and thyroid hormones (the keys) bind to these receptors, causing a ripple effect of responses throughout the body. Nearly every cell and tissue in the body has receptors for thyroid hormones, so these chemical messengers directly or indirectly influence virtually every cellular process.

Thyroid hormones influence the body's basal metabolic rate, which is the amount of energy the body uses when at rest. Thyroid hormone binds to receptors in cells to control gene regulation and the production of hormones, enzymes, and tissues. Thyroid hormones bind to receptors located on the mitochondria, the powerhouses of all cells, and increase nutrient breakdown to produce adenosine triphosphate (ATP). That's a fancy way of saying that thyroid hormones increase your metabolism. ATP is your body's energy currency; it's like the gas that powers your car. Thyroid hormones even turn on genes that regulate how you burn the calories, in a process known as glucose oxidation.

Thyroid hormones are required for normal fetal and childhood growth and development. They are vital for proper nervous system development in the fetus, throughout early childhood, and into adulthood. Thyroid hormones regulate healthy levels of reproductive hormones. That is why deficiencies and abnormalities in thyroid hormone levels may lead to infertility and other adverse effects on reproduction. In addition, these powerful thyroid hormones help maintain the body's sensitivity to other hormones that are involved in different biological processes, such as epinephrine (adrenaline) and norepinephrine. To put it simply, optimal thyroid hormone regulation is critical to your good health and function.

SYNTHESIS AND RELEASE OF THYROID HORMONES

The thyroid gland synthesizes thyroid hormone. Here's how it happens: signals from the body stimulate a small structure at the base of the brain called the hypothalamus to produce a hormone called thyrotropin-releasing hormone (TRH).

TRH is released into blood vessels that transport it to another area in the brain called the anterior pituitary gland. There, activated cells called thyrotropes produce a hormone called thyrotropin-stimulating hormone (TSH). TSH is released into the bloodstream and carried to its primary target, the thyroid gland.

In the thyroid gland, TSH binds to receptors in its follicles to trigger a series of events that ultimately synthesize and release thyroid hormone from the thyroid gland.

Those steps include the following:

- transport of iodide into the thyroid follicular cells, where iodide undergoes oxidation, resulting in the production of iodine (I_2), which passes through the follicle cell membrane into the colloid
- production of thyroglobulin (Tg), the backbone of thyroid hormones, and its transport into the follicle colloid
- linking of the iodine by thyroid peroxidase enzymes (TPO) in the colloid to thyroglobulin to produce iodinated thyroglobulin
- transport of the iodinated thyroglobulin back into the thyroid follicular cells
- breakdown of the iodinated thyroglobulin into the individual thyroid hormones thyroxine (T4) and triiodothyronine (T3)
- release of T4 and T3 into the blood by the thyroid gland to be delivered to cells throughout the body

T3 and T4 are bound to carrier proteins in the bloodstream for delivery to body tissues. The binding also prevents T3 and T4 from being misused or broken down on the journey. The liver produces carrier proteins, such as thyroid-binding globulin (TBG), transthyretin, and albumin.

When thyroid hormones bound to carrier proteins reach the cells and tissues, the T3 and T4 are separated from the protein to become free T3 and free T4. These free hormones can bind to thyroid hormone transport proteins to be carried into the cells, where they have a physiological effect. Less than 1 percent of the circulating T3 and T4 in the body is unbound, or "free." The remaining 99 percent of circulating T3 and T4 remains bound to TBG, transthyretin, or albumin and acts as a thyroid hormone reserve.

CELLULAR REGULATION OF THYROID HORMONES

There is minimal discussion between allopathic doctors and their patients regarding how thyroid hormones work in the cells, yet that is where they make an impact. As a student of allopathic medicine, I was taught that the transportation of thyroid hormone into the cells is a passive process called "simple diffusion." That means thyroid hormones move from areas of high concentration (the blood) to areas of low concentration (the cells) as cells use their supply of thyroid hormones. But, as Dr. Eric discusses in part 2, this is not entirely true, and the discrepancy makes a world of difference.

I now believe that this misunderstanding is the basis for the allopathic idea that "as long as there is enough thyroid hormone (T3 and T4) in the blood, there is enough hormone inside the cells to drive cell metabolism and other actions."

Another major challenge of my allopathic training was a lack of education on other aspects of thyroid physiology within the cells. For example, a critical factor in the cells is the action of deiodinase enzymes. These enzymes either activate or deactivate thyroid hormones.

Much of medicine's understanding of the thyroid transporters, deiodinases, and receptors is only a few decades old. This seems like a long time, but as I pointed out previously, it can take time for science to show up in textbooks and professors' lectures.

My training explained that thyroid hormone passively diffuses into cells, converts into the active hormone (T3), and binds to receptors. I was taught that one blood test for TSH was the best, and often the only, test needed to evaluate thyroid physiology. This philosophy has not changed.

I was not taught very much, if anything, about the complexity of cellular control of thyroid physiology. I was not taught that the deiodinase enzymes could activate or deactivate thyroid hormones except in critical illness. I was not taught that there are different thyroid hormone receptors or that the type and concentration of the receptors varies from tissue to tissue.

What I was taught was very basic thyroid physiology. My professors explained that the thyroid gland controls thyroid physiology and that all tissues respond to thyroid hormone in the same way. They said that classic hypothyroid symptoms were not caused by a thyroid problem unless TSH was above the lab reference range. I was taught that if TSH was high and T4 was low, a medication would fix the deficiency. Most of my allopathic brethren were taught the same thing. Today science shows that this simple allopathic model of thyroid physiology is *too* simple.

This is why Dr. Eric and I wrote *The Thyroid Debacle*. We want to bring some of this science to you, the person struggling with chronic thyroid problems, as well as to you, the doctor who hasn't learned the new paradigm and science of thyroid physiology.

WHERE WE ARE HEADED

In the chapters to come in part 1, you will learn how this simplistic approach to thyroid physiology affects allopathic medicine's evaluation and treatment of thyroid disorders. Even though the science and understanding of thyroid physiology's complexity has grown dramatically in the past few decades and continues to evolve, the treatment model in allopathic medicine has changed very little.

Because thyroid hormones play such an essential and influential role throughout the body, learning how to optimize your thyroid gland function and physiology is imperative for your health.

Coming up in part 2 is a discussion of issues regarding thyroid physiology that often begin at a cellular level, not in the thyroid gland itself. As Dr. Eric will explain, having a comprehensive understanding of the complicated thyroid hormone physiology at the cellular level is essential to approaching how to amend what may have gone awry. Because of this complexity, treatment is not as easy as simply saying, "Your thyroid gland isn't working well. Let's just medicate you with synthetic thyroid hormone."

The body knows what it is doing; it may shut down the production of thyroid hormones for a specific reason that I will dig deeper into in the next chapter. Now that we have gone over the basics of thyroid anatomy and physiology, I will take a look at the allopathic perspective of thyroid pathology—that is, what happens in the body when the thyroid gland is not working properly.

CHAPTER 3

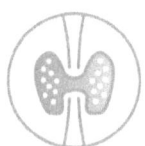

PATHOLOGIES OF THYROID PHYSIOLOGY

THE NUMBERS

Diabetes is considered the most common endocrine disorder in the United States, with over 10 percent, 34 million people, of the US population being impacted. However, when we add the numbers of people believed to have prediabetes, the precursor to type 2 diabetes, we see the number of people affected balloons to 122 million people, or 37 percent of the US population.

By contrast, thyroid disorders are estimated to impact about 20 million Americans, or 6 percent of the US population. So it's no wonder diabetes seems to get most of the attention. However, we think these estimates are likely much lower than the actual number of people impacted by altered thyroid physiology. This is because reduced thyroid hormone inside your cells, a condition called cellular hypothyroidism, plays a crucial role in developing insulin resistance, prediabetes, and diabetes.

As you will learn in this chapter and throughout the book, it's allopathic medicine's lack of consideration regarding cellular regulation of thyroid physiology that results in likely underreported levels of people impacted by alterations in thyroid physiology.

In this chapter, we will focus on the classification of thyroid disorders from the traditional allopathic perspective. These are the concepts I learned in medical school and the concepts that drove the medical management of my patients. In part two, Dr. Balcavage will introduce you to a different way of looking at thyroid physiology. Although all the ideas and concepts he discusses are backed by scientific literature and clinical experience, they are not part of allopathic medicine's current medical training or treatment paradigm.

According to the American Thyroid Association's website, www.thyroid.org, one of the most prominent resources on thyroid physiology, one in eight women will develop a thyroid disorder during her lifetime. And while men are not immune to thyroid disorders, women are five to eight times more likely to develop a thyroid disorder.

THYROID DISORDERS

Allopathic medicine breaks the disorders of thyroid physiology down into two main categories: disorders of the gland and disorders away from the gland. The three primary disorders of the gland include hypothyroidism, hyperthyroidism, and thyroid cancers. The disorders of thyroid physiology away from the gland are central hypothyroidism and euthyroid sick syndrome (also called nonthyroidal illness syndrome and low T3 syndrome).

Disorders of the Thyroid Gland

I will cover thyroid cancer in a bit. For now, let's discuss the two primary thyroid disorder classifications: hyperthyroidism (a condition where too much thyroid hormone is produced) and hypothyroidism (a condition where too little thyroid hormone is produced).

Before I cover both these disorders, I need to give you a bit of background on some terms used to describe tissue changes that can occur at the thyroid gland.

Goiter

A goiter is an enlargement of the thyroid gland. There are two general classifications of goiters: diffuse and nodular. A diffuse goiter is a general enlargement of the whole thyroid gland devoid of lumps or nodules. A nodular goiter is an enlargement of the thyroid gland caused by the growth of one nodule (uninodular goiter) or multiple nodules (multinodular goiter).

When someone has a goiter and thyroid hormone production is still within a normal range, the goiter is called a euthyroid, or nontoxic, goiter. However, when thyroid production increases or decreases out of the standard lab range, it is called a toxic goiter.

A goiter can be caused by multiple factors, including iodine deficiency or access, thyroiditis, Graves' disease, thyroid cancer, and pregnancy. Common signs and symptoms of a goiter include enlargement of the gland, difficulty swallowing or breathing, hoarseness of the throat, and coughing.

A medical doctor will often confirm the diagnosis with thyroid labs, ultrasound, and biopsy. Medical treatment is determined by the cause, size, and type of goiter. Interventions may include medications to shrink the goiter, surgery to remove the thyroid, and radioactive iodine treatments to destroy overactive thyroid tissue.

Thyroid Nodule

A thyroid nodule is a solid or fluid-filled lump or mass that forms within the thyroid gland. Thyroid nodules are relatively common, with most being detected incidentally during ultrasound evaluation for other conditions. It is thought that up to 68 percent of the general population may have a thyroid nodule. Most often, the nodules are benign. But in 7 to 15 percent of the cases, the nodules are either malignant or suspicious of potential malignancy. Ultrasound and fine-needle aspiration biopsy are used to determine the risk of cancer.

Thyroid nodules can develop due to overgrowth of normal thyroid tissue (called a thyroid adenoma), too much or too little iodine, inflammation of thyroid tissue, and cancer. Thyroid nodules are often asymptomatic but can cause symptoms similar to those experienced by people with goiters. Diagnosis and treatment of thyroid nodules are similar to those used for goiters.

Thyroiditis

Thyroiditis is the inflammation of the thyroid gland. Thyroiditis can result in both overproduction and underproduction of thyroid hormone. It is not unusual that a person with thyroiditis may experience episodes of hyperthyroidism followed by episodes of hypothyroidism.

Allopathic medicine differentiates thyroiditis into several different types:

- Hashimoto's thyroiditis
- silent thyroiditis
- postpartum thyroiditis
- subacute thyroiditis
- acute thyroiditis
- drug-induced thyroiditis
- radiation-induced thyroiditis

By far, Hashimoto's thyroiditis is considered the most common. Hashimoto's, silent, and postpartum thyroiditis are all deemed to be caused by a disorder of the immune system resulting in damage to the thyroid gland. In some cases, thyroiditis is short-term and the thyroid gland recovers. However, in many cases, the thyroiditis results in significant damage to the thyroid gland, rendering it unable to produce appropriate levels of thyroid hormone, resulting in a diagnosis of hypothyroidism and requiring thyroid hormone replacement therapy.

Subacute and acute thyroiditis are thought to be caused by infectious organisms. Radiation and medication-induced thyroiditis are caused by medical intervention.

Thyroiditis symptoms can vary depending on whether a person is experiencing too much or too little thyroid hormone release as a result of the inflammatory damage.

Hyperthyroid symptoms may include the following:

- irritability, anxiety, nervousness
- insomnia
- increased heart rate
- heart palpitations
- fatigue
- weight loss
- increased sweating and heat intolerance
- increased appetite
- tremors

Hypothyroid symptoms may include the following:

- weight gain
- constipation
- depression
- fatigue
- dry skin
- brain fog
- reduced libido

Allopathic evaluation of thyroiditis includes thyroid blood tests, ultrasound, and radioactive iodine uptake test. Treatment is based on symptoms and underlying cause. When one is experiencing hyperthyroid signs and symptoms, beta-blockers are often used.

In addition, anti-inflammatory medications may be used to reduce pain and inflammation. If thyroiditis is drug-induced, a change in the offending medication usually occurs. For those with hypothyroid symptoms, thyroid hormone replacement therapy may be prescribed.

It is not unusual that thyroiditis can result in permanent destruction of the gland, requiring long-term treatment.

Hyperthyroidism

Although diving deeply into every facet of hyperthyroidism is beyond the scope of this book, I think it's essential to be aware of the allopathic perspective of the condition. Hyperthyroidism is characterized by an overactive thyroid gland that is producing abnormally high amounts of thyroid hormones. Symptoms may include tachycardia, weight loss, nervousness, and tremors. The diagnosis is clinical, meaning that it is based on signs and symptoms as well as abnormal thyroid function tests.

The most common cause of hyperthyroidism is Graves' disease. In this autoimmune disease, autoantibodies directed against the TSH receptors on the thyroid follicular cells are responsible for the overproduction of thyroid hormone. The hyperthyroidism of Graves' disease can be life-threatening if not treated.

A radioactive iodine uptake (RAIU) test differentiates Graves' disease from Hashimoto's thyroiditis. First, a minimal amount of radioactive iodine is given orally or intravenously. A scanner then detects the amount of radioiodine that is absorbed by the thyroid. (This test can also be used to calculate the dose of radioactive iodine that may be needed to treat hyperthyroidism.)

Areas of the thyroid that show an increase (hot) or decrease (cold) in radioactive iodine uptake on the scan help distinguish areas of possible cancer. Thyroid cancers exist in less than 1 percent of hot nodules compared with 10 to 20 percent of cold nodules. Therefore, the doctor is likely to biopsy cold nodules to investigate whether or not cancer cells are present.

The American Association of Clinical Endocrinology (AACE) classifies hyperthyroidism based on the RAIU test and whether or not circulating thyroid-stimulating antibodies to the TSH receptor are present. Graves' disease can be treated with antithyroid medications, such as methimazole and propylthiouracil; radiation therapy; or surgical removal of the gland. (Radiation therapy, or radioactive iodine ablation, is the use of radioactive iodine to destroy the thyroid gland and is the most commonly used treatment in the United States.)

Hyperthyroidism can be fatal, so if you have this condition, it is important to be under the care of a health-care practitioner to ensure your safety.

Hypothyroidism

Most thyroid disease involves inadequate production of the thyroid hormones T3 and T4, or hypothyroidism. ("Hypo" means "low.") By definition, hypothyroidism "can be caused by any structural or functional abnormality that interferes with the production of adequate levels of thyroid hormone."[3]

Hypothyroidism can be caused by problems with the thyroid gland (primary hypothyroidism), the pituitary gland (secondary hypothyroidism), or the hypothalamus (tertiary hypothyroidism).

In secondary and tertiary hypothyroidism, reduced function of either gland can result in reduced TSH production and therefore reduced levels of circulating thyroid hormones. Secondary and tertiary hypothyroidism are often classified together as central hypothyroidism.

The National Health and Nutrition Examination Survey, which collected data from 4,392 participants, reflecting 222 million individuals, during 1999–2002, found a prevalence of hypothyroidism in the general population of 3.7 percent, and hyperthyroidism prevalence was 0.5 percent. Among women of reproductive age, hypothyroidism prevalence was 3.1 percent.[4] Pregnant women with undiagnosed or inadequately treated hypothyroidism have an increased risk of miscarriage, preterm delivery, and severe developmental problems in their children.

Ethnicity is also a possible risk factor for thyroid disease. For example, non-Hispanic whites are at higher risk for hypothyroidism than non-Hispanic Blacks, but at a lower risk for hyperthyroidism. In comparison, Mexican Americans have the same risk as non-Hispanic whites for hypothyroidism but are at higher risk for hyperthyroidism.[5]

Primary Hypothyroidism

Approximately 95 percent of all hypothyroidism cases are primary hypothyroidism, making it the most common thyroid pathology. It's so common that the medical community says its prevalence is akin to that of heart disease and cancer.

The most common cause of primary hypothyroidism is Hashimoto's thyroiditis. Some 10 to 14 million Americans have it. Outside the United States, however, iodine deficiency is considered by allopathic medicine to be the primary cause of hypothyroidism.

Two other common but much less frequent causes of primary hypothyroidism are radiation therapy to the thyroid and thyroid removal (thyroidectomy). Radiation and thyroidectomy are typically done to treat resistant hyperthyroidism (too much thyroid hormone production).

Clinical Vs. Subclinical Primary Hypothyroidism

Primary hypothyroidism may be clinical or subclinical, according to the levels of TSH and T4 in the blood. Interestingly, the severity of signs and symptoms, such as weight gain, cold intolerance, and depression, are not used as part of the diagnostic distinction between clinical and subclinical hypothyroidism.

With clinical primary hypothyroidism, the amount of TSH in the blood is higher than the lab reference range, and T4 is below the lab reference range. As a result, people with clinical primary hypothyroidism often have dry skin, hair loss, and weight gain. However, even when T4 is normal, a person can experience these symptoms. Dr. Eric explains why this happens in part 2. For now, suffice it to say that even if you are experiencing symptoms, your allopathic doctor will likely rely on your T4 level to determine whether you have clinical or subclinical hypothyroidism. This is important because the guidelines doctors follow on diagnosing, treating, and managing hypothyroidism do not always encourage treatment for subclinical hypothyroidism.

With subclinical primary hypothyroidism, the level of TSH in the blood will be elevated, but the free T4 level will be in the lab reference range. Therefore, the clinical management is not straightforward, because allopathic medicine typically doesn't indicate hormone replacement therapy with T4 unless the T4 level is lower than the lab reference range. (Treatment of primary hypothyroidism is thyroid hormone replacement therapy.)

Subclinical primary hypothyroidism may advance, as it does more often than not, to primary hypothyroidism. This happens when the T4 level finally falls below the lab reference range. At that point, a doctor usually formally diagnoses primary hypothyroidism and offers treatment with synthetic T4 medication. In the meantime, if you have subclinical primary hypothyroidism (remember: high TSH but normal T4), recent research shows that you still may experience various widespread negative consequences, such as hypertension, elevated cholesterol, and cardiovascular abnormalities.

> **Subclinical Hypothyroidism**
>
> Subclinical hypothyroidism is a mild elevation in TSH levels despite normal T4 levels and is associated with hypertension, elevated cholesterol, and cardiovascular abnormalities. If not treated, the progression rate to overt hypothyroidism is between 2 percent and 5 percent per year.[6]

Despite the risks, there still remains quite a bit of controversy within allopathic medicine regarding whether or not subclinical primary hypothyroidism should be treated with thyroid hormone replacement therapy. In addition, since the T4 level in the blood is normal in subclinical disease, there may be some concern about causing other problems by driving T4 levels too high with supplemental T4.

Nonetheless, if you have subclinical primary hypothyroidism, you may be experiencing symptoms but are left in the wasteland until your T4 level drops below normal. Or you may have a practitioner that takes the risks seriously and treats you with supplemental T4 medication, which may ease your symptoms for a while but isn't treating the root cause of your thyroid problems.

Hashimoto's Thyroiditis

Hashimoto's thyroiditis is a chronic autoimmune thyroiditis in which the body's own immune system attacks the gland, causing inflammation and thyroid damage. (*Chronic* means long-term; *autoimmune* means the body's own immune system is causing the attack and destruction, and *thyroiditis* means the thyroid gland is in a state of inflammation.)

Hashimoto's thyroiditis is the most common type of primary hypothyroidism. It occurs most often in those of age forty-five to sixty-five and is five to eight times more likely to affect women than men. It affects about 14 million people in the United States, including myself and Dr. Eric. So chances are that you or someone you love has this diagnosis too.

As with most autoimmune diseases, Hashimoto's thyroiditis has a component linked to HLA–DR3, a histocompatibility complex gene group in DNA. This gene group provides instructions for making a protein known as the human leukocyte antigen (HLA) complex. Some histocompatibility complex genes have hundreds of identified versions (alleles), each of which is given a particular number, such as HLA-DR3. HLA complexes help the immune system distinguish the body's own proteins from the kinds of proteins made by pathogens. This is extremely relevant in autoimmune diseases that occur when the body fails to distinguish its own proteins from those of pathogens and sets off an attack on itself. Thus, HLA-DR3 may be associated with the aberrant immune response in Hashimoto's thyroiditis.

Although it is a generally accepted fact in allopathic medicine that Hashimoto's thyroiditis is idiopathic, meaning the cause is unknown, practitioners acknowledge that a combination of factors are likely to play a role in its development. Those factors include genetic predisposition to hypothyroidism and exposure to triggers, such as a toxin, infection, or trauma. In addition, most autoimmune thyroid diseases are lifelong conditions and will likely need to be managed with medication in the form of hormone replacement and continued medical evaluation.

The guidelines that medical doctors follow on how to diagnose, treat, and monitor primary and central hypothyroidism come from the American Association of Clinical Endocrinologists (AACE). The AACE guidelines agree that autoimmune thyroiditis seems to have a genetic component, stating, "Autoimmunity to the thyroid gland appears to be an inherited defect in immune surveillance, leading to abnormal regulation of immune responsiveness or alteration of presenting antigen in the thyroid."[7] This means that the body's attack on itself involves protein-producing genes that aren't as good at telling self from nonself, which predisposes the body to abnormal responses, such as abnormal antibody production to one's own tissues.

Antibodies are blood proteins typically produced in response to a specific antigen. (An antigen is anything that your body considers foreign, such as bacteria or a virus.) The immune system recognizes the antigen and creates antibodies to attach to it and eliminate it from the body. Autoantibodies are antibodies to proteins in the body, such as those in the thyroid (Hashimoto's thyroiditis), brain myelin (multiple sclerosis), or joint tissue (rheumatoid arthritis).

Autoimmune thyroiditis can be diagnosed with tests that detect thyroid autoantibodies circulating in the blood. These autoantibodies include antimicrosomal/antithyroid peroxidase antibodies (TPOAb), antithyroglobulin antibodies (TgAb), and TSH receptor antibodies (TSHRAb). However, even when tested for, antibodies are not always found.

Ord's Thyroiditis

Ord's thyroiditis, also known as Ord's disease, is a less common form of autoimmune thyroiditis than Hashimoto's thyroiditis. It is named after the physician William Miller Ord, who first described it in 1877. In this disease, antibodies to thyroid peroxidase enzyme (TPO) or thyroglobulin protein (TG) cause gradual destruction of follicles in the thyroid gland, and so the gland atrophies and becomes smaller. This is the key distinguishing feature between Ord's and Hashimoto's thyroiditis: Hashimoto's thyroiditis does not result in gland atrophy but more often causes the gland to become larger than normal.

However, more recent research would suggest that the thyroid atrophy seen in Ord's disease versus the hypertrophy found in Hashimoto's thyroiditis are only extremes within the same disease process and do not represent separate disorders. Nonetheless, their allopathic management is the same—that is, when T4 is low, it is replenished with supplementary T4.

Like Hashimoto's thyroiditis, Ord's is more common among women than men of the same age. It is characterized by the invasion of the thyroid tissue by white blood cells. Eventually the destruction of the thyroid gland in Ord's thyroiditis typically results in primary hypothyroidism. However, unlike Hashimoto's thyroiditis, a transient hyperthyroid state in the acute phase of Ord's disease is thought to be rare.

Thyroid Cancer

Thyroid cancer is a condition where abnormal thyroid cells grow uncontrolled. Thyroid cancer is relatively rare but does impact women more than men at a ratio of 3:1. Thyroid cancer is typically divided into three types; differentiated, medullary, and anaplastic or undifferentiated.

Differentiated Thyroid Cancer

Differentiated cancer is broken down into three types: papillary, follicular, and Hurthle cell cancers.

Papillary cancer is the most common form of thyroid cancer. Eight out of ten cancers are papillary cancer. Papillary cancer tends to impact one side of the thyroid gland and is slow growing but can spread to surrounding lymph tissue. While very common, it is rarely fatal.

Follicular cancer is caused by abnormal cell growth of the follicular cells of the thyroid gland. It is the next most common form of cancer and accounts for about 10 percent of thyroid cancers.

Hurthle cell cancer is the least common of the differentiated cancers, accounting for 3 percent of thyroid cancers.

Medullary Thyroid Cancer

Medullary cancer develops in the parafollicular cells of the thyroid gland. It is relatively uncommon, accounting for 4 percent of thyroid cancers. Medullary thyroid cancer has two types: sporadic and familial. The sporadic type tends to be found in older populations, and the familial in younger populations.

Anaplastic or Undifferentiated Thyroid Cancer

This is the least common form of thyroid cancer. It accounts for 2 percent of the cases of thyroid cancer.

Non-Thyroid Gland Disorders Causing Hypothyroidism

Central Hypothyroidism

Central hypothyroidism refers to low thyroid hormone production that stems from disorders of the hypothalamus or pituitary gland. As you learned in chapter 2, the hypothalamus releases thyrotropin-releasing hormone (TRH), which stimulates the pituitary gland to secrete TSH, which stimulates the thyroid to produce thyroid hormones. In central hypothyroidism, the thyroid gland is normal but is not adequately stimulated to produce sufficient thyroid hormones.

As I mentioned earlier, central hypothyroidism is separated into secondary and tertiary types. Secondary hypothyroidism is caused by inadequate TSH secretion from the pituitary gland. Tertiary hypothyroidism results from inadequate TRH secretion from the hypothalamus.

In children, a brain tumor, previous radiation therapy for a brain tumor, or blood cancer is often the cause of central hypothyroidism. In adults, it is usually due to pituitary macroadenomas (tumors), pituitary surgery, or radiation therapy. Fatigue and swelling of the legs and feet are the most common symptoms. Typically, TSH is in the normal or low–normal range, and thyroid hormones are low–normal. A TRH stimulation test confirms the diagnosis. Therapy includes the use of synthetic T4 to relieve symptoms.

Unlike primary hypothyroidism, central hypothyroidism cannot be monitored with a TSH test. The test that identifies hypothyroidism is a TSH test with reflex to fT4, which means that a TSH test is done first, and if it is abnormal, the lab will automatically test for fT4. If your TSH is normal, no fT4 test is done. This can make identifying secondary or tertiary central hypothyroidism very difficult, and even the best practitioners may miss it.

For example, if you report to your doctor that you've recently felt more tired than usual, he or she will order a TSH test to rule out hypothyroidism. If the TSH is normal, no fT4 test is done, and central hypothyroidism, if you have it, may be missed. In a busy medical practice, your doctor is unlikely to have your complete file spread out on the desk, so lab test results that might have been a red flag to look for central hypothyroidism may be missed. On the other hand, the doctor may see that your TSH is normal, assume your thyroid physiology is fine, and consider that your fatigue and other complaints are the result of some situation not related to thyroid physiology.

Euthyroid Sick Syndrome

The *Merck Manual* defines euthyroid sick syndrome as "a condition in which serum levels of thyroid hormones are low in clinically euthyroid patients with nonthyroidal systemic illness. Diagnosis is based on excluding hypothyroidism. Treatment is directed toward the underlying illness; thyroid hormone replacement is not indicated."[8]

Euthyroid Sick Syndrome (ESS) is also called nonthyroidal illness syndrome or low T3 syndrome (because there are low levels of T3 in the blood). It is not the result of a problem with the thyroid gland, but of some other acute or chronic illness or condition, such as prolonged fasting and starvation, protein-energy malnutrition, severe trauma, myocardial infarction, chronic kidney disease, diabetic ketoacidosis, anorexia nervosa, cirrhosis, and sepsis.

A decrease in T3 is more common than a decrease in T4 in ESS. However, low T4 levels sometimes occur. In ESS, it is also common to see an increase in serum reverse T3 (rT3). Reverse T3 is another, less common, form of thyroid hormone made from T4 in the peripheral tissues, which will be covered in more depth in subsequent chapters. Importantly, people with ESS can have a normally functioning thyroid gland and still have symptoms of hypothyroidism.

The exact mechanism of ESS is unknown; however, according to the *Merck Manual*, this condition may involve "decreased peripheral conversion of T4 to T3, decreased clearance of rT3 generated from T4, and decreased binding of thyroid hormones to thyroxine-binding globulin (TBG). In addition, proinflammatory cytokines (for example, tumor necrosis factor-alpha, IL-1) may be responsible for some changes."[9] This may sound complicated, but what it means is that during ESS, normal thyroid metabolism beyond the thyroid gland is altered.

Euthyroid sick syndrome, or low T3 syndrome, can result from the following:

- modifications to the hypothalamic-pituitary axis
- altered binding of thyroid hormone to carrier proteins
- modified entry of thyroid hormone into tissue
- changes in thyroid hormone metabolism due to altered expression of the deiodinases (See chapter 2.)
- changes in thyroid hormone receptor (THR) expression or function

While you may not be clear about how these mechanisms work, the important point to understand is that when someone has ESS, nearly every aspect of thyroid physiology beyond the thyroid gland can become compromised.

The difficulty for allopathic doctors lies in deciphering whether or not a patient has actual hypothyroidism or ESS. From a medical perspective, a TSH test is best. In ESS, the TSH level is low, normal, or slightly elevated but not as high as it would be in hypothyroidism. The blood level of rT3 is usually elevated too. However, in the allopathic model for thyroid care, doctors rarely measure rT3.

Allopathic doctors learn in medical school that thyroid tests such as TSH are not reliable in severely acute or chronically ill people and cannot be relied on to diagnose thyroid physiology problems. For example, one study that monitored thyroid function tests of intensive care unit patients found the prevalence of abnormal thyroid function tests to be remarkably high. More than 70 percent of the patients had low T3 levels, and around 50 percent had low T4 levels. Therefore, unless thyroid dysfunction is highly suspected, doctors don't order thyroid function tests for acutely ill patients that could be experiencing ESS.

Treatment of ESS does not involve thyroid replacement therapy, even if the T4 level is low in an ill person. Replenishing thyroid hormone doesn't improve the outcome, except for those with cardiovascular disease. In other words, when a person has ESS, treating him or her with thyroid hormone doesn't help. If a sick patient has ESS, treatment should focus on resolving the cause, such as septic shock or meningitis.

A FEW FINAL THOUGHTS

Medical doctors do their best to identify and address thyroid disorders and help their patients. Medical intervention is often critical to rule out pathology and manage acute situations. It is not our intent to disparage the work of allopathic physicians. Instead, we want to clear up some of the confusion regarding allopathic thyroid care.

Many people who struggle with chronic hypothyroid and hyperthyroid symptoms while being managed by allopathic physicians become frustrated. Despite family practitioners and endocrinologists following medical guidelines, patients' chronic signs and symptoms lead them to start doing their own research, and they find out that there are additional thyroid tests and alternative forms of thyroid medication their allopathic physician has not offered. They become frustrated and angry. They wonder why these tests are not run and why alternative medication options are not offered.

Our goal is to help you understand that this is not the result of the allopathic doctor not doing his or her job. Instead, the allopathic doctor *is* doing his or her job. The doctor is following the guidelines for allopathic treatment. The problem lies in the current allopathic paradigm of what hypothyroidism is and the tools available to address and manage hypothyroidism in the allopathic model. I had the same education and followed the same guidelines.

It was not until I developed hypothyroidism that I became fully aware that what the allopathic model had to offer was limited. Allopathic medicine was able to help manage my condition, my TSH, but not get me well. Allopathic medicine was able to help me achieve normal TSH and T4 levels with medication, resulting in biochemical euthyroid, but it could not provide well-being.

Because of this, I, like you, became frustrated. I could not envision living the rest of my life managing my blood tests with thyroid medication and not feeling well. I needed to find a solution. I needed to find answers to why I wasn't feeling healthy and well despite thyroid medication and normalized TSH and T4 levels.

In the next chapter of part 1, I explain how allopathic medicine evaluates, diagnoses, and treats thyroid physiology based on the medical guidelines. I also discuss some of the failures and shortcomings of the allopathic model. Finally, in part 2, Dr. Balcavage will discuss a new paradigm for understanding thyroid physiology.

While allopathic medicine may not change its medical intervention guidelines, we hope to provide a better understanding of why chronic symptoms persist and describe how a functional medicine approach can provide the answers and support that the current allopathic medicine model does not have the tools to address.

CHAPTER 4

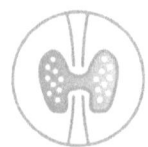

THYROID EVALUATION AND TREATMENT

After doctors have learned about the structure and function of the thyroid gland (as explained in chapter 2) and the pathologies in thyroid physiology (discussed in chapter 3), they apply this knowledge to real-life patients. This interaction begins while they are still in medical school and continues throughout their entire careers. The application of medical knowledge has a steep learning curve. It takes years to learn the signs and symptoms of various diseases, such as thyroid dysfunction, and select the proper tests, including labs and imaging techniques like CT scans, to reach appropriate diagnoses. When a diagnosis is made, it typically leads to interventions, such as drug therapy or surgery.

Clinical guidelines help make medical practice more manageable and provide more uniformity in how various diseases are managed. In addition, guidelines offer recommendations on diagnosing and treating various conditions; they are commonly formulated by scientific evidence (of varying degrees) and expert opinion. This chapter focuses on the steps your medical doctor takes in evaluating, screening, and managing hypothyroidism, as directed by the most recent published guidelines of the American Academy of Clinical Endocrinologists.

These guidelines dictate doctors' clinical decisions regarding hypothyroidism. They are (an updated version of) the guidelines that I was taught to rely upon and upon which I was to base management of my patients suffering from hypothyroidism. Specifically, these guidelines give recommendations on when and in whom to screen for thyroid problems, how to screen (with labs), the lab reference ranges to consider normal versus abnormal, and, finally, how and when to use medication to treat hypothyroidism. The guidelines, as stated, are more recommendations than they are hard, fast rules; nor are they by any means perfect. Doctors can use their own judgment if they find the recommendations not to fit their patient's needs.

THYROID PHYSICAL EXAM EVALUATION

When meeting with patients in a clinical setting, doctors are taught to do a thorough history and physical (H&P). A typical medical H&P consists of subjective questions (history); a physical examination; studies, such as laboratory blood work; and scans, such as ultrasounds, CTs, and MRIs. The history is broken up into sections:

- **Presenting symptoms (a.k.a. "chief complaint"):** Depending on the type of visit, a patient may or may not present with a chief complaint. (He or she may just be visiting the doctor for an annual physical.) If a patient does have complaints, the doctor initiates a discussion about those symptoms, asking questions such as when the symptoms started, what activities or events may have occurred when they began, and how long the symptoms typically last. The physician uses these questions to determine which labs or studies to proceed with following the visit, especially if the patient complains of hypothyroid symptoms.
- **Medical history:** This is a review of past diagnoses going all the way back to birth. This history may or may not include other

medical problems that have not been formally diagnosed, such as intermittent back pain from a car accident.
- **Pharmaceutical and supplement history:** This includes doses, timing, and length of treatment.
- **Family medical history:** This includes a review of the maternal and paternal history of diseases such as cancer, diabetes, depression, hypertension, and heart disease. It will also include inquiring about a family history of thyroid disease if the doctor suspects thyroid disease.
- **Social history:** This includes information about employment, hobbies, marital status, sexual orientation, number of children, living conditions, diet, alcohol consumption, drug use, and tobacco use. It generally involves a safety precaution review to assess whether the patient feels safe at home and takes precautions like regularly wearing a seatbelt.
- **Review of systems:** As the name implies, this is where a large amount of information regarding the other systems (e.g., the gastrointestinal system, cardiovascular system, and musculoskeletal system) in the body that are not covered in the presenting symptoms section are surveyed by asking the patient questions like "What are your bowel movements like?"
- **Allergies (both drug and environmental):** Lastly, the doctor asks if the patient has any medication or environmental allergies, when these allergies began, and what happens if the patient is exposed to the allergen.

In regard to thyroid health, if a doctor suspects a patient may be experiencing hypothyroidism, he or she may ask and record in the medical record if a patient has been experiencing dry skin, cold sensitivity, fatigue, muscle cramps, voice changes (hoarseness), depressed mood, constipation, carpal tunnel syndrome, hair loss, brittle nails, or sleep apnea.

After a thorough history is obtained, a physical exam is performed. *Bates' Guide to Physical Examination and History Taking* is the text that most physicians initially rely on for learning how to perform a proper physical exam. They also learn this information from attending physicians in residency and medical school training. In terms of the actual physical thyroid assessment, the doctor stands behind the patient, places both fingers on the gland, and then instructs the patient to swallow while he or she feels for any abnormal nodules or movement of the gland.[10]

A properly performed exam can indicate several possible abnormalities. If the doctor feels diffuse enlargement of the gland, this may indicate Graves' disease, Hashimoto's thyroiditis, or an endemic goiter. If the doctor feels a single solid nodule, this could be a cyst, benign tumor, or malignant growth. If the doctor feels multiple nodules, this is most like a multinodular goiter from iodine deficiency. Other significant findings of note when this exam is performed are that if the nodule is soft, this can be associated with Graves' disease; if it is firm, this is more suspicious for Hashimoto's thyroiditis and malignant and benign nodules. Tenderness can be elicited in patients with thyroiditis. And lastly, the doctor will use his or her stethoscope to listen to the blood flow in the thyroid gland for what is called a bruit, which indicates abnormal blood flow and can be associated with hyperthyroidism and Graves' disease.[11]

During the physical, the doctor will look for other signs of a low-functioning thyroid, such as dry skin and hair, hair loss or thinning, cracked nails, hoarseness of voice, visible goiter, and a high or low heart rate. The AACE guidelines also state that "recent studies strongly correlate the degree of hypothyroidism with a slow ankle reflex relaxation time, a measure rarely used in current clinical practice today."[12]

Your doctor may or may not be using this ankle reflex assessment as part of your physical exam if he or she suspects hypothyroidism symptoms. The AACE guidelines state it is "rarely used." I first read about this reliable test in my Bates physical exam textbook, but I did not see many physicians performing it in my training in residency. In fact, I would say I was never taught to perform it while in residency. I believe this is because it can be challenging to ascertain the degree of reflex time and perhaps also because the practice of medicine seems to be moving away from physically laying hands on patients and more toward reading numbers in lab reports and looking at scans (MRI, CT) to determine health or illness. In other words, we have more sophisticated ways of diagnosing hypothyroidism than the ankle relaxation time, especially in developed countries like the United States.

If after a full H&P a doctor is suspicious for thyroid dysfunction, or if a patient meets screening guidelines, which are discussed in the following section, the doctor will order a blood TSH (also referred to as "thyrotropin") level as a screening test for thyroid pathology/dysfunction. Whether a thyroxine (T4) blood level is measured as well is up to the doctor, but this is typically done when a TSH comes back high to determine whether the patient has clinical or subclinical hypothyroidism. This is called "TSH with reflex to fT4." The reflex means that if TSH is abnormal, the lab will automatically measure the levels of fT4, which stands for free T4, because this is vitally important information in the diagnosis of hypothyroidism.

THYROID LABORATORY TESTING

As mentioned previously, the guidelines on when to use laboratory testing to screen, diagnose, and monitor hypothyroidism come from the American Association of Clinical Endocrinologists (AACE). How and when your doctor uses thyroid tests such as TSH and T4 is likely to be based on the AACE guidelines unless the doctor has had outside training (or experience that suggests the guidelines are not always appropriate). Examples of outside training include courses or certification from the Institute of Functional Medicine (IMF) and the American Academy of Anti-Aging Medicine (A4M), to name two of the most popular. "Experience" refers to a doctor having learned that, in some instances, solely relying on TSH (as dictated by the AACE guidelines) to initially screen for hypothyroidism can be inadequate.

The word "guidelines" is often called out as a misnomer, even by allopathic doctors, and makes what the AACE has laid out sound like hard, fast rules when they are more akin to suggestions in the art and practice of medicine. An even better word to describe the AACE guidelines would be "recommendations"; the doctor is free to go outside of them (or not follow them at all) when he or she feels it is appropriate. An example of this would be where the guidelines say to screen with TSH, but the doctor feels that his or her patient should also have his or her free T4 drawn regardless of the TSH.

The following quote is direct from the guidelines, detailing who wrote the guidelines and what information they used to create them. "The development of these guidelines was commissioned by the American Association of Clinical Endocrinologists (AACE) in association with American Thyroid Association (ATA). AACE and the ATA assembled a task force of expert clinicians who authored this article. The authors examined relevant literature and took an evidence-based medicine approach that incorporated their knowledge and experience to develop a series of specific recommendations and the rationale for these recommendations."[13]

I include this information regarding thyroid laboratory testing and management because I think it is important to understand why your doctor does what he of she does—in other words, how he or she makes decisions about when to use thyroid labs to screen and monitor. For example, I have had many patients come in and tell me that they went to their doctor complaining of multiple symptoms consistent with hypothyroidism. The doctor used only a TSH to rule in or out hypothyroidism. When their TSH came back normal, they were told their thyroids were fine. Patients often feel testing their TSH only is insufficient. And when their TSHs come back normal, they often feel their doctors dismiss their symptoms. All the while, their doctors were following the guidelines, never intending to dismiss or mistreat their patients.

[13]

SCREENING

Following a complete history and physical (medical evaluation), your doctor will decide whether to screen you for hypothyroidism. Screening is meant to rule in or rule out hypothyroidism (i.e., to diagnose it or not [black and white]). Screening consists of a TSH with reflex to free T4 (fT4). The reflex means that if the TSH comes back high (outside the reference range), then your blood sample will automatically be tested for free T4 levels.

If, during your appointment, you complain of symptoms of hypothyroidism, you will automatically qualify to be screened.

Symptoms of Hypothyroidism

Feeling cold when other people do not
Constipation
Muscle weakness
Weight gain despite eating the same foods
Joint or muscle pain
Feeling sad or depressed
Feeling very tired
Pale, dry skin
Slow heart rate
Less perspiring than usual
Puffy face
Hoarse voice
Heavier than usual menstrual flow
Insomnia
Reflux
Elevated cholesterol and low-density lipoprotein cholesterol
Fatty liver disease
Insulin resistance
Gallbladder disorders
Palpitations
Sore throat
A feeling of being choked
Thinning hair and eyebrows
Irregular menstrual cycles
Low libido
Brain fog
Gas
Bloating
Poor memory

If you have been diagnosed with any of the following conditions, you should also be screened automatically, even if you do not complain of hypothyroid symptoms:

- adrenal insufficiency—when steroid hormone levels (mainly cortisol) are found to be low
- alopecia—hair loss
- anemia
- cardiac dysrhythmia—irregular heartbeat
- congestive heart failure
- changes in skin texture
- constipation
- dementia
- dysmenorrhea—pain during menstruation
- hypercholesterolemia—high cholesterol
- hypertension—high blood pressure
- mixed hyperlipidemia—high blood lipids (triglycerides)
- malaise and fatigue
- myopathy—diseases of muscle tissue
- prolonged QT interval—abnormal repolarization of the heart after a heartbeat
- type 1 diabetes
- vitiligo—autoimmune loss of pigment of the skin
- weight gain

Additionally, the AACE recommends screening those with

- any autoimmune disease;
- pernicious anemia;
- a first-degree relative with autoimmune thyroid disease;
- history of neck radiation to the thyroid gland, including radioactive iodine therapy for hyperthyroidism and external beam radiotherapy for head and neck malignancies;
- prior history of thyroid surgery or dysfunction;
- abnormal thyroid examination;
- psychiatric disorders; and
- amiodarone or lithium carbonate use.

If you are asymptomatic, meaning that you do not have any symptoms of hypothyroidism or diagnoses that fit the criteria for screening, you may or may not be screened, depending on which organization's screening recommendations your doctor follows. If your doctor follows the American Thyroid Association's recommendations and you are over the age of thirty-five, you should be screened every five years. If he or she follows the American Academy of Family Physicians, regular screening of hypothyroidism begins when you are sixty or older. It just depends on your doctor's preference for one of the six organizations' recommendations.

As stated, if your doctor does decide to screen you for hypothyroidism, he or she will do so with a TSH with reflex to free T4. The AACE guidelines state, "A serum thyrotropin [TSH] is the single best screening test for primary thyroid dysfunction for the vast majority of outpatient clinical situations." This means that your doctor will (most likely) rely on the results of your TSH test to determine your diagnosis and course of treatment if need be.

In our opinion, this method of screening may miss some diagnoses of hypothyroidism. There are two major problems. The first is that your TSH level is only a measure of the hypothalamic-pituitary response to thyroid hormones, meaning that the TSH produced by your pituitary gland in response to your hypothalamus is only a reflection of the levels of thyroid hormone detected by this tiny gland in your brain, not of thyroid hormone effects throughout your entire body. (This will be extensively covered in depth in part 2).

The second problem is that reference ranges for what is considered normal and abnormal for TSH have been criticized for being too broad. The predominant issue is how high the TSH cutoff is on the range.[14]

TSH Normal Range

Laboratory reference ranges (considered the acceptable range for health or lack of disease) are supposed to be formulated from "healthy" populations of people. In most cases, the reference range takes the lab results of this healthy population of people, finding the average value and allowing two standard deviations of variance high or low. This creates the laboratory reference range. By definition, 5 percent of all results from healthy people will fall outside of the reported reference interval (range) and, as such, will be flagged as being "abnormal."[15]

Reference lab ranges are typically used for both diagnoses and treatment. If your lab value is outside the accepted reference range, then your lab value is considered abnormal. For example, a TSH level two standard deviations above the mean (denoted by an *H* on your lab report) would indicate possible hypothyroidism, a TSH level two standard deviations below the mean (denoted by an *L* on your lab report) would indicate likely hyperthyroidism.

However, the glaring problem is that when creating reference ranges, the assumption is made that the average is being generated from those who are healthy and without thyroid disease or any other disease for that matter. Yet when I learned about reference ranges in medical school, this is what I was taught—that reference ranges are generated from a normal, disease-free, healthy population using the same methods.

Unfortunately, what I was taught in school and what today's reality in determining reference ranges is based on are quite different. The first issue is the term "healthy." There is no clear-cut, universally agreed-upon definitions or criteria of what "healthy" is. How do we define what the healthy range is if there is no universal definition of "healthy"? How can someone poll a population of people to determine the reference range if we can't define who is healthy? As you will learn if you dig into this topic further, lab ranges are not necessarily based on healthy populations of people but on other criteria, such as the general population of people reporting to a given lab. This is one reason the laboratory reference range from one laboratory can differ from the lab reference range at a different laboratory.

You can see how confusing this can be for a medical doctor to determine the appropriate normal reference range for TSH and other lab tests. This may be why there are multiple sets of recommendations regarding the cutoff for TSH; we aren't sure because we aren't basing it on good data.

A review of data from NHANES III suggests that the upper limit of the reference interval is close to 4 mIU/L.[16] The National Academy of Clinical Biochemists has suggested a much lower cutoff of 2.5 mIU/L.[17] The American Association of Clinical Endocrinologists (AACE) and the American Thyroid Association (ATA) suggested using the reference interval established by any given laboratory using a third generation TSH assay. If this is not available, the next option would be to use the NHANES III range of 0.45-4.12 mIU/L.[18]

Table 7 from the guidelines, "Thyrotropin Upper Normal," has varying levels of "TSH upper normal" from various groups, studies, and societies.

Various Upper Normal Limits of TSH

Most clinical laboratories have not lowered the upper cutoff for TSH to comply with NACB guidelines based on observations that "22 to 28 million more Americans would be diagnosed with hypothyroidism without any clinical or therapeutic benefit from this diagnosis."[19] Now, whether there would be a clinical or therapeutic benefit is hard to determine, but it would likely lead to more people being diagnosed and treated with thyroid medication. Two of the biggest labs in the United States, Labcorp and Quest Labs, use a reference range for TSH of 0.450–4.500 mIU/L.

In my practice, I prefer to use a reference range for TSH of 1.8–3.0 mIU/L. However, I also run a full thyroid panel that includes free

T4, T4, free T3, rT3, and tests for antibodies. This is because I have spent time learning above and beyond what I was taught in medical school and residency training about thyroid physiology. Testing more comprehensively enables me to understand better what is going on so I don't miss a problem with the thyroid gland or thyroid physiology. The upper range for TSH is only one piece of the puzzle, and I recognize its limitations. I acknowledge that a TSH can be considered normal in my own accepted functional range of 1.8–3 mIU/L but that it may not be appropriate considering a patient's signs and symptoms. Dr. Eric will cover this in part 2.

ALLOPATHIC INTERPRETATION OF THYROID SCREENING TESTS

Most guidelines recommend that if TSH is within normal lab range (and I already discussed how those lab ranges may vary and that there is mixed consensus in regard to what the normal lab range should be), patients be diagnosed as *not* having a thyroid disorder by medical standards.

The AACE guidelines state, "An elevated TSH, usually above 10 mIU/L, in combination with a subnormal free T4 characterizes overt hypothyroidism."[20] So if you don't meet these criteria, you may not be considered to have a hypothyroid condition by an allopathic doctor until those numbers change.

Symptomatic with Normal TSH and T4

Let's say that you have a plethora of hypothyroid symptoms (such as weight gain, dry skin, and depressed mood). You and your doctor might consider you have a hypothyroid condition. However, if your doctor runs a screening thyroid test and your TSH and T4 are within normal limits (meaning possibly up to 10 mIU/L for TSH) based on the guidelines, you will likely be told a hypothyroid condition is not causing your symptoms. Instead you may be instructed to reduce your food intake (go on a diet), exercise more, and perhaps even take an antidepressant for signs of depression.

This was often an experience I had with patients when I practiced as a traditional allopathic physician. Many of my patients would come and see me with symptoms that I, right in line with my patient, considered hypothyroidism symptoms. I would often run thyroid screening tests on these patients who had the signs and symptoms of hypothyroidism, only to be surprised when the results would come back normal. In these instances, I had to say things like "I know you have experienced weight gain and dry skin and feel depressed, but your thyroid seems fine because your TSH and free T4 are within the normal range."

My hands were tied in that I had no justification for prescribing thyroid hormone for what seemed to be symptoms of hypothyroidism. My only recourse was to provide generic lifestyle recommendations and medications to manage their symptoms. I knew their symptoms were real, but until their labs became abnormal and indicated hypothyroidism, thyroid hormone replacement therapy was not a recommended option.

Patients often met such recommendations with eye-rolls, disbelief, and feelings of hopelessness. However, the guidelines supported my (and most likely your doctor's) clinical decision to consider that their symptoms were most likely due to poor lifestyle choices, habits, and stress if the labs were normal, not due to problems with their thyroids. "Treat the paper, not the patient" was really what I felt I sometimes had to do.

This is because, as I mentioned, there are no tools in the allopathic toolkit to address situations like this. If our tool is medication to increase T4, but the T4 is normal, we as doctors have nothing to offer. If your thyroid lab values (TSH and T4) are normal, then there is nothing to treat, per se, in the allopathic model. In most cases, doctors are forced to send patients out the door without treatment (such as a prescription) until their pathological process does enough damage to cause the labs to become out of range. Then, at last, medication can be started.

The allopathic model has no options for treating the actual cause of thyroid dysfunction. The typical process is to let the destruction of the gland continue untreated and provide thyroid hormone replacement therapy only once the damage has reached a level of destruction where the thyroid gland can no longer produce sufficient thyroid hormone, driving TSH and T4 out of the lab reference range. It may take up to 90 percent of the thyroid gland to be damaged before lab values indicate hypothyroidism.[21] It is not the doctor's fault that some treatment for your thyroid condition isn't offered sooner; they are working within the allopathic model. The doctor is just doing what they were taught; I was doing what I was taught as per the guidelines. The medical model is off, not the doctor.

I was never taught in any of my traditional medical training what is actually happening in these patients with chronic hypothyroid symptoms but normal TSH. I was not taught the concept of cellular hypothyroidism (what is causing hypothyroid symptoms) and that standard thyroid tests can completely miss this. I was not taught that giving synthetic T4 does not address the underlying cause of a hypothyroid problem!

Because I have been extensively trained on cellular hypothyroidism by Dr. Eric, I look back, and hindsight is 2020. I know what I did wrong - how I erroneously relied on TSH for screening, how I waited while destructive processes continued in my patients because I did not know what else to do, how I prescribed medication to normalize labs but rarely helped a person in my care become healthier. You, too, will learn about cellular hypothyroidism as it is our focus in part 2 of this book. You will get the opportunity to learn what I learned, and our hope is that it will change your life as it did for me, both personally and professionally.

Symptomatic with High TSH and Low T4 = Clinical Hypothyroidism (a.k.a. Overt Hypothyroidism)

If a patient presents with symptoms that correlate with a low-functioning thyroid gland (or is asymptomatic but meets screening criteria), and if their TSH is elevated and their T4 is low, a formal diagnosis of Clinical (aka Overt) hypothyroidism can be given, along with a prescription for synthetic T4, such as levothyroxine. (Brand names include Synthroid, Tirosint, Levoxyl, Unithroid, and Levo-T.) That is it. Diagnosis. Medication. Forever.

The goal of treatment with medication is to normalize TSH. Medical doctors are taught that when TSH is normalized, thyroid physiology is restored in the body. Voila! Once this normalization is established, a state called euthyroidism, any other symptoms a patient may still be having are considered not to be associated with hypothyroidism but to be caused by something else. Again, in medicine, we don't give a whole lot of attention to the why; rather, we direct most of our attention (treatment) at the what. For example, if a patient with diagnosed hypothyroidism is being treated with levothyroxine, and this brings his or her TSH down to 2.0 (which is normal) but he or she is still experiencing depression, the patient may be offered an antidepressant. The symptom of depression would not be attributed to thyroid dysfunction but rather to some unknown root cause. The allopathic model's strategy is to once again provide lifestyle recommendations (diet and exercise) and treat symptoms.

Symptomatic with High TSH and Normal T4 = Subclinical Hypothyroidism

If a patient presents with symptoms that correlate with a low-functioning thyroid gland (or is asymptomatic but meets screening criteria) and his or her TSH is above the normal limit but his or her T4 is normal, then a diagnosis of subclinical hypothyroidism (SCH) is given. This condition occurs in 3 percent to 8 percent of the general population. It is more common in women than men, and its prevalence increases with age. Of patients with SCH, 80 percent have a serum TSH of less than 10 mIU/L. The most important implication of SCH is the high likelihood of progression to clinical hypothyroidism.[22] As per the guidelines, doctors can treat this condition with medication or wait until the patient's T4 finally falls below normal. Once the decision to treat is made, it's—you guessed it—levothyroxine.

Another interesting point that the guidelines state regarding SCH is "The decision to treat subclinical hypothyroidism when the serum thyrotropin is less than 10 mIU/L should be tailored to the individual patient." They go on to describe the "beneficial response" regarding cardiovascular (heart) health in treating patients with subclinical hypothyroidism: "A substantial number of studies have been done on patients with TSH levels between 2.5 and 4.5, indicating beneficial response in atherosclerosis risk factors such as atherogenic lipids, impaired endothelial function, and intima-media thickness." Atherosclerosis is a disease of the blood vessels that can cause heart attacks and strokes.

Based on this recommendation, treating SCH in those with TSH levels of between 2.5 and 4.5 to lessen those aforementioned cardiovascular risks seems like a good idea. However, this is a very controversial issue. Some doctors will treat these cases because the guidelines specifically tell them that studies show benefits from treatment. Some doctors do not. One reason doctors may be hesitant to treat a patient with normal TSH is that patients may experience signs and symptoms of hyperthyroidism.[23]

Treating people with SCH with synthetic T4 therapy may provide some initial symptom relief, but it can make the underlying process of cellular hypothyroidism worse in the long run. Addressing the cause (or more likely causes) of cellular hypothyroidism is covered in part 3.

The description of subclinical hypothyroidism from the AACE guidelines raises some interesting questions. "Hypothyroidism may be either subclinical or overt. Subclinical hypothyroidism is characterized by a serum TSH above the upper reference limit in combination with a normal free thyroxine (T4). This designation is only applicable when thyroid function has been stable for weeks or more, the hypothalamic-pituitary-thyroid axis is normal, and there is no recent or ongoing severe illness. An elevated TSH, usually above 10 mIU/L, in combination with a subnormal free T4 characterizes overt hypothyroidism."[24]

What this is saying is that a diagnosis of SCH is appropriate only if (1) something hasn't caused thyroid function to be unstable—recent acute illness, new drug therapy with amiodarone or lithium or acute trauma—(2) the patient's hypothalamic-pituitary-thyroid connection and communication hasn't been determined to be abnormal, and (3) the patient does not have a severe illness that is long-standing. Number 1 is pretty straightforward, but determining numbers 2 and 3 is not as straightforward, which brings up some valid questions:

- How is a normal hypothalamic-pituitary-thyroid axis determined in clinical practice?
- What does it mean to have a severe illness?
- What are the subjective and objective parameters for subclinical hypothyroidism? Do they even exist? Or do we assume that one has no problems until one has a sudden and severe onset of disease?

Spoiler alert: These questions don't have good, solid answers for anyone, including the best, most caring allopathic doctors. Without good answers and explanations, the default is to wait on treatment until labs are abnormal. I recall being frustrated as a doctor when dealing with SCH because I felt that I could not provide my suffering patients with the help they were looking for. Doctors are not trained on what to do when a person doesn't have full-blown disease. It is a very black-and-white system, but the majority of us live in the gray zone—somewhere between being healthy and being in a hospital bed. We weren't provided with the system to evaluate and treat the gray zone, other than providing symptom-suppressing medication—as in the case of SCH. Instead we are taught that SCH can be temporary and one can go back to normal. We are also taught that it can and often will progress to clinical or overt primary hypothyroidism. But, as physicians, we are taught to wait and see. In part 3, we will cover reasons that can cause the abnormalities in the gray zone so that we can prevent patients from ever getting to the black diagnosis of disease. Maybe you have a doctor who is frustrated with the current guidelines and their lack of clarity too.

WHICH LABS ARE NOT RUN BY ALLOPATHIC DOCTORS AND WHY

T3, fT3, T3U, RT3

From the standpoint of an allopathic doctor, the measurement of total T3 (T3), free T3 (fT3), T3 uptake (T3U), and reverse T3 (RT3) are irrelevant when it comes to diagnosis and treatment of hypothyroidism. The diagnosis and treatment of hypothyroidism revolve around two values in the allopathic model. First, since only TSH and T4/fT4 are needed to diagnose and treat hypothyroidism, the other available tests are irrelevant. Second, if a test does not help diagnose and manage a condition, it is considered to be medically unnecessary. Medical doctors shy away from running tests that are deemed not medically necessary. Why? Because insurance companies often deny paying for tests that are deemed not medically necessary, causing their patients to receive unexpected bills.

The guidelines a traditional doctor follows go so far as to recommend specifically *not* use either total T3 or free T3 to diagnose or monitor hypothyroidism. This recommendation gets a really good grade (grade A), meaning it is based on sound scientific evidence. You may be confused because you may believe or have heard that a complete thyroid evaluation must include total T3, free T3, T3U, and RT3. How can the recommendation not to use total T3 or free T3 get such a good grade?

Doctors have been taught, and evidence suggests, that T3 and free T3 values rarely leave the lab reference range. So why run them? The body maintains T3 and fT3 within the reference range as a biologic priority.[25] I agree that T3 and fT3 rarely leave the lab reference range, but we often see them out of the optimal range. I also agree with the recommendations not to use total or free T3 to diagnose primary hypothyroidism. However, I can't entirely agree that they should never be tested. Total and free T3 are very important pieces of the proper evaluation of thyroid physiology, as are T3U and RT3.

Even more controversial is the testing of reverse T3. When this test was originally established, many allopathic doctors providing T4 thyroid hormone replacement therapy did run this test. It is known that T4 can be converted into T3, an active thyroid hormone, or rT3, an inactive thyroid hormone, by the cells of the body. Doctors wanted to know if the thyroid hormone they provided (T4) was converting into T3 or rT3. If they saw reverse T3 levels going up due to T4 hormone therapy, they assumed the patient had a polymorphism (a gene defect) that slowed their conversion of T4 to T3, resulting in increased reverse T3. The solution was to provide more T4 therapy to these patients. The result, unfortunately, in many led to a hyperthyroid state, which was not what the doctors wanted. In time, the idea of using reverse T3 as a test to evaluate thyroid hormone replacement therapy was scrapped. Since the test was no longer of value to diagnose or treat hypothyroidism, it, too, was determined to be "not medically necessary." Once again, Dr. Eric will discuss the significance of reverse T3 in functional medicine in part 2.

FOLLOW-UP EVALUATION OF HYPOTHYROIDISM

The AACE guidelines state that hypothyroidism should be monitored in follow-up evaluations with TSH alone. "Measurement of serum TSH is the primary screening test for thyroid dysfunction, and for evaluation of thyroid hormone replacement in patients with primary hypothyroidism."[26] Recall that the goal of treatment is to normalize

TSH, which is thought to reflect normalized thyroid hormone physiology, which then assumes that hypothyroid symptoms should also normalize. Seems like a lot of assumptions to me.

Interestingly, the guidelines also state that "TSH levels vary diurnally by up to approximately 50 percent of mean values, with more recent reports indicating up to 40 percent variation on specimens performed serially during the same time of day."[27] This means that TSH levels can vary widely based on the time you have your blood drawn. Knowing this and that the reference ranges for TSH may not be very accurate, we must consider that TSH may not be the most reliable and accurate test for diagnosis or, specifically, for monitoring thyroid disease.

We will show you research in part 2 that explains why TSH, the gold standard test in allopathic medicine, may not be as reliable as once hoped. Learning this information allowed me to better understand why a normal TSH value did not always correlate with what my patients were experiencing. I just wish I had known this information sooner. But as the saying goes, when you know better, you (hopefully) do better!

To recap, TSH levels can vary up to 40 percent even when drawn on a patient at the exact same time of day. However, doctors are directed to use it to evaluate thyroid hormone replacement in patients with primary hypothyroidism (except if you are pregnant or severely ill). Based on the guidelines, free T4 can be used selectively if the doctor chooses to do so. He or she very well may not, and by allopathic standards, that is okay. If this approach sounds strange to you, you are not alone. It reminds me of this quote by Confucius: "The man who asks a question is a fool for a minute; the man who does not ask is a fool for life." I believe I started to question what I was doing while practicing allopathic medicine because I experienced firsthand the guideline-led treatment for hypothyroidism. And even though my TSH normalized, I still felt terrible. Asking questions may come across as challenging the norm, but all I ever wanted was to feel better. I think that's all anyone ever wants. My doctor brethren do the best they can with the information they are given. Dr. Eric and I hope to provide them with new information to process and utilize in practice.

WHACK-A-MOLE MEDICINE

Whether or not you get a formal diagnosis of clinical hypothyroidism or subclinical hypothyroidism, and whether or not you are placed on synthetic T4 replacement therapy, rarely will anyone in the allopathic model ever ask, "Why is this occurring? Why does this patient have thyroid disease?" But for those who do ask the questions, there are very few answers in allopathic medicine. We use terms like "idiopathic," meaning the cause is unknown. And with this one word, doctors are expected to move on and just treat the symptoms. It can be a very frustrating occupation. It can be even more frustrating for a patient. I know; I have been both.

Root causes of disease are often unaddressed or overlooked because of two important factors:

- Allopathic doctors are not trained to ask "Why?"
- Even if they knew the answer, they are not trained or paid to fix it.

Administering synthetic thyroid hormones may normalize lab ranges and may provide some symptom relief for some people, but drugs do not fix the underlying problem in cases of hypothyroidism. Instead, giving thyroid hormone alone lets the root cause or causes continue to smolder, which may shut down other processes and essential functions in the body, leading to other, often more severe, medical diagnoses for which drugs are the typical allopathic answer. This is what we refer to as "whack-a-mole medicine."

Because prescription drugs are typically the only treatment for primary hypothyroidism, it unfortunately keeps patients returning to their allopathic practitioner for multiple reasons. The first is that since the cause of hypothyroidism is never addressed, there is a lifetime need for thyroid hormone replacement that often needs to be adjusted. The second reason is that since the cause of hypothyroidism is not addressed, the cause or causes can persist, resulting in other symptoms, conditions, and disorders that ultimately require more medical treatment and medication. The third is that each medication has effects and side effects. Many of those side effects require more medications to manage.

As we have said and as I have experienced, the doctor is not to blame; the model needs an upgrade. This is reflected by the staggering stats on the amount of prescription medication used in the United States. In a recent study from the *Journal of the American Medical Association* (JAMA), nearly three in five American adults are taking a prescription drug. That is pretty darn high. What is worse is that the number keeps getting higher! This same study found that prescription medication use had risen from 51 percent to 59 percent when comparing use in 2000 to 2012. During the same period, the percentage of people taking five or more prescription drugs nearly doubled, to 15 percent from 8 percent.[28] You read that right—five or more medications, and it doubled. Again this points to the model needing some major attention.

Let's take a look at an example of the allopathic model in action. Jenny Doe comes in for her yearly physical. She is a forty-two-year-old mother of two with a high-stress job and little emotional support at home. She tells her physician that lately she's gained weight, feels cold all the time, is losing hair, and feels depressed. Her doctor documents her complaints and does a thorough physical exam, which includes palpating her thyroid gland, which he says "seems normal."

Because Jenny fits the screening criteria, her doctor agrees to run some labs to screen her for hypothyroidism. Her TSH comes back at 4.8 µIU/mL (with a normal range of 0.45 to 4.5 µIU/mL); this abnormally high TSH reflexively prompts her free T4 to be run, which comes back to be 0.84 ng/dL (with a normal range of 0.82 to 1.77 ng/dL). Her doctor tells her that her TSH is just above normal but her free T4 is normal, so her thyroid "seems fine right now," and instructs her to cut calories and exercise more.

She returns in six months and reports a worsening of her symptoms. The labs are repeated, and her TSH is now 5.0 µIU/mL (high), and her free T4 is now 0.7 ng/dL (low). The doctor officially diagnoses her with primary hypothyroidism. He places her on Synthroid, a synthetic T4 drug.

Jenny starts to take the medication as prescribed, and she feels better for a period of time. Her mood is better, she feels less cold, and she has more energy, but the improvement in her symptoms ends fairly quickly—it is what's called a "honeymoon period." She goes back to her doctor. He checks her TSH, which is again found to be above normal, so he increases the dose of her medication but does nothing else. He is following the guidelines and treating her disease as he should in the allopathic model.

A couple of years pass, and Jenny is still on Synthroid and has "normal TSH and free T4," as her dose has increased a little each year. Yet she is still gaining weight and has terrible brain fog and depression, for which she takes an antidepressant. She notices that she has to urinate a lot more often than usual and is constantly thirsty. So she goes back to her doctor, who runs some standard labs and tells her that she now has prediabetes. She is placed on Metformin and told to cut more calories and exercise. Time has passed since her initial visit at age forty-two, when she complained of hypothyroid symptoms. But now, at age forty-eight, she has the same symptoms as she did when she originally went in but also has two medical diagnoses and is on three pharmaceutical medications. She's asked her doctor why her body seems to be falling apart, but he has no answers. Hypothyroidism is considered idiopathic, so he, unfortunately, has nothing more to offer but is very sympathetic toward her.

This whack-a-mole description is not in any way intended to disparage allopathic doctors. It's just what happens when the root causes are not addressed; more medications are needed to treat more diseases. I know doctors, including myself, are good people who are doing their best. I used this model, and I was doing my best. Was I frustrated? Yes, but I didn't have any other options. Now that I have learned about cellular hypothyroidism from Dr. Eric, I have a whole new understanding of hypothyroidism. I get to see people get off medications instead of playing whack-a-mole! What is exciting is that, in part 2, Dr. Eric will teach you too!

CHAPTER 5

CHALLENGES WITH THE CURRENT THYROID MODEL

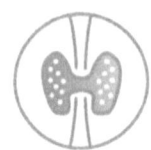

It's Not All Bad

Before I delve into the problems Dr. Eric and I see with the medical model of thyroid care, I must say that allopathic medicine plays an invaluable role in diagnosing and treating thyroid disorders. Make no mistake, the ability of allopathic physicians to provide thyroid hormone replacement therapy to those with primary hypothyroidism or to provide medical care to those in a hyperthyroid crisis can be lifesaving and life-changing. This doesn't mean, however, that acute treatment in times of crises will be the best long-term solution for a person's health and well-being.

In the allopathic model of thyroid care, once a person has been diagnosed with primary hypothyroidism, doctors prescribe thyroid hormone replacement therapy. The goal of a daily supplement of thyroid hormone (T4) is to normalize the person's TSH level and becomes the long-term management strategy. While this approach often works well in normalizing TSH, it often fails to provide what most patients are looking for—that is, elimination of hypothyroid signs and symptoms and restored health. The initial boost in metabolism provided by thyroid hormone replacement therapy may improve many chronic symptoms. But for many people, the improvement can be short-lived. Chronic hypothyroid symptoms are rarely completely eliminated with hormone replacement therapy. And, for some people, not only does the supplemental T4 not improve their symptoms, it makes them feel worse.

You might ask how many people are dissatisfied with the current allopathic model of thyroid care. Is it just a few? Is there any evidence? There is quite a bit of evidence. A study was conducted in 2018 to investigate the patient level of satisfaction with the current allopathic model. A total of 12,146 individuals diagnosed and treated for hypothyroidism completed a satisfaction survey. The overall degree of satisfaction with their therapy was rated a 5/10. We think this study confirms the point.

Candace was at a point of utter frustration when Dr. Eric and I met her. She had been to quite a few endocrinologists who had tried everything to address her primary hypothyroidism. She had been placed on all forms of hormone replacement therapy—T4 therapy, T3 therapy, and T4/T3 combination therapy. Each form of supplemental thyroid hormone lowered her TSH, but all of them created significant side effects.

"It didn't matter what form of thyroid hormone replacement therapy the endocrinologists prescribed, I never felt well. Small amounts of any form of thyroid hormone would improve some symptoms. But doses large enough to bring my TSH to the desired level, always made me feel worse. When the endocrinologists were happiest with my TSH test, I felt my worst. It was crazy! I would have symptoms of hyperthyroidism and hypothyroidism at the same time. I was anxious, edgy, and irritable. I couldn't sleep. My mind would not shut down. Yet I was gaining weight and chronically fatigued. I had no libido, super dry skin, and irritable bowel syndrome.

The higher the thyroid hormone dose, the worse I felt. The lower the dose the better I felt, but the less pleased my endocrinologists were. At one point I was on multiple medications to treat the side effects of the thyroid hormone dose that kept my TSH in the normal reference range. The medications caused more symptoms, and I could feel my life spinning out of control. I begged each endocrinologist to reduce my thyroid medication dose. They always did, and I immediately started feeling better. I stopped all the additional medications, and while I still wasn't well, I felt better.

That's when I found you. What happened next was nothing short of amazing. You listened to my story. You believed what I was telling you about how thyroid hormone replacement therapy made me feel. You said it is not unusual, and that many people have the same experience. We got to work identifying and addressing what was causing my hypothyroidism. In my case, it was nutrient deficiencies and chronic infections. Addressing those conditions changed dramatically.

My chronic symptoms are gone. My weight is back to what it was before I had children. I have energy and a libido. I'm back. The most important thing I learned was that the way to fix my chronic thyroid condition and relieve the symptoms had less to do with my thyroid and more to do with fixing everything else."

Could it be possible that the dose of thyroid medication Candace's doctors prescribed could make her feel worse even if her TSH was normal? If the TSH levels are normal can people still experience hypothyroid symptoms? If TSH is restored with thyroid hormone replacement therapy, how can symptoms persist? Is it be possible that thyroid hormone replacement can make a person feel worse? It is not only possible, but probable.

Candace's experience raises several other questions. Were her symptoms not caused by hypothyroidism? Maybe the chronic symptoms thought to be due to hypothyroidism were really caused by another disorder or condition. Or maybe, there was a disconnect between what hypothyroid is or isn't. Or maybe there is a disconnect between how allopathic medicine defines and identifies hypothyroidism and how thyroid physiology works in the body. Are people like Candace are few and far between? Dr. Eric's and my experience is that Candace is not an anomaly and neither are you. And neither are the thousands of people who seek out functional medicine care every year to address their chronic hypothyroid symptoms.

IS THERE EVIDENCE OF A PROBLEM?

Since you're reading *The Thyroid Debacle*, you probably suspect there is a problem with the medical model of thyroid care you or a loved one is receiving. Is Candace's experience common? Are there enough people complaining to warrant concern? There are, especially when scientific papers are being written on the topic. Continually more evidence suggests a significant proportion of patients treated with thyroid hormone replacement therapy (levothyroxine or branded drugs such as Synthroid and Tirosint) continue to experience residual hypothyroidism symptoms.[29,30,31]

Despite these patients achieving euthyroidism—that is, their TSH returns to the reference range with thyroid hormone replacement therapy--an estimated five to ten percent of hypothyroid patients continue to struggle with persistent symptoms.[32,33,34,35] Given the overall satisfaction rating found in the study I discussed previously, I feel the estimate of five to ten percent is low. There are likely even more patients who complain of persistent hypothyroid signs and symptoms, but doctors either dismiss their complaints or tell them another condition is at fault.

In spite of achieving normal TSH levels, many patients continue to complain of persistent hypothyroid symptoms like an inability to lose weight or continuous weight gain. A common complaint is that they just don't feel normal. They don't feel like they did before their hypothyroidism developed.[36]

There has been a long-raging battle within allopathic medicine about why some patients continue to struggle when thyroid replacement therapy restores their TSH to normal. The phenomenon is questioned, regardless of the fact that multiple scientific papers have been published describing patients experiencing chronic hypothyroid symptoms even when their TSH levels are suppressed to a point of being barely detectable.[37]

This has led to spirited discussions about whether or not T4/T3 combination therapy is a better treatment for those continuing to experience symptoms on T4-only therapy. There is no clear-cut answer. There are many potential reasons and hypotheses for why thyroid hormone replacement therapy fails to restore optimal thyroid physiology.[38]

There is disagreement, too, about what the normal, TSH reference range should be for those with and without hypothyroidism. There is also continuing debate about what is the best form of thyroid replacement therapy.

A growing population of people are struggling under the current standard of care for hypothyroidism. You are likely one of them. I don't think we need to draw this point out any longer. A problem exists with the current model, but why?

WHY IS THYROID CARE FAILING?

Some of the major reasons why the current model of thyroid care is failing. Among them is believing that:

- normal labs values are more indicative of successful treatment than how a patient is feeling.
- TSH is the best and sometimes only test needed to assess thyroid physiology.
- TSH is an early indicator of thyroid gland dysfunction.

- no symptom can be the result of insufficient thyroid hormone unless TSH is out of the reference range.
- thyroid hormone regulation is the same in all tissues.
- thyroid hormone regulation is the same in states of high stress as it is in low stress.
- use of thyroid replacement therapy to return TSH to normal indicates that thyroid physiology is restored to its optimal state for health.
- most hypothyroidism is caused by an autoimmune condition (which is true, at least in the US), and since it is idiopathic, there is nothing that can be done to limit the damage.
- the only solution for hypothyroidism is thyroid hormone replacement therapy.
- bio-individuality doesn't play a role among patients who don't respond to hormone replacement therapy.

The best thing to do is to take these beliefs one by one and see what the current science is showing. It's one thing to tell you why Dr. Eric and I think the current model of thyroid care is not working, it's another to show you that there is science to back up what we are saying.

Prioritizing Lab Values Over How You Feel

Dry skin, thinning hair, weight gain, fatigue, constipation, brain fog, abnormal menstrual cycles, and constipation are all symptoms commonly associated with hypothyroidism. They are so well established that if you walk into a medical doctor's office with these complaints, the immediate assumption is that you had a thyroid condition, and the doctor will order a TSH with reflex to fT4 tests to confirm the diagnosis.

However, if the TSH value turns out to be within the reference range, the doctor is likely to say that you don't have hypothyroidism, and your symptoms are the result of something else. But scientific research is showing that you can have a normal TSH, normal thyroid gland function, normal levels of thyroid hormone in your blood, but low thyroid hormone in your cells is creating the symptoms.[39, 40,41,42,43]

The reason for this is that while the production of thyroid hormone by the thyroid gland is important, thyroid hormone is mostly active inside your cells.

Your cells and tissues have an ability to regulate how much free thyroid hormone enters your cells, and what happens once it's there. If the cells want or need to increase their metabolism, they will bring free thyroid hormone into the cell and convert it to the more active form, triiodothyronine (T3). If cells want to slow down their metabolism, they will bring less free thyroid hormone into the cell, and deactivate both T4 and T3 that is reaching the cell. The ability of your cells to control thyroid hormone regardless of how much is circulating in the bloodstream is critical to our survival.

The TSH Fallacy

The gold standard test of thyroid physiology is TSH. Almost every set of guidelines considers this the definitive measure of thyroid physiology. Many allopathic physicians consider a TSH test not only to be the best test but the only one needed to evaluate thyroid physiology.[44] Yet nearly all of the medical organizations providing diagnosis and treatment guidelines disagree on what the TSH reference range is. You would think that if one test is going to be used as the gold standard test to assess thyroid status, there would be no disagreement or uncertainty what is a normal TSH level.

You would also think that if one test determines such an important aspect of our physiology that it would not be influenced by other factors. And yet there are multiple things from when the blood sample is withdrawn to whether it's from a man or woman that can influence TSH, either raising or lower it. Of course, that makes the significance of questionable. Multiple papers in the last decade question whether TSH on its own can always reflect thyroid status.[45] In fact, diseases, medications, supplements, age, gender, ethnicity, iodine status, time of day, time of year, autoantibodies, heterophilic antibodies, smoking, and other factors influence the level of TSH.[46]

Chronic inflammation is the greatest health challenge we are facing today. Research shows it is responsible for a host of disorders and diseases. A 2014 Rand research report estimates that 61 percent of the US population struggles with at least one chronic inflammatory condition.[47] Chronic inflammation lowers TSH levels, despite low levels of thyroid hormone in the blood and peripheral tissues.[48,49]

This begs the question, "How accurate can TSH be if it can be influenced by so many factors, including chronic inflammation, the number one health problem in this country? How many people have a hidden hypothyroid condition because inflammation is suppressing their TSH level? How would your doctor know whether or not you have hidden hypothyroidism, if inflammatory tests are not run along with your TSH?" If your only thyroid test is for TSH, and you have chronic inflammation, your TSH will appear normal or even low. Your doctor will diagnose you as not having a thyroid disorder because that is what the diagnosis and treatment guidelines dictate. Instead you will likely be told your weight gain, fatigue, and depression are caused by factors unrelated to your thyroid. This may result in you being diagnosed with a disorder caused by tissue hypothyroidism (diabetes, a fatty liver, or an intestinal disorder) and the "disorder" being treated instead of the root cause of the disorder, tissue hypothyroidism.

Is TSH the most sensitive test of thyroid dysfunction?

In the allopathic model of thyroid care, measuring the amount of TSH in the blood is the most sensitive test to suggest thyroid dysfunction.[50] A rise in TSH is supposed to be the earliest indicator of thyroid disease. But how sensitive a test is it? If it is the most sensitive test of thyroid dysfunction and thyroid disease, then we should expect the TSH levels would rise when the thyroid gland is beginning to show signs of dysfunction. Yet, the literature indicates that more than 90% of the thyroid gland must be destroyed before TSH and T4 leave the reference ranges and allow for a hypothyroid diagnosis. Dr. Eric and I believe an elevated TSH may be a better indicator of late-stage thyroid dysfunction then the most sensitive early indicator.[51,52] If TSH is the most sensitive test of thyroid gland dysfunction, we should expect to see it elevated BEFORE disease sets in, since disease develops as a result of dysfunction. For example, one or more *thyroid nodules*, an abnormal growth of thyroid cells that forms a lump within the thyroid gland, are a form of thyroid gland dysfunction. If TSH is the most sensitive test of thyroid gland dysfunction, the level of TSH in the bloodstream should move out of the reference range as nodules start to develop. However, research shows that 68 percent of the general population have thyroid nodules,[53] despite normal TSH levels.

How about thyroid cancer? The incidence of thyroid cancer has increased at an alarming rate in both men and women in the United States. The etiology of this epidemic is unclear.[54] Can TSH be an early predictor? You would think that if TSH is the most sensitive test of thyroid gland dysfunction, surely it would be out of the reference range in a person with thyroid cancer. But that does not appear to be the case. Experts in thyroid cancer say that most of those with thyroid cancer will have normal TSH levels.[55]

So, if the TSH level may not be elevated until at least 90% of the thyroid gland has been damaged, and that it is often normal in those with thyroid nodules and thyroid cancer, how sensitive can a TSH test be?

Can Hypothyroid Symptoms Exist in the Absence of An Elevated TSH?

I can't tell you how many people have come to me saying that because their TSH was normal, their doctors told them that since their TSH test was normal, their classic hypothyroid symptoms could not be caused by a thyroid condition. Instead their symptoms are blamed on other conditions or disorders not related to thyroid physiology. Could you have hypothyroid symptoms despite a normal TSH? The answer is absolutely. Hypothyroid symptoms are caused by a reduced amount to active thyroid hormone inside your cells. This could obviously occur in primary hypothyroidism where the gland can't make enough thyroid hormone. But it can also occur when TSH secretion is normal, because cells and tissues can regulate thyroid hormone to some degree independently of TSH, blood levels of T4 and T3, and other tissues.[56] Dr. Eric discusses this in great detail in Part 2.

Do All Tissues of the Body Regulate Thyroid Hormone the Same?

This is a concept that I think is rarely ever explained to people with thyroid disorders as a reason why they have chronic hypothyroid symptoms despite a normal TSH. Every tissue in the body needs thyroid hormone but nearly all tissues can regulate thyroid hormone differently but at the same time. Each tissue can fine tune thyroid physiology, based on the needs of that particular tissue independently of the other tissue types. Your liver can regulate thyroid hormone independently of the heart, GI tract, or brain. Dr. Eric will discuss the cellular regulation of thyroid hormone in Part 2, but for now, understand that research shows that there are variations in cellular thyroid hormone transport proteins, cell deiodinase enzymes, and thyroid hormone receptors, and the central (think brain) and peripheral (non-brain and thyroid tissues) thyroid systems regulate differently.[57]

Is Thyroid Physiology Regulated the Same in Stressed and Non-stressed States?

One of the amazing things about the body is how it regulates itself in different situations. Your physiology works one way when you are lying on a beach with not a care in the world but is able to switch how it works on a dime if your body is threatened. Much of that change in physiology is controlled by thyroid hormones.

Today's research is indicating that thyroid physiology has two main operating systems. One system for low-stress situations (*homeostasis*) and one for high-stress situations (*allostasis*).[58,59] This means that we can't expect your thyroid physiology to work the same way in both situations. Based on the type of stress imposed on a person, their TSH could be high, normal, or low. The high or low level may not be the result of a dysfunction of the gland. Not understanding a person's level of stress of can and often does lead to misdiagnosis.

An elevated TSH may be the result of glandular dysfunction and an inability to produce thyroid hormone or it could be the bodies protective response to protect itself. Without a more complex thyroid and metabolic blood panel, the right interpretation may not be made.

Does Thyroid Hormone Replacement Therapy Restore Normal Thyroid Physiology?

"The dogma in clinical thyroidology that LT4 (L-thyroxine the most common form of thyroid replacement medication) monotherapy at doses that normalize serum TSH is sufficient to restore euthyroidism has come into question because evidence suggests a significant proportion of patients treated with LT4 continue to experience residual symptoms of hypothyroidism, including psychological) and metabolic effects."[60]

Initially it was thought that if a person suffers from hypothyroidism and takes a thyroid hormone drug in a sufficient dose to bring TSH into the reference range, thyroid physiology will would be restored in all body tissues.

Today, functional medicine doctors know that for a growing number of people in of the hypothyroid community receiving thyroid replacement therapy, this just isn't the case. Many people continue to struggle with hypothyroid symptoms despite T4 medication. This belief has led to great controversy in medicine, regarding what the appropriate TSH level should be for those on thyroid hormone replacement therapy. What makes the challenge even harder is that apparently the TSH level and the dose of thyroid replacement therapy needed to have the greatest impact on symptoms and functions is extremely variable and specific to the individual.

The lack or limited improvement of many hypothyroid patients while taking thyroid medication despite having their TSH restored to normal or even lower has resulted in growing patient dissatisfaction with the allopathic model of thyroid care.

Of equal importance to Dr. Eric, me, and others, is that there must be more to thyroid regulation than TSH and the amount of thyroid hormones in the blood. It points to what science is now confirming, that thyroid physiology is complex, is regulated by multiple factors, and cannot be simplified with just one or two tests.

"TSH has gained a dominant but misguided role in interpreting thyroid function testing in assuming that its exceptional sensitivity thereby translates into superior diagnostic performance."[61] Can it be that TSH doesn't have value? Absolutely not. TSH clearly has an important value for diagnosis of altered thyroid physiology, disorders, and disease, but Dr. Eric and I don't use one test to assess the complexity of a person's thyroid physiology. Due to the complexity of thyroid physiology and its different regulatory mechanisms during stressed and non-stressed states, "pituitary TSH cannot be readily interpreted as a sensitive mirror image of thyroid function…"[62]

The Primary Cause of Hypothyroidism Is Autoimmunity so There is No other Option but To Provide Thyroid Hormone

Allopathic practitioners consider two primary causes of hypothyroidism: iodine deficiency or autoimmunity. Iodine deficiency is thought to be the major cause of primary hypothyroidism worldwide, especially in areas of iodine deficiency. In the US and other areas where iodine is sufficient, autoimmune attack is most often to blame. Up to 90% of cases of primary hypothyroidism in the US is a result of autoimmunity.[63]

You might wonder if autoimmunity is at fault, why don't medical doctors look for what is prompting the autoimmune attack on the thyroid gland. Wouldn't it make more sense to use thyroid hormone medication in the short run to restore sufficient thyroid hormone levels in the body, while at the same time looking for and addressing the autoimmune attack? Many of us in the functional medicine field believe that to be the best strategy, but allopathic practitioners have a different philosophy. Since researchers can't identify a cause for the autoimmunity linked to Hashimoto's disease, the allopathic solution is to manage the damage the autoimmune attack causes. Since autoimmune conditions have no clear cause and no specific treatment, the allopathic model assumes the ultimate outcome is the destruction of the gland. To prevent this, allopathic practitioners attempt to flood the body with thyroid medication. The thought is that it is the production of thyroid hormone by the thyroid gland is what causes more immune damage. If thyroid medication is provided, then the gland does not need to produce thyroid hormone, and the immune attack and damage to the gland will be slowed. They focus on diagnosing the disorder and prescribing the peer-reviewed, recommended treatment to manage the condition. For most people who don't choose a functional medicine model of thyroid care, that means a lifetime of thyroid hormone medication. The good news is that there is another option.

Treating the Diagnosis, Not the Individual

If you were having a heart attack, would you want a group of doctors to stand around in that moment and discuss why you were having a heart attack? Would you want them to consider in that moment whether or not your heart attack was caused by your diet and some other lifestyle factors? Or your genetics? Probably not. In that moment you want your doctors to focus on keeping you alive. In that moment, who cares what caused the heart attack? You want your doctor to manage the crisis at hand with whatever means are necessary.

As I explained in Chapter 1, allopathic medicine is a very structured system where attention is given first to the symptoms, then the focus is on diagnosing the disorder or disease causing your complaints, and finally determining the approved treatment for that disorder or disease. Too often this system has led treating the "diagnosis" and the individual with the disease. The term for individualized health care is *bio-individualized medicine*. While the concept of bio-individualized medicine is not new to functional medicine, it is a rather new and controversial concept in allopathic medicine, especially allopathic thyroid care.

Today, there are well-respected individuals and groups that are calling for "individualized requirements for optimum treatment of hypothyroidism."[64] Why? Because science seems to be indicating that "each individual appears to have his/her own, unique relationship between TSH and T3 or T4".[65] What this means is that each of us may have a different optimal range for TSH, T4, T3 and other markers that are unique to us and influenced by our genetics, metabolism, life stress and trauma, diet, and lifestyle.

The controversy and discussions in allopathic medicine are happening because of the frustration of doctors and patients regarding the current model of thyroid care.[66] Too many people are complaining of persistent symptoms despite their TSH being normalized with thyroid replacement therapy. There seems to be no rhyme or reason for who does better on T4 vs T4/T3 vs T3- therapy. There seems to be no uniform dose of thyroid hormone replacement regardless of the form, that is appropriate for everyone. And, there seems to be no consensus as to what the optimal TSH reference range is for those on thyroid hormone replacement therapy.

To say that the current model does not help many of those diagnosed with hypothyroidism would be a mistake. However, there are some significant flaws. The purpose of *The Thyroid Debacle* is to help you understand some of them so that you can make sense of why you feel the way you do. The information in this book will help you understand why your doctors don't seem to listen to you, are not willing to order more extensive testing than TSH and fT4 tests, and may not be willing to offer you more than thyroid hormone supplements. Dr. Eric and I also explain the new science of hypothyroidism as well as some of new hypotheses regarding thyroid physiology. We are in the trenches every day and see what our model, the *Strategic Thyroid Solution* model, is able to do in improving symptoms, hypothyroidism, and reducing the amount of thyroid hormone medication our patients need.

A CASE IN POINT

Meet Joy. When she first came to see me, she me she was 35 years old. She had been diagnosed with primary hypothyroidism three years earlier. She was told she had Hashimoto's autoimmunity, but no thyroid antibodies were ever tested. Despite three years of thyroid medication, she continued to gain weight and had more then 15 classic hypothyroid symptoms. She had bounced around to a few different endocrinologists who suggested that despite her TSH level being normal, she needed a stronger dose of thyroid hormone. Each time her thyroid hormone supplement was increased, her symptoms worsened. Her biggest complaint regarding hormone replacement therapy was that as soon as a doctor increased the dose, the aches and pains in her body became worse, limiting her ability to exercise and be active. She was told by multiple doctors that the aches and pains were caused by arthritis and had nothing to do with the thyroid medications or her thyroid condition. Desperate for help she reached out to my office.

Within two months of following the principle of the Strategic Thyroid Solution, Joy was able to see a 6 percent improvement of her symptoms. She lost 12 pounds and four inches from her waist and hips. On a return visit to her endocrinologist, she was even more excited. Her endocrinologist explained to her that she no longer needed more thyroid hormone medication, she actually needed less. Her prescription was reduced to .88 mcg/day of her T4 medication. Her endocrinologist was shocked at the transformation in her body and that her symptoms were relieved. Most of this transformation occurred without supplemental thyroid hormone. Most of her protocol revolved around modification in diet and lifestyle.

> Thyroidologist: A medical doctor who has special training in diagnosing and treating thyroid diseases.
>
>> *"Recent surveys have highlighted considerable dissatisfaction with the standard LT4 treatment of hypothyroidism and indicated a willingness of most thyroidologists, depending on case presentation, to circumvent treatment recommendations endorsed by current guidelines. Expression of strong diverging patient and expert opinions coincides with recent advances in our understanding of thyroid hormone regulation in health and disease.*
>>
>> *A long-held tenet has been falsified that replacing only the prodrug LT4 in the treatment of primary hypothyroidism in a dose guided by the TSH reference range in thyroid health, would under all circumstances guarantee derivation of adequate amounts of T3 by various organs for their autonomous utilization and proper functioning. The unexpected collapse of the conventional reference system, particularly for TSH, in the treatment situation makes current biochemical definitions of hypothyroidism unreliable tools for guiding substitution therapy of the deficiency. This requires a thorough reassessment of basic principles applicable to LT4 use in patient care, extending statistical aggregation of population results obtained from many epidemiological studies that are not readily applicable to the individual level. Trait-like personal markers such as setpoints, together with a renewed focus on clinical disease definition and tissue markers of*

> *hypothyroidism, may offer a future perspective for making personalized treatment decisions. Apparent shortcomings in the standard therapy with LT4, discussed in this and other reviews, should stimulate more interest in the development of modern T3-based drugs, such as slow-release T3 preparations."*[67]

[67]

What this well written but complex conclusion points out is that there are some significant flaws with the current model of thyroid care based on our current understanding of thyroid physiology. Doctors need better evaluation tools that take into consideration what is happening beyond what can be identified with a TSH test.

PART 2

HYPOTHYROIDISM SEEN THROUGH A NEW LENS

Part 2 introduces you to a new paradigm regarding thyroid physiology. This paradigm views thyroid physiology as a regulator of cell metabolism. It asserts that an alteration in thyroid physiology is often not a mistake or dysfunction (at least not at the onset) but is an adaptive, defensive, and protective function.

The concepts in part 2 result from thousands of hours of research and study of the scientific literature and patient interactions. They result from being in the trenches with hundreds of people with hypothyroidism over the last twenty-plus years.

Much of the content of part 2 flies in the face of the current allopathic paradigm of thyroid physiology and hypothyroidism. The concepts and ideas presented in these chapters result from needing a different strategy to help ourselves and our patients with hypothyroidism—people like you, who are struggling with symptoms because of the current allopathic paradigm of thyroid care.

Dr. Kelly and I feel strongly that there will be a paradigm shift in how medical professionals approach thyroid physiology and thyroid disorders in time. While this book is primarily written about thyroid physiology, the concept that most dysfunctions begin at the cellular level holds true for all health conditions.

The human organism is complex and poorly understood. Many of the early concepts and hypotheses regarding human physiology have proven to be too simplistic or inaccurate. As science progresses, it becomes increasingly apparent that human physiology is more intricate and integrated than we ever imagined.

The future of health care lies in understanding the concept of emergentism. Emergentism is the concept that all parts combine and integrate to make a complex system like the human body. Reducing human physiology to its individual parts does make it easier to understand basic structure and function. Still, we must not lose sight of the significance of the emergent properties at the cellular level. Accepting that concept is essential if we are to do more than simply attempt to manage illness and disease.

CHAPTER 6

A PARADIGM PAST ITS PRIME

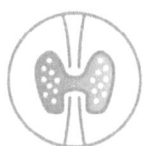

"What's in a name? That which we call a rose by any other name would smell as sweet." This line from Shakespeare's *Romeo and Juliet* is one of my favorite quotes. What Juliet is asking is, Does the name really matter? It's the experience the rose provides that matters, not the name. But what about in hypothyroidism? What matters more—the symptoms (the experience) or the diagnosis (the name)?

WHAT DOES HYPOTHYROIDISM REALLY MEAN?

In allopathic thyroid care, the definition of hypothyroidism matters most. This is how allopathic medicine defines it: "Hypothyroidism, also called underactive thyroid, is when the thyroid gland doesn't make enough thyroid hormones to meet your body's need."[68] The tool used in allopathic medicine to determine whether the thyroid gland isn't making enough thyroid hormone to meet the body's needs is a TSH test. In chapter 5, Dr. Kelly pointed out some of the flaws of the allopathic model of thyroid care and the reliance on TSH as a screening test of the cellular status of thyroid hormone.

The definition of hypothyroidism matters. Perhaps this is one reason why there is such a disconnect between what hypothyroidism is and what it isn't. Unfortunately, in allopathic medicine, the diagnosis (based on the definition of the disease) often trumps one's symptomatic experience.

In the allopathic model of hypothyroidism, your signs and symptoms will lead your doctor to suspect hypothyroidism and order a TSH test. If your TSH is elevated, your doctor will likely consider an underactive thyroid as the cause of your complaints. If your TSH is normal, he or she will likely consider some other dysfunction, disorder, or disease. This puts most of the responsibility for evaluating the state of your thyroid physiology on one screening test, TSH. (A blood test for free T4 [fT4] is routinely done to confirm the screening TSH test results.)

But does TSH alone reflect the state of thyroid physiology in your body's cells? Dr. Kelly and I would argue the answer is often no. A normal TSH level cannot rule out hypothyroidism. Thyroid physiology is too complex for TSH only to be an accurate indicator. So, how and why has TSH become the de facto test? The test has gained prominence because of the reductionist allopathic definition of hypothyroidism and the misconception of what TSH truly reflects.

A REDUCTIONIST VIEW OF THYROID PHYSIOLOGY

The current allopathic model is very linear and reduces thyroid physiology to the following simplistic steps:

1. When the body needs to increase metabolism, signals are sent to a gland in the brain called the hypothalamus.
2. The hypothalamus then increases the production of thyrotropin-releasing hormone (TRH).
3. TRH stimulates the pituitary gland to produce thyrotropin-stimulating hormone (TSH).
4. TSH then stimulates the thyroid gland to produce the thyroid hormones triiodothyronine (T3) and thyroxine (T4). (T4 predominates.)

5. Most T4 (and to a lesser degree T3) circulates in the blood bound to carrier proteins.
6. When thyroid hormones are needed by the body's cells, some T3 and T4 separate from their carrier proteins, becoming free of the carrier protein and available to be transported into cells (hence the terms "free T4" [fT4] and "free T3" [fT3]).
7. These free hormones then diffuse from high concentration in the blood to low concentration in the cells.
8. Free T4 is converted to active T3 inside the cells.
9. T3 then binds to receptors inside the cell and increases cell metabolism.
10. When the cells' needs have been met, signals are sent to the brain to reduce TSH production, slowing the release of thyroid hormones from the thyroid gland.

While it sounds straightforward, these steps simply are not accurate. This narrow view of thyroid physiology is referred to as reductionism. Scientific reductionism is the idea of simplifying complex biologic interactions and summarizing them either by choosing one or two components of an interaction that appear to have an overarching or controlling role, or by reducing the interaction to the overall outcome of the process. Reductionism makes studying and learning a complex interaction like thyroid hormone physiology more accessible, but it does not mirror the complexity of how the body actually works.

While the medical community may realize that thyroid physiology is much more complex than the simplistic reductionist model suggests, current evaluation and treatment of hypothyroidism are still based on a reductionist model. The allopathic model assumes that hypothyroid symptoms occur only if the thyroid gland doesn't produce enough hormones. It assumes that the full complexity of thyroid physiology can be reduced to the assessment of TSH.[69,70,71,72]

IF IT SOUNDS TOO SIMPLE, IT IS PROBABLY NOT ACCURATE

Although the allopathic model of thyroid physiology is basic and simplistic, it does work well for screening primary hypothyroidism, the end stage of thyroid disease, and managing thyroid hormone replacement therapy. But you might be wondering how good the model can be if hypothyroidism has become one of the most frequently diagnosed diseases of the modern world. Likewise, how accurate can the model be if levothyroxine is one of the most commonly used drugs worldwide?

Patients, functional medicine practitioners, and a growing number of medical doctors are beginning to question the validity of the allopathic model of thyroid care. One of its most significant flaws is the high priority placed on one test as the de facto test of thyroid physiology, TSH. Dr. Kelly alluded to increasing amounts of research recognizing that TSH is less reliable as a definitive screening tool than previously assumed.[73,74,75]

According to a 2019 paper in the *Journal of Thyroid Research* titled "Individualized Requirements for Optimum Treatment of Hypothyroidism: Complex Needs, Limited Options," the point is abundantly clear: "It has become increasingly apparent that a historic experiment using an ill-founded 'one size fits all' approach and a simplistic TSH-centered method for defining a prevalent disease such as hypothyroidism has failed."[76]

Furthermore, allopathic doctors often don't consider that multiple factors influence TSH. These factors include medication, disease, age, ethnicity, iodine availability, toxins, and chronic, low-grade inflammation, the latter of which is the most prominent condition plaguing modern society.[77] So how can TSH possibly be as reliable as the current model suggests? It can't.

Other concerns regarding a TSH-driven model of thyroid assessment include

- a continuing disagreement as to what the optimal TSH reference range should be[78],
- what TSH truly represents,
- when to prescribe thyroid hormone replacement therapy,
- what the optimal TSH level is for those receiving thyroid hormone replacement therapy, and
- what to do for those who continue to complain of persistent hypothyroid symptoms despite undergoing thyroid hormone replacement therapy and achieving a euthyroid state, meaning the restoration of TSH to the reference range.

It's clear that patients are increasingly dissatisfied with the diagnosis and treatment they've received.[79,80] This chapter will reveal new concepts of thyroid physiology that will help you understand why the allopathic model of thyroid care is failing, frustrating you and your doctors. And you'll see why doctors need a paradigm shift in their view of thyroid physiology.

A PROBLEM WITH PERSPECTIVE

One of the issues with the allopathic definition of hypothyroidism is that it doesn't consider what is happening beyond the thyroid gland. It misses a massive piece of the thyroid physiology picture, which is what is happening in the cells and tissues. The definition assumes that thyroid physiology is solely dependent on the production of thyroid hormones by the thyroid gland and considers no other factors. It assumes that TSH represents thyroid hormone status in all the tissues of the body. These assumptions are false, but that hasn't changed thyroid care.

It is essential to understand is that hypothyroid symptoms occur because there is insufficient thyroid hormone (T3) reaching the thyroid receptors inside your cells. So yes, reduced thyroid hormone production by the thyroid gland can cause hypothyroidism. But ultimately, hypothyroid symptoms and hypothyroidism result from reduced thyroid hormones within the cells. So maybe a better definition would be "Hypothyroidism is a state of undersupply of the body with thyroid hormones and/or a resulting lack of response of the organism to hormonal actions."[81]

Ironically this isn't a new definition, but it's one you'll find in older textbooks describing hypothyroidism. The old-school definition considers that hypothyroidism could result from a lack of thyroid hormone production or a reduced impact of thyroid hormone activity within the cells or both. If any physiological alteration or adaptation prevents thyroid hormone from reaching the thyroid receptors in your cells, thyroid signaling will be altered, leading to the hypothyroid signs and symptoms you experience. In Dr. Kelly's and my opinion, the old definition of hypothyroidism is much more fitting than the one in use today.

Why is the definition of hypothyroidism so important? Because unless your situation fits the current definition of hypothyroidism that allopathic medicine follows, it's likely your doctor will say you don't have a thyroid disorder. Instead, chances are he or she will tell you your symptoms are related to stress or are all in your head, or that you are just overeating, not exercising enough, or are depressed.

Allopathic medicine has a very narrow view of hypothyroidism. Allopathic medicine defines it as a condition that occurs only when the thyroid gland doesn't produce sufficient hormones. But the question that your doctor should ask is "What is causing your hypothyroid symptoms?"

If you pressed any physician involved in thyroid care about why you have hypothyroid symptoms, the general agreement would be that they result from insufficient levels of T3 reaching the thyroid receptors inside your cells and tissues. If that is the case, the doctor should ask the following questions:

1. Is there any situation in which the thyroid gland could produce sufficient thyroid hormone yet low levels of T3 could be reaching the thyroid receptors?

2. Do the cells of all body tissues regulate thyroid hormones in the same way?
3. Does the body have the same regulatory system when you are in a state of homeostasis (balance and low stress) versus a state of allostasis (stress and danger)?
4. Can one test, TSH, reflect the thyroid physiology in all cells and tissues simultaneously?
5. Can TSH be an accurate diagnostic tool in both the homeostatic and allostatic states?
6. Is there a situation in which TSH could be elevated not because of a disease of the thyroid gland instead as an appropriate adaptation to metabolic demand?
7. Is there a situation where TSH could be normal or low despite disease or dysfunction of the thyroid gland, resulting in insufficient T3 reaching the cellular thyroid receptors?

These are crucial questions that recent research answers, helping Dr. Kelly and I understand why the current allopathic model of thyroid care is failing.

GLAND-CENTRIC VERSUS HOLISTIC VIEW OF THYROID PHYSIOLOGY

The idea that thyroid physiology works optimally as long as the thyroid gland is secreting sufficient thyroid hormones has been debunked. Research shows that the amount of thyroid hormone produced by the thyroid gland is important but is only a part of the complex puzzle that is thyroid physiology.

Once thyroid hormones (T3 and T4) enter the bloodstream, multiple factors influence how much reaches your cells and eventually how much T3 is available to bind with thyroid receptors inside your cells, allowing for optimal thyroid physiology. For this reason, we must look at thyroid physiology from a holistic perspective.

When someone like you struggles with chronic symptoms consistent with low levels of thyroid hormones in your cells and tissues, your doctor must be willing to investigate whether something is preventing enough of those hormones from reaching the thyroid hormone receptors inside your cells.

Just as a full tank of gas does not ensure your car will perform optimally, a TSH within the lab reference range does not ensure optimal thyroid physiology in your body or the absence of hypothyroid signs and symptoms. Let me walk you through the multiple ways thyroid physiology can be less than optimal despite a normal TSH, healthy thyroid gland function, and no thyroid disease.

CARRIER PROTEINS

Once the thyroid gland makes thyroid hormones and releases them into the bloodstream, the hormones bind to proteins in the blood, which carries them to your body's cells and tissues. Think of the binding proteins as a car. Your car takes you to the places you want to go. Likewise, the binding, or carrier, proteins deliver thyroid hormones to your cells and tissues.

There are three primary carrier proteins in your blood: thyroid-binding globulin (TBG), transthyretin, and albumin. These carrier proteins play an essential role in getting thyroid hormone to your cells and tissues, but they also fulfill other significant roles in thyroid hormone physiology.

Without carrier proteins, the optimal distribution of thyroid hormones to all your cells and tissues would be virtually impossible. The vast majority of thyroid hormones, T4 (99.97%) and T3 (99.7%), are bound to these proteins. The carrier proteins

- distribute thyroid hormones throughout the body,

- provide a ready-on-demand reserve of thyroid hormones independent of the thyroid gland,
- protect thyroid hormone reserves from degradation, and
- prevent excessive levels of free thyroid hormones from circulating and inducing tissue hyperthyroidism.

Anything that increases or decreases the number of carrier proteins can result in hypothyroid or hyperthyroid symptoms despite normal thyroid gland function. Therefore, if you have actual thyroid gland disease, plus alterations of thyroid-hormone-binding carrier proteins simultaneously, your condition (hypothyroidism or hyperthyroidism) could be masked or augmented, complicating diagnosis and treatment.

Thyroid-binding globulin (TBG) is the dominant thyroid-hormone-binding protein. One of the most common factors impacting TBG levels is the amount of circulating estrogen, a hormone found in women and men, though in much smaller amounts in men. As estrogen levels rise, TBG levels rise as well. And as TBG levels rise, free T4 and free T3 levels in the blood drop, resulting in less thyroid hormone being available to move into cells and tissues. For thyroid hormone to get into your cells and tissues, it must be released from its carrier proteins.

If you drove to the mall but never left your car, you would not be able to shop. If estrogen levels are elevated because of birth control, hormone replacement therapy, poor detoxification pathways, or bacterial imbalances in your intestinal tract, you could have normal thyroid gland function but chronic hypothyroid signs and symptoms.

THYROID-HORMONE CELL TRANSPORTERS

For thyroid hormone to manifest its dominant actions, it must get into the cells of your body. In the allopathic model of thyroid physiology, it is considered a foregone conclusion that thyroid hormones in your blood separate from the carrier proteins and move effortlessly into your cells and tissues in a uniform fashion. For a while, it was thought that the movement of thyroid hormones from the blood into the cells was the same for all body tissues. It was also believed that it required no energy but occurred via simple diffusion.

However, today's science indicates that the movement of thyroid hormone into your cells is quite energy dependent. It occurs via specific transport proteins. The types and quantities of thyroid hormone cell transport proteins vary in different body tissues.[82]

Why is this important? This means that the cells of different tissues don't all receive thyroid hormones in the same manner. An in-depth understanding of the various cell membrane transport types (MCT8, MCT10, OATP, LAT, and NTCP) is not essential for this discussion. What is important and relevant is that your brain's cells, muscles, intestines, heart, and other tissues can have all types of transporters, just a few, or just one type. The number of transporters of each type varies wildly between different tissues.

Think about transporters like doorways or access points to get into a mall. A mall has many access points. There are main entrance doors that allow everyone in and out. There are doors for service employees only. Some doors allow access only to employees of specific stores. The different doors enable the mall to precisely control who comes in and how they gain access. In your cells and tissues, the cell transporters control thyroid hormone access. Each transporter type has a preference for a different form of thyroid hormone. The diversity of transporter types and the differing quantity of each type in your cells and tissues make it impossible for a single test like TSH to gauge what is happening throughout your body.

Many factors affect thyroid hormone transporters. Genetic defects in particular transporters can lead to significant developmental disorders. The most prevalent is a defect of the MCT8 transporter, which is specific for transporting T3. It causes a serious though rare condition affecting brain development called Allan-Herndon-Dudley syndrome.[83] Other factors influencing thyroid hormone transport include common medications and nutritional supplements. Any one of these influences can lead to hypothyroid signs and symptoms despite normal thyroid gland function and hormone production.

DEIODINASES ENZYMES

The third level of thyroid hormone control that can be independent of thyroid gland function and hormone production is the action of intracellular enzymes called deiodinases enzymes. Cells produce deiodinase enzymes to convert T4 and T3 into various substances. Thus, the deiodinase enzymes give cells another control point to influence their metabolism independent of thyroid gland production and thyroid hormone concentrations in the blood and tissues.

There are three forms of deiodinase enzymes: deiodinases 1 (D1), deiodinases 2 (D2), and deiodinase 3 (D3). Some cells and tissues have all three forms, some have two types, and some only one. This again means that the regulation of thyroid hormone is specific to cells and tissues and is another reason why TSH alone cannot reveal the thyroid hormone status of all tissues.[84,85]

THYROID HORMONE RECEPTORS

Thyroid hormone receptors are similar to electrical outlets in your home. For an appliance to work, it must plug into the receptacle. For thyroid hormones to impart biological actions, they, too, must plug into receptors. Hormone receptors provide the last step of independent control that cells and tissues can use to regulate thyroid hormone activity.

As you may have guessed already, there is more than one thyroid hormone receptor type. And yes, the type of receptor, the quantity of each type, and the function of each type vary from tissue to tissue in your body.

Some receptors are significantly more sensitive to thyroid hormone than others. Thyroid hormone receptors in the hypothalamus, for instance, are ten times more sensitive to thyroid hormones than receptors outside the hypothalamus.[86] This means that small amounts of T3 will quickly satisfy the hypothalamus long before other areas in the body. This is why you can have a low TSH but still have chronic hypothyroid symptoms.

When thyroid hormones plug into some cell receptors, activation occurs, while plugging into other receptors turns activity off. When people think of hypothyroidism, they think low thyroid hormone levels reduce activity, but in some cells, lack of T3 increases specific activities. It all depends on the types of receptors in that cell.

There are thyroid hormone receptors located in your cells' nuclei, mitochondria, and plasma membranes. Each type of thyroid hormone receptor imparts specific actions unique to a specific tissue type's cells.

I hope this section gives you a sense of the complexity of thyroid hormone physiology. You don't need to remember the exact details, but you should now understand the following:

- Thyroid physiology is too complex to be assessed by one lab test.
- There are multiple levels of thyroid hormone control.
- How much thyroid hormone reaches your cells and tissues can be influenced by more than the amount of thyroid hormone your thyroid gland produces.

While a reductionist, gland-centric linear view of thyroid hormone physiology provides a simple explanation to students and patients and allows for a simple way to diagnose and manage hypothyroidism, it is a model that fails in many ways.

What Dr. Kelly and I propose is a holistic view of thyroid physiology, taking into consideration these facts:

- Hypothyroidism can occur with normal thyroid gland function.
- Signs and symptoms of hypothyroidism result from what is and isn't happening in the various body cells and tissues independent, many times, of thyroid gland production and the amount of thyroid hormone in the bloodstream.
- Primary hypothyroidism is often not diagnosed until more than 90 percent of the thyroid gland tissue is destroyed. Therefore, primary hypothyroidism is not the beginning of altered thyroid physiology but often the end stage of that alteration.
- At least at the onset, hypothyroidism may not be a mistake of the immune system but a protective mechanism.

Dr. Kelly and I invite you to view thyroid physiology and hypothyroidism from a holistic perspective. We want you to consider that hypothyroidism often starts in your cells and is not a mistake but a protective mechanism. We would like you to consider the possibility that the damage to your thyroid gland is probably not the result of an out-of-control immune system initially but is part of a protective mechanism.

The information I present in the following chapters is backed by scientific research. Some of it is Dr. Kelly's and my hypothesis based on years of caring for patients and reviewing thousands of research papers. The ideas, concepts, and the perspective of thyroid physiology that we discuss are the backbone of our Strategic Thyroid Solution protocol, which has dramatically improved our patients' thyroid physiology, signs and symptoms, and quality of life.

A FRESH LOOK AT THYROID PHYSIOLOGY

This chapter points out the challenges facing the current allopathic model of thyroid physiology. When reading the chapters in part 2, I ask that you open your mind. Forget everything you think you know about thyroid physiology and consider the ideas and perspectives I put forward. I want to walk you through a new perspective and hypothesis regarding thyroid physiology. Where possible, I will blend long-held beliefs and relatively new science with our perspectives and theories.

The following chapters present some of the most complex concepts in *The Thyroid Debacle*. But if you hang in there, I promise you will gain a clear understanding of the new view of thyroid physiology. It is one that I think clarifies what we see in our patients. If you are a healthcare practitioner, this new concept about thyroid hormone activity explains why your patients don't feel better when thyroid hormone replacement therapy restores their TSH levels to normal. If you are struggling with chronic hypothyroid symptoms despite having a normal level of TSH due to thyroid hormone replacement therapy, the following chapters should help you understand that your hypothyroid symptoms are real. The information I present in part 2 explains why it may seem your doctor is unable to help you truly feel well.

CHAPTER 7

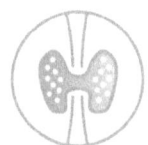

A NEW PERSPECTIVE

A lot of fuss is made about how much TSH and thyroid hormones are circulating in the blood, assuming that the level of these substances in the blood reflects the amount of T4 and T3 inside the cells. This chapter digs deeper into this concept and expands the idea that what is inside the cell counts the most.

IT'S WHAT'S INSIDE THAT COUNTS

Hypothyroid symptoms occur when the amount of thyroid hormone (primarily T3) reaching the thyroid hormone receptors inside the nuclei and mitochondria of your cells is inadequate. It would be nice if the levels of T4 and T3 in the blood accurately reflected the amount of thyroid hormone inside your cells, but they just don't.[87] Even when blood tests also measure the levels of free T4 (fT4) and free T3 (fT3), the numbers cannot precisely convey the amount of these hormones inside your cells.

Why? Thyroid hormones in the blood, whether made by the thyroid gland or coming from thyroid hormone replacement therapy, have three fates: they enter the cells and convert to active forms, they reach the cells and are deactivated, or they are broken down (a.k.a.

metabolized) and removed from the body without ever reaching most of your cells and tissues. Just because there is a normal level of T4 in your blood, that does not mean that enough T4 makes its way into all of your cells evenly, converts to T3, and binds to receptors within your cells.

T4 circulates in the blood at significantly higher levels than T4 inside cells. Most of the T4 (and T3, for that matter) circulates in the blood, bound to carrier proteins. This essentially maintains a circulating reserve of both T4 and T3 that is available when needed by cells and tissues. When triggered by cell signals, T4 and T3 can become "free" of the carrier proteins, becoming available to be transported into cells. Small amounts of T4 move into cells and tissues as they require it. The body maintains T3 circulating in the blood at much lower levels than T4 and defends it vigorously. In individuals with normal thyroid physiology, the thyroid gland produces less than 20 percent of the T3 circulating in the bloodstream. The bulk of it comes from peripheral cells. Deiodinase 1 in the plasma membrane of peripheral cells converts T4 to T3 which directly enters the bloodstream. Deiodinase 2 inside peripheral cells converts T4 to T3, which enters the bloodstream after binding to T3 receptors inside peripheral cells. Both contribute to maintain a healthy reference range of T3. Maintaining the T3 level is a biologic priority, since some tissue cells cannot convert T4 to T3.[88]

The biologic stability of T3 in the blood is one reason allopathic doctors rarely order blood tests for T3 or free T3 levels. This is because the reference ranges are set in such a way that T3 or fT3 rarely fall below or rise above their reference ranges. However, functional medicine practitioners do measure T3 and fT3 because levels below the optimal reference range are a good indicator that T3 levels inside some of the cells are low as well, causing hypothyroid symptoms.

Many cells have the ability to convert T4 to T3 via an enzyme called deiodinase 2. When activated, this enzyme allows cells to dramatically increase their T3 level compared to the amount of fT3 outside the cells. When cells have optimal thyroid physiology, the T3 concentration inside the cells may be similar to T3 levels in the blood. However, in times of altered thyroid physiology, the level of fT3 inside the cells can be significantly higher or lower than blood levels.[89]

CELLULAR HYPOTHYROIDISM

Hypothyroid symptoms result from reduced levels of thyroid hormones (primarily T3) reaching the thyroid receptors inside your cells. When receptors inside your cells lack sufficient T3 to bind to them, cellular hypothyroidism occurs. When many cells of a specific tissue have reduced T3 inside the cells, you have tissue hypothyroidism. I refer to it as cellular hypothyroidism.

Cellular hypothyroidism (which I refer to as CHT) is not a new concept. It has been discussed quietly in the scientific literature for decades with very little fanfare.[90] It can arise despite any of the following situations:

- a normally functioning thyroid gland
- normal levels of TSH, T4, and T3 in the blood
- normal reverse T3 (rT3) in the blood.
- thyroid hormone replacement therapy

Cellular hypothyroidism may not occur in all tissues simultaneously or to the same degree. Since the effects of hypothyroidism on cell metabolism and function depend on the extent to which levels of thyroid hormones fall and which tissues are impacted the most, hypothyroidism cannot be a single condition.[91] Rather, hypothyroid symptoms are specific to tissues affected, depending on how your body regulates thyroid physiology in response to the stresses and strains your cells and tissues are facing.

So that we are all on the same page, here's a brief review: If you have primary hypothyroidism (what I refer to as glandular hypothyroidism) and your thyroid gland is not producing a healthy supply of thyroid hormones, you will ultimately have widespread cellular hypothyroidism. You cannot have primary hypothyroidism without cellular hypothyroidism. But you can have cellular hypothyroidism without glandular hypothyroidism.

To return to our car analogy, if there is no gas in your car, your engine will not run. However, you could have plenty of gas in your car and the car might not run well, if it runs at all. For your car, gas is a critical component but not the only component. For healthy thyroid physiology, thyroid hormone production is important. But multiple other factors may prevent thyroid hormones from working appropriately once they are produced by the thyroid gland or taken as a medication. As pointed out throughout *The Thyroid Debacle*, the current challenge is that allopathic medicine disregards the concept of cellular hypothyroidism.

The assumption has long been that if TSH is within the reference range, you do not have hypothyroidism and do not need medical treatment with thyroid hormone replacement therapy. It has also been assumed by many in the allopathic medical community that if a doctor prescribes thyroid hormone replacement therapy to bring a patient's TSH to within the reference range, the treatment restores a level of biochemical euthyroidism, meaning healthy thyroid physiology in all tissues throughout the patient's body. However, the scientific literature continues to grow, discussing the lack of patient and doctor satisfaction with medically restored euthyroidism.[92] The reality is that there is a massive community of people struggling with symptoms despite thyroid hormone replacement therapy and a TSH level within the reference range.

One of the biggest challenges to accurate diagnosis and helpful therapy is the fact that there is no direct measure of thyroid hormone status within the cell. Nor is there a test that specifically assesses thyroid hormone status in all the body's cells, let alone the cells in one type of tissue. Instead, health-care providers must use signs, symptoms, and indirect, nonspecific tests to diagnose thyroid problems. The diagnostic process is not simple and straightforward.[93]

I describe in upcoming chapters how Dr. Kelly and I evaluate cellular hypothyroidism. But, for now, just realize that if you are struggling with hypothyroid symptoms despite a normal TSH level or the use of thyroid hormone replacement therapy, you are likely struggling with cellular hypothyroidism. Cellular hypothyroidism, in our opinion, is happening in epidemic proportions and is woefully underdiagnosed and underappreciated. This is because the focus in allopathic medicine is often on managing hypothyroidism and its symptoms, not on identifying and removing its root causes. Too often, when people don't understand something or know how to solve a problem, they either ignore its existence or identify a controllable aspect of the problem, redefine the symptoms as the problem, and manage those symptoms. This is where most physicians are with thyroid care. Many are not even in agreement on how to identify or treat hypothyroidism.[94,95,96] They are unaware of cellular hypothyroidism, how to evaluate it, and how to address it. So instead, cellular hypothyroidism continues to be virtually ignored.

The definition of hypothyroidism has been modified to fit what can be measured and managed—overt glandular hypothyroidism. Doctors can determine when the thyroid gland loses 90 percent of its function with some accuracy by using TSH. Allopathic medicine's solution is just to replace what the gland can no longer make. This strategy has resulted in millions of people having their thyroid condition managed with medication for the rest of their lives.

WHAT CAUSES CELLULAR HYPOTHYROIDISM?

There is a constant flux of thyroid physiology within cells and tissues. There is an increase in the amount of T3 available to reach receptors when metabolism needs to increase and a reduction of T3 when metabolism needs to be turned down. Each tissue (pancreas, lung, liver, gut, brain, and so forth) regulates thyroid hormone a bit differently, and to some degree independently of each other. When there is a significant, persistent drop in fT3 reaching your nuclear and mitochondrial thyroid hormone receptors, you start to experience the signs and symptoms of hypothyroidism.

What triggers cellular hypothyroidism? I will discuss this in greater detail in the next chapter, but for now I will simplify it and narrow it down to these three factors:

- lack of thyroid hormone in the body as a result of loss of thyroid gland function
- reduced amounts of thyroid hormones entering the cells
- the cells actively deactivating thyroid hormones before they can bind to receptors

The third mechanism is often the primary, initial driver of hypothyroidism. Something triggers the cells to prevent thyroid hormone entry or favors the deactivation of thyroid hormones inside the cells over activation to T3.

But what is the trigger? It's the cell danger response to excessive cellular stress, such as the stress that microbes, physical stressors, chemical stressors, toxins, radiation, or lack of oxygen cause. The cell danger response inside the cells shifts cell metabolism away from growth and development, and toward self-defense. As a result, the cells actively attempt to slow metabolism to address and control the threat, whatever it may be.

I will cover this more in chapter 8, but for now, here's an analogy to help you understand the cell danger response. If you were cooking a meal for your family and someone broke into your home and started threatening or assaulting all of you, would you continue to cook, or would you shift your attention to defending yourself and your family? You would likely change from nurturer to defender.

Your cells do the same. When there is excessive stress on your cells, they shift to self-defense mode. Growth, repair, and development slow to put effort into defending against the danger. The deactivation of thyroid hormone controls the slowing of cell metabolism. With less T3 binding to receptors inside cells, growth and development are turned down, and cell defense is ramped up. Yes, it may result in unpleasant symptoms, but it's not a mistake. It's a calculated response to danger.

WHEN DOES HYPOTHYROIDISM START?

This is where everything gets a bit messy. There is an age-old question: "Which came first; the chicken or the egg?" The same could be asked of hypothyroidism: which comes first, cellular hypothyroidism or glandular hypothyroidism?

Hypothyroidism starts when your TSH level rises above the reference range and your T4 level drops below it in the allopathic model. Another diagnosis often occurs before a doctor diagnoses primary hypothyroidism, called subclinical hypothyroidism. (See chapter 3.) This is when your TSH level is elevated but your T4 level is still within the lab reference range. In subclinical hypothyroidism, many people struggle with chronic hypothyroid symptoms. Most guidelines recommend against thyroid hormone replacement therapy for those with subclinical hypothyroidism. However, there is a hot debate in allopathic and functional medicine communities about treating subclinical hypothyroidism.[97,98,99]

The big question is, When does hypothyroidism actually start? Does it start when you begin to experience classic hypothyroid symptoms? Does it start when blood tests reveal signs of hypothyroidism, such as elevated lipids or when insulin resistance appears, stomach acid decreases, skin becomes dry, and hair thins? Or does it start only when TSH rises above the reference range and T4 drops below it? Does hypothyroidism occur only when medicine has something to treat or manage?

Let's say you have a water heater in your home. You are used to the water heater producing enough hot water for your family of five to take showers one right after another with no drop in water temperature. If suddenly only four people in a row can take a hot shower, wouldn't you think there may be a problem with your water heater? Or would you assume there is no problem until there is no hot water at all? I would say that as soon as you notice the water heater cannot supply the same quantity of hot water it once did, there is a problem with its function.

Dr. Kelly and I suggest that hypothyroidism often starts long before your doctor says you have primary hypothyroidism. It begins long before taking thyroid hormone medication becomes necessary. This is not unlike nearly every disorder in which altered function starts long before tissue damage or organ disease occurs. For example, diabetes is a blood sugar regulation disorder that starts decades before your doctor diagnoses it. Cardiovascular disease, Alzheimer's disease, fatty liver disease, renal disease, Crohn's disease, and colitis are all the end stages of long-term altered function affecting tissues or organs. Your diagnosis of a disorder or disease is not the beginning of a problem, but the end stage of one.

Glandular hypothyroidism, in which your gland can no longer produce sufficient thyroid hormone to support your body, is the end stage of hypothyroidism, not its beginning. Scientific research shows that by the time your blood test results indicate you have primary hypothyroidism, you've lost greater than 90 percent of your thyroid gland function. Does that sound like the beginning of a problem or its end? We argue that hypothyroidism starts before the signs and symptoms of hypothyroidism are noticed by you or your doctor. And we believe that hypothyroidism begins long before your TSH level rises.

The challenge is how to treat cellular hypothyroidism—or, for that matter, almost any phase of hypothyroidism—before the massive loss of thyroid gland function. Rather than prescribing thyroid hormone replacement therapy, we focus on identifying and removing as many stressors driving the cells to deactivate thyroid hormones as possible. This type of treatment falls outside the current paradigm of allopathic care for hypothyroidism, but it is how both Dr. Kelly and I resolved our own hypothyroid conditions and how we help our patients restore their thyroid physiology and overall health.

HYPOTHYROIDISM IS A SPECTRUM DISORDER

In our model of hypothyroidism, it is a spectrum disorder. What this means is that there are many levels or phases of hypothyroidism. It may start as a thyroid gland disorder first, but that is not what we often see in our practices after reviewing hundreds of patient histories and blood test results.

We see hypothyroidism starting initially at the cell and tissue level, prompting signs and symptoms that may or may not even be attributed to hypothyroidism. For example, you may complain of weight gain, fatigue, and other hypothyroid symptoms. But, because your TSH is within normal range, many allopathic doctors would dismiss your complaints entirely or chalk them up to some other disorder or condition. Instead you may be diagnosed with elevated cholesterol, diabetes, obesity, adrenal fatigue, reflux, or depression, and yet the hidden cause is some form of hypothyroidism, often cellular hypothyroidism.

As I described above, hypothyroidism starts as cellular hypothyroidism due to the activation of the cell danger response signals caused by excessive cell stress. In time, if cell stress is persistent, those stresses activate immune reactions at the thyroid gland, triggering a disorder called Hashimoto's thyroiditis. The more prolonged the excessive cell stress and the longer the thyroid gland is under attack, the more likely you will eventually develop glandular, or primary, hypothyroidism. If you look at hypothyroidism as a progressive spectrum disorder, glandular hypothyroidism no longer seems to be primary.

When you look at hypothyroidism as a spectrum disorder often starting in the cells and progressing to all-out destruction of the thyroid gland, it starts to make sense that you can have chronic hypothyroid signs and symptoms—cellular hypothyroidism and thyroid gland damage—long before you have high TSH and low T4 levels. You can also understand why allopathic thyroid care leaves patients and doctors dissatisfied. No treatment is recommended until a patient loses greater than 90 percent of his or her thyroid gland function. Flooding the body with thyroid hormone replacement therapy does not address the root cause of how the process started at the cellular level in the first place. This is why so many people receiving thyroid hormone replacement therapy continue to complain of chronic symptoms despite biochemical euthyroidism being achieved.

This perspective of hypothyroidism fits more in line with nearly every other disorder and disease that impacts humanity. Some form of stress activates a cell danger response and alters normal physiology. Sustained altered physiology results in dysfunction. Dysfunction eventually results in disease.

But what is causing the hypothyroid spectrum? Is it a mistake of the body? Is the immune system out of control? Or is it triggered as a protective mechanism? I will delve into these questions in the next chapter.

CHAPTER 8

LOOKING BEYOND TSH

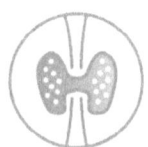

In previous chapters, I discussed the reductionist allopathic view of thyroid physiology. Its premise is to simplify or reduce complex physiology to basic individual parts. Doing so makes it easier to diagnose hypothyroidism and prescribe a treatment. This reductionist approach is not unique to thyroid physiology; it's the allopathic paradigm of all conditions and diseases.

The allopathic approach to thyroid physiology has been to simplify it to one thing—thyroid hormone production (T4) by the thyroid gland. This reductionist approach breaks down the complexity of thyroid physiology to the amounts of two thyroid hormones, TSH and T4, both of which can be measured with a simple blood test.

The allopathic view of thyroid physiology has made the diagnosis and treatment of thyroid conditions elementary and straightforward. The problem, however, is that this view and the two blood tests used to evaluate thyroid function can't assess the complexity of thyroid physiology.

This chapter will explain why the reductionist view isn't complete and describe a different approach to evaluating thyroid physiology. This chapter will be a bit technical and challenging at times, but do your best to follow along. And don't hesitate to reread each section until you understand it. I believe knowing this information is vital because it clarifies why you may not feel well despite a doctor saying, "Your thyroid function is fine" or "The thyroid medication has brought your thyroid hormone level back to normal."

If you are a health-care provider reading *The Thyroid Debacle*, understand that what you are learning may be quite different from what you learned in school. Research is changing the traditional allopathic view and introducing a different paradigm that is still evolving.

The new paradigm takes a broader "systems" approach to understanding thyroid physiology. Hypothyroid symptoms result from low levels of thyroid hormone (mainly T3) reaching the thyroid hormone receptors inside your cells. The new paradigm considers the complexity of factors that influence that process, including the following:

- thyroid hormone production
- release of thyroid hormones from the thyroid gland into the bloodstream
- the amounts of bound and free thyroid hormones circulating in the bloodstream
- transport of thyroid hormones into the body's cells and tissues
- conversion of thyroid hormones into active and inactive metabolites
- binding of thyroid hormones to receptors on the surfaces of cells and within them

In chapter 7, I describe a state called cellular or tissue hypothyroidism, and I use the terms interchangeably throughout the book. Dry skin, weight gain, fatigue, sensitivity to cold, and other symptoms (see chapter 4) are indications of cellular hypothyroidism. These symptoms occur because there is not enough T3 reaching the thyroid receptors in your cells' nuclei and mitochondria. In over twenty years of helping people with chronic hypothyroid symptoms regain their health and vitality, I have found that most of my patients have cellular hypothyroidism.

WHAT THE ALLOPATHIC MODEL IS MISSING

The allopathic model of thyroid care focuses on the thyroid gland. Accordingly, if you have what seem to be hypothyroid symptoms but have a normal TSH blood level, your doctor is likely to say your symptoms are not due to hypothyroidism but to something else. Your doctor may diagnose your signs or symptoms, such as high cholesterol, weight gain, insulin resistance or diabetes, or fatty liver disease, as the problem. Your doctor may not be aware that cellular hypothyroidism is often a common cause of many common diagnoses. Allopathic physicians have been taught that as long as the TSH blood level is within the reference range, your thyroid is secreting sufficient thyroid hormones and there is adequate thyroid hormone reaching your cells and tissues.

In contrast, the functional medicine view of thyroid physiology opens a range of possibilities. For instance, you can have low levels of T3 reaching the thyroid receptors inside your cells even though your TSH, T4, and even T3 are within their reference ranges. The actual amount of T3 in your cells may be inadequate even though you have a perfectly functioning thyroid gland. The thyroid gland's role is to produce thyroid hormones, but it is the individual cells and tissues that fine-tune thyroid hormone physiology.[100] The individual cells control how much T3 binds to their thyroid hormone receptors.

Functional medicine practitioners learn that thyroid physiology is not thyroid gland–centric, as was previously thought. Research shows that thyroid physiology is much more complex than the allopathic model. While allopathic medicine remains stuck in the old paradigm, here is what today's science reveals:

- Symptoms associated with hypothyroidism or hyperthyroidism occur because of cellular events—that is, what is happening within the cells.[101]
- Thyroid hormone production is just *one* part of thyroid physiology, not *the* part.[102]

- Thyroid hormones enter the cells through active transport. Therefore, if your cells are low on energy, they may not be able to transport thyroid hormone into your cells no matter how much T3 and T4 are in your blood.[103]
- Thyroid gland production does not determine the fate of thyroid hormones. Instead, forces within individual cells and tissues determine their fate.[104] (I describe some of the forces later in this and the following chapters.)
- Events within the cells affect the conversion of T4 to active T3 or inactive reverse T3 (rT3).[105,106]
- T3 binds to thyroid hormone receptors or is deactivated based on what is happening within the cells and tissues.[107]
- T3 can be directly used by most cells. However, most cells prefer to control the conversion of T4 to T3 internally.[108] This means taking T3 hormone medication may not eliminate hypothyroid symptoms. Instead it can make you feel worse by flooding your body with T3, which signals your hypothalamus and pituitary glands that you are in a hyperthyroid state. That message prompts the pituitary gland to suppress TSH, and the thyroid gland cuts back on the production of thyroid hormones. As a result, some cells and tissues may be in a hypothyroid state despite a normal or low TSH blood level.
- Your body fights to maintain healthy levels of T3 in the blood, often at the expense of the T3 in peripheral cells. Defending blood levels of T3 is a biologic priority. Your doctor may tell you that T3 testing is not important when research shows that your T3 level is of significant importance.
- The levels of T4, fT4, T3, and fT3 in your blood do not always correlate with the levels in your cells.[109,110] Therefore, you can have hypothyroid symptoms even when your thyroid hormones' blood levels are normal.
- Your TSH does not represent the thyroid hormone status of all the cells of your body, especially in times of stress.[111] Instead it more accurately represents the thyroid hormone status of the hypothalamus and pituitary glands.

- Thyroid hormone transporters (the mechanisms by which thyroid hormone enters your cells), deiodinase enzymes (the enzymes that either activate or deactivate thyroid hormones), and thyroid receptors (the binding sites for T3 in the nuclei and mitochondria of your cells) vary from tissue to tissue. For this reason, your TSH blood level cannot represent the thyroid hormone status of all cells.
- Your thyroid hormone physiology is always changing, depending on the stress placed on individual cells, tissues, and the body as a whole.[112] In most cases, physiological changes and the symptoms they cause are not mistakes but result from adaptations the cells make to protect themselves.[113,114]
- Bringing TSH into its reference range with thyroid hormone medication does not always restore normal thyroid physiology in all cells, a state known as euthyroidism.[115]
- Hypothyroidism's effects on your metabolism depend on the tissues impacted and the level of hypothyroidism they are experiencing. In addition, not all tissues undergo the same thyroid hormone deactivation level, and symptoms vary from person to person, depending on their cellular responses to stress.[116]
- People with Hashimoto's thyroiditis often experience symptoms of hypothyroidism and hyperthyroidism.

The reality is that thyroid physiology is even more complex than even this overview suggests. The point is that thyroid physiology is simply too complex to be assessed with just TSH and T4 blood tests. When there is not enough T3 reaching the appropriate receptors inside your body's cells, you have hypothyroidism symptoms. That's it. And if you have chronic hypothyroid symptoms, you could have one or all of the following problems with your thyroid physiology:

- a lack of thyroid hormone in the body due to loss of thyroid gland function

- reduced thyroid hormones entering the cells
- active deactivation of thyroid hormones by cells before the hormones can bind to receptors

Thyroid physiology could be compromised anywhere along the path from TRH production in the hypothalamus to the binding of T3 to receptors in your cells. The allopathic model assumes that if TSH is normal, the thyroid gland is working appropriately. And if the thyroid gland is producing sufficient thyroid hormone, then the thyroid hormone must be getting to the right place in all the cells and tissues of the body. However, this often isn't the case. Think of it this way: just because you donate money to a charity doesn't necessarily mean the money is used appropriately.

If you've been told your blood tests show that your thyroid hormone levels are normal but you have classic hypothyroid symptoms—your skin is as dry as the Sahara Desert, your hair is thinning, your bowels aren't moving as they should, and your libido left and hasn't come back—then the problem is likely deactivation of thyroid hormones in your cells. Similarly, if your doctor diagnoses primary hypothyroidism and prescribes thyroid hormone medication, bringing your blood levels of thyroid hormones (TSH and fT4) to their reference ranges, but you still have hypothyroid symptoms, then the problem is likely that thyroid hormones are being deactivated inside your cells. On the other hand, if you are diagnosed with primary hypothyroidism and prescribed thyroid hormone but do not have cellular hypothyroidism, your symptoms are likely to go away in a short time, your good health will resume, you will return to your fighting weight, and your libido will come back from hiatus. But if the medication helps you only partially or temporarily, you likely have cellular hypothyroidism, and excessive cellular stress is to blame.

Our job as doctors is to figure out what is causing your cellular stress and address it. We must help restore your optimal cellular thyroid physiology so your cells begin healing and you regain your health.

The guidelines your primary care doctor and endocrinologist follow recommend testing only TSH and fT4 levels in your blood. There is little, if any, discussion of thyroid hormone transport into your cells, deiodinase enzyme activity, or thyroid hormone deactivation within those guidelines. However, Dr. Kelly and I believe these three factors are critical for assessing thyroid physiology. (I explain each of these factors in detail later in this chapter.)

As Dr. Kelly explained in chapter 5, allopathic physicians generally believe that if a patient doesn't have primary hypothyroidism (elevated TSH levels and low fT4), there is no need for thyroid hormone replacement therapy. They also think that hypothyroid symptoms and clinical signs of hypothyroidism, such as elevated cholesterol, do not result from hypothyroidism until the thyroid gland is dysfunctional. This is like saying that nothing should be done to support or address insulin resistance or cardiovascular disease until diabetes develops or a heart attack occurs. It's ludicrous.

I agree that prescribing thyroid hormone replacement to people with TSH and T4 measures in the reference range is ineffective in most cases. The cells may be deactivating thyroid hormones, and therefore, prescribing thyroid hormone often only makes patients feel worse. In such cases, thyroid hormone replacement therapy can induce a hyperthyroid state at the hypothalamic-pituitary-adrenal axis and a hypothyroid state in the peripheral tissues.

Worse yet, many doctors merely prescribe medications to suppress symptoms instead of looking for their causes. The idea that symptoms stemming from compromised thyroid physiology in the cells don't represent a true thyroid condition until the thyroid gland becomes dysfunctional ignores the fact that most thyroid hormone activity often occurs within the cells.

Instead of looking at hypothyroidism as a condition that develops only if the thyroid gland is dysfunctional or diseased, doctors need to understand that thyroid hormone alterations at the cellular level are the cause of hypothyroid symptoms and can begin long before the thyroid gland becomes diseased. Physicians must understand this concept to help people.

In most cases, hypothyroidism starts as a cellular event due to some form of excessive cellular stress or danger. In times of stress, the body shifts its thyroid hormone use to manage that stress. This shift in thyroid hormone physiology does not occur uniformly across all body cells and tissues. The tissues, organs, and systems that play an essential role in addressing excessive cellular stress upregulate, or increase, the activity of their thyroid hormone physiology. In contrast, other tissues, organs, and systems that play less significant roles downregulate their thyroid hormone physiology. Even within individual cells, the processes change. The cells support activities that are most critical to their defense and protection, while less essential functions for cell defense are downregulated, or become less active.

For example, being chased by a tiger stresses your body, and getting away requires a lot of energy. Your brain and muscle thyroid physiology upregulates under this acute stress, and the energy production of those organs increases. Simultaneously, less critical thyroid physiology, such as that which affects sex hormone production, sleep, digestion, and cellular repair, downregulates.

The intelligence of the human body is incredible. In the split second you notice the tiger coming after you, your body is capable of dramatically changing its physiology to adapt to that stress. Instantaneously, it shuts down or deprioritizes noncritical systems, alters energy production, and shifts thyroid physiology in trillions of cells to drive reactions that enhance your ability to escape the tiger and survive.

This design is fantastic in crisis situations where the stress is short-term. The problem occurs when you are bombarded with chronic stressors, such as infection, excessive exercise, or insomnia, that keep your body in danger mode. Chronic stress leads to a chronic cellular danger response (see the Introduction), which alters thyroid physiology, creating hypothyroid symptoms, thyroid autoimmunity, and, eventually, primary hypothyroidism.

YOUR CELLS ARE IN CHARGE

At one point, scientists understood that the thyroid gland controlled thyroid physiology throughout the body. The assumption was that the thyroid hormone released by the thyroid gland solely determined how much of those hormones reached peripheral cells. If high amounts of thyroid hormone were released from the thyroid gland, a person would have a higher metabolism. If lesser amounts of thyroid hormone were released from the thyroid gland, a person would have a slower metabolism.

The movement of thyroid hormone into the cells was believed to be caused by simple diffusion. Simple diffusion occurs when solutes are moved along a concentration gradient in a solution or across a semipermeable membrane. In the case of thyroid hormone movement into cells, the theory was that thyroid hormone in the blood (an area of high concentration) moved into cells (an area of lower concentration) by diffusion, which is a passive phenomenon. Scientists now understand that this is not the case. Thyroid hormone transport into cells is actually an active process and requires energy.[117] And because thyroid hormone transport into your cells and tissues does not occur through diffusion but by active transport, the level of thyroid hormone circulating in your bloodstream may not represent what is in your cells and tissues.

Scientists also thought that once thyroxine (T4) entered the cells, it always converted to triiodothyronine (T3) and that the cells had little control of their own thyroid physiology. But, again, scientists now know this is not true. Rather, the cells of your body have a significant influence on the fate of T4 and T3.[118]

Current research tells us that earlier theories are too simplistic and inaccurate. For some reason, however, allopathic medicine seems to be stuck in the old reductionist paradigm that hypothyroidism is caused by factors outside of our control and nothing can be done about them. Allopathic medicine relies on the dogma that the only solution is to manage primary hypothyroidism; it can't be corrected. The management strategy relies on prescribing medication, since the thyroid gland is too dysfunctional to make enough on its own. The assumption is that if a patient receives enough thyroid medication to restore his or her TSH blood level to the reference range, he or she will regain thyroid physiology throughout the body.

That's the bad news. The good news is that research is showing thyroid physiology is much more complex than was initially thought. An appreciation of this complexity allows patients and doctors to understand how a person can have perfectly normal TSH and T4 blood levels and still struggle with chronic hypothyroid symptoms. It also makes it possible to understand the probable cause of hypothyroidism in all its forms and know how to correct it.

Those of us in functional medicine pay close attention to what researchers are reporting. New studies continue to provide a wealth of information about thyroid physiology's complexity. We're learning the cells aren't passive bystanders but rather are critical components in the process of thyroid hormone signaling in the body.[119,120,121]

The current thinking is that the thyroid gland releases spurts of thyroid hormones T4 and T3 but it is up to the peripheral cells to determine what happens to those hormones. The peripheral cells decide whether or not thyroid hormones

- enter the cells via active transport,
- cannot enter the cell,
- convert to active thyroid hormone (T3), and
- convert to less active thyroid hormones (rT3 and 3,3' T2).

I believe doctors need to consider each of these possibilities. I feel it is fair to say that doctors don't consider them in the allopathic model of thyroid care because TSH and T4 levels alone can't evaluate each option. Looking at all of the variables does not fit well in the reductionist allopathic model of thyroid care.

Physicians must stop looking at hypothyroidism as a singular condition. The various tissues of the body regulate thyroid hormone differently because they use different transport mechanisms to allow thyroid hormones into their cells, different deiodinase enzymes, and different thyroid receptors.[122,123]

I don't want to go too far down the rabbit hole into the details of thyroid hormone transport and thyroid receptor mechanisms. I do, however, want to explain these key components of cellular thyroid physiology. Later I will discuss the cellular enzymes called deiodinases. They play an essential role in the fate of thyroid hormone, and their action is a foundational premise of *The Thyroid Debacle*.

THYROID HORMONE TRANSPORT

Thyroid hormone imparts most of its actions inside the cells of your body. As a result, several cellular transport molecules have been identified, including MCT8, MCT10, LAT2, and OATP. I won't bore you by discussing the detailed mechanisms by which each of these transporters works. Instead my goal in this section is to give you a general understanding of them.

For some people struggling with hypothyroidism, there is a reduced ability of transporters to bring thyroid hormones into the cells. Some people have genetic defects in one or more of these transporters, but in those cases, severe hypothyroidism typically develops early in life; this is known as congenital hypothyroidism. The primary factor influencing how these transporters work in people without congenital defects is the amount of energy the peripheral cells produce.

The types and numbers of thyroid hormone transporters vary throughout the body.[124] Some tissues' cells may have all types, while other tissues' cells have only one transporter type. In addition, some cells may have many thyroid transporters, while others have only a few. These variations regarding transporters significantly impact the flow and control of thyroid hormone into cells. These concepts also explain why the amount of thyroid hormone in the blood may not represent how much is in the cells and why all cells may not contain the same amount of thyroid hormone.

Think of transporters of thyroid hormones into cells as the doors that let people into a store. If one store has four doors to let people in and the other store has only one door, the number of people entering the store within a specified time may differ. Likewise, if one store has a security person checking everyone's bags and personally escorting them into the store and the other store has no guard, there is also a difference in how many people are inside one store at any one time.

Different tissue types also require different amounts of energy to transport thyroid hormones. For example, some tissues, like those of the hypothalamus and pituitary gland in your brain, require less energy to transport thyroid hormone than peripheral tissues do. Why is this important? Because certain tissues become saturated with sufficient thyroid hormone more quickly than others. This is especially true of the hypothalamus and pituitary gland. Thus, tissues critical for addressing stress responses tend to require less energy for thyroid hormone transport into the cells. Conversely, tissues that are less critical for responding to stress require more energy for thyroid hormone transport.

This energy-dependent transport system results in thyroid hormone being regulated differently throughout the body—a factor that can't be fully recognized by measuring TSH blood levels alone. Any condition that interferes with the energy-producing power plants of your cells, the mitochondria, reduces the cellular energy available to transport thyroid hormone into the cells. Eventually mitochondrial dysfunction leads to cellular hypothyroidism. The degree of reduced thyroid hormone transport in cells and cellular hypothyroidism varies, depending on the tissues involved.

Multiple conditions are associated with mitochondrial dysfunction and reduced thyroid hormone transport, including the following:

- aging[125,126]
- anxiety[127,128]
- cardiovascular disease[129,130]
- chronic and acute or crash dieting[131,132]
- chronic fatigue syndrome[133,134,135]
- chronic infections[136]
- depression[137,138,139]
- fibromyalgia[140,141,142]
- high cholesterol and triglyceride levels[143,144]
- inflammation[145,146]
- chronic illness[147]
- insulin resistance[148,149]
- prediabetes and diabetes[150,151]
- migraine headaches[152,153]
- neurodegenerative disease, such as Parkinson's[154]
- obesity[155,156]
- physiological stress, such as starvation, cold exposure, noise, and hemorrhage[157,158]

Researchers do not know precisely how or why a compromise in the transport of thyroid hormone into the cells occurs, but it appears that most, if not all, of the possible mechanisms result from cellular stress and reduced cellular energy. For example, it has been established that the transport mechanisms for the hypothalamus and pituitary gland are affected less than peripheral cells by medications, environmental toxins, and inflammatory substances released under cellular stress.

What this means for you is that in times of cellular stress, the hypothalamus and pituitary gland, which have the most significant impact on TSH blood levels, receive thyroid hormones more quickly than the peripheral cells. As a result, receptors in these areas of the brain receive adequate levels of T3 and produce less TSH long before the peripheral cells receive sufficient thyroid hormones. This is why you may have peripheral cellular hypothyroidism and chronic hypothyroid symptoms while your blood levels of TSH and thyroid hormones remain normal. T4 and T3 levels may even be elevated in a situation of cellular stress because the thyroid hormones aren't reaching the peripheral cells in sufficient amounts. One of the few ways to see the effect of reduced cell transport is to look at rT3 in conjunction with total and freeT4 and T3, a test that few allopathic doctors run.

When stress affects peripheral cells and tissues, the primary thyroid hormone deactivating enzyme, deiodinase 3, moves from inside the cell to the cell membrane, deactivating T4 and T3 before these hormones ever have a chance to enter the cell.[159] Unfortunately, Deiodinase 3 can also deactivate T4 and T3 inside the cell, limiting the amount of T3 available to bind to nuclear and mitochondrial thyroid receptors, resulting in hypothyroidism symptoms. As a result, rT3 rises. If rT3 is not measured, your doctor would never know that this is occurring. However, you might feel the effects of this process because you may be struggling with hypothyroid symptoms.

To summarize thyroid hormone transport:

- Thyroid hormone transport into the cells is energy-dependent.
- The energy required to transport thyroid hormone varies among tissue types.
- The *types* of thyroid hormone cell transporters on the cells of all the body tissues are not uniform.

- The *quantity* of thyroid hormone cell transporters on the cells of all the body tissues is not uniform.
- The hypothalamus and pituitary gland require less energy for thyroid hormone transport than most peripheral cells. Hence, their cells receive thyroid hormone much more readily in low-energy or stressed states. Therefore, the hypothalamus and pituitary gland are much more sensitive to small fluctuations in thyroid hormone levels than the peripheral cells.
- Owing to variations in both quantity and type of thyroid hormone cell transporters on cells throughout the body's tissues, one blood test value, such as TSH, cannot represent the quantity of thyroid hormone in all your cells.

INTRACELLULAR THYROID HORMONE ACTION AND THE DEIODINASES

There is a misconception that thyroid hormone availability in the blood equates to thyroid hormone utilization in the cells. Unfortunately, this is not always the case. For example, having sufficient T4, fT4, T3, and fT3 in your blood does not necessarily correlate with T3 reaching the receptors inside the cells where the hormone acts.

Once thyroid hormone reaches your tissues and cells, the individual tissues and cells determine what happens to the thyroid hormone. It can be:

- activated,
- deactivated, or
- metabolized and excreted by the body.

For thyroid hormones to have their classic effects, they must separate from the carrier proteins escorting them throughout the body and be actively transported into the cells. (See chapter 6.) According to the current paradigm, thyroid hormones have only one fate: the hormones simply diffuse into the cells without resistance. T4 is converted to T3, which comes into the cell ready to be used. T3 binds to receptors inside the cells without anything getting in the way.

This couldn't be further from the truth.

The tissue / cellular-regulating system plays the most significant role in thyroid physiology.[160] Why do I say that? Because if your thyroid gland had a problem and could no longer provide your body with sufficient thyroid hormone, you could replace it with thyroid hormone medication and maintain healthy blood levels. But it is up to the tissues and cells to determine what happens when the thyroid hormones get to them, regardless of the source. All the thyroid hormones in the world will have little benefit if they can't get into your tissues and cells to do their jobs.

The underlying mechanism by which the level of thyroid hormones in the cells differs from levels of plasma, the liquid portion of your blood, is the tissue / cellular-regulating system, which is significantly influenced by deiodination.[161] Deiodination is the process of removing iodine molecules from thyroid hormone molecules. It is the primary fate of thyroid hormones once they reach the cell. Deiodination can result in thyroid hormone activation (T4 converting to T3 or thyroid hormone deactivation (T4 converting to rT3 and T3 to T2).

(There are active forms of T2, which once were thought to be inactive metabolites of thyroid hormone. They aren't truly inactive but may play an essential role in the regulation of cell activity, metabolism, and function. A discussion of T2 is beyond the scope of this book.)

Including deiodination, there are at least six biochemical activities that may affect thyroid hormones after the thyroid gland releases them and they enter the blood and cells:

- deiodination
- sulfation
- glucuronidation
- deamination

- decarboxylation
- ether-link cleavage

Deiodination is the most significant in the context of our discussion of cellular hypothyroidism; however, I will provide a brief introduction to all six of these actions.

DEIODINATION

Deiodination involves removing an iodine molecule from either the inner or the outer ring of a thyroid hormone molecule, transforming it into a different thyroid hormone. Depending on the deiodinase enzyme, this may happen outside the cell, within the cell membrane, or inside the cell.

- Iodine molecule removal from the outer ring of a T4 molecule creates T3.
- Iodine molecule removal from the inner ring of a T4 molecule creates rT3.
- Iodine molecule removal from the outer ring of an rT3 molecule creates T2.
- Iodine molecule removal from the inner ring of a T3 molecule results in the production of T2.

Figure 1: Deiodination of thyroid hormones.

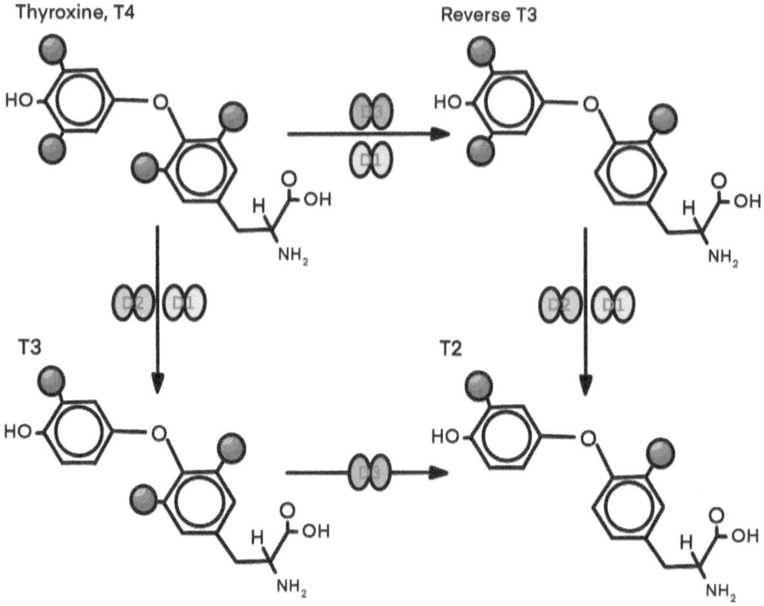

The enzymes that perform deiodination are called deiodinase enzymes, or selenoproteins. They require attachment to the mineral selenium for optimal function. There are three deiodinases: deiodinase 1, deiodinase 2, and deiodinase 3.

Each tissue in the body has a different number of deiodinases. Some tissues have only one or two deiodinases, while others can have all three. Thus, each deiodinase enzyme plays a unique role in regulating thyroid hormone physiology at the cellular level.

Deiodinase 1

Deiodinase 1 (D1) is primarily found in the cells of the liver, kidneys, thyroid, and pituitary gland. D1 is located at or near the plasma membrane of the cell. Its primary role is to degrade rT3 via deiodination.[162] Its secondary role is to convert T4 to T3.

Figure 2: Cellular regulation of thyroid hormones.

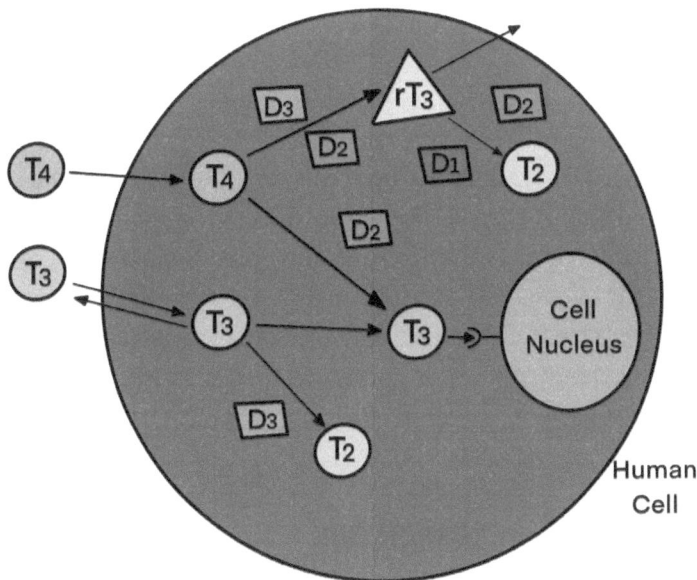

At one point, it was thought that D1's primary role was converting T4 to T3 in the liver and kidneys to maintain optimal levels of T3 in the plasma. However, current science indicates that of the 30 mcg of T3 made daily, approximately 5 mcg is made by D1 in the liver and kidneys, 5 mcg by the thyroid gland, and the remaining 20 mcg by the D2-producing cells of the body.

Deiodinase 2

Deiodinase 2 (D2) is found in most tissue types throughout the body but is most highly active in the brain, pituitary gland, brown fat, placenta, innate immune cells, and skeletal muscle. In addition, D2 is found in the endoplasmic reticulum within cells, where it removes iodine from the outer ring of thyroid hormones. Its primary role is the conversion of T4 to T3.

When there is a need for increased metabolism within the cells, D2 activity rises to increase the conversion of T4 to T3. Conversely, when there are sufficient levels of T3 binding to thyroid receptors, D2 activity slows.

Deiodinase 3

Deiodinase 3 (D3) is found in most tissues. The primary role of D3 is the deactivation of thyroid hormones T3 and T4 by removing iodine from the inner ring of the thyroid hormone molecule. In states of cellular homeostasis, D3 concentrations are typically low. However, under cellular stress, D3 activity increases to reduced cell metabolism. D3 typically performs its action at the plasma membrane or just outside the cell.

SULFATION AND GLUCURONIDATION

Sulfation is the process of adding a sulfur group to a thyroid hormone molecule. Sulfation blocks outer-ring deiodination. Thus, it is a means of deactivating thyroid hormone and making it more water soluble so your body can excrete it. In addition, sulfatase enzymes and gut bacteria can reactivate T4 and T3 when thyroid hormone production slows.

Glucuronidation is the process of adding glucuronic acid to a thyroid hormone molecule. It is another way in which the body can deactivate thyroid hormones. Glucuronidation also makes thyroid hormones more water soluble for excretion.

Both sulfation and glucuronidation are part of the body's detoxification process, which is why they are called phase II detoxicants. When glucuronidated metabolites are excreted into the gastrointestinal tract, they can be reactivated (much like sulfated thyroid hormone) by healthy bacteria in the GI tract. For example, some GI bacteria produce an enzyme called beta-glucuronidase, which can pull the glucuronic acid molecule off the thyroid hormone, reactivating it. In addition, certain medications, such as antiepileptics, can increase T4 glucuronidation, resulting in low levels of circulating and cellular T4.

DEAMINATION, DECARBOXYLATION, AND ETHER LINK CLEAVAGE

All three of these reactions are typically minor ones that occur in a nonstressed (homeostatic) state. Inflammation and oxidative stress increase these reactions. Further research is needed to understand the impact these reactions have on cellular thyroid physiology.

The most significant reason to list all the possible pathways that T4 and T3 may take is to emphasize that most of these reactions occur away from the thyroid gland. They have an impact on cellular thyroid hormone levels of T4 and T3, which affects whether you feel normal, hyperthyroid, or hypothyroid. All of these reactions can occur without a significant change in TSH or any dysfunction of the thyroid gland. This is another reason why the level of TSH in the bloodstream does not and cannot fully indicate the thyroid status of one's cells. It also points out that the thyroid gland is not the sole determinant of how much thyroid hormone reaches cells and tissues.

Now that you have a general understanding of the possible fates of T4 and T3 once they reach your cells and tissues, we can circle back to the deiodinases. Understanding deiodinase function is critical to comprehending cellular or tissue hypothyroidism. In addition, once you understand the significance of deiodinases, it is easier to grasp how you can have chronic hypothyroid symptoms even if your TSH level is normal.

REVERSE T3, THE MISSING TEST

Understanding the concept that the regulation of thyroid hormones in blood differs from the regulation of thyroid hormones in tissues[163] is essential for comprehending cellular hypothyroidism. Thyroid hormone levels in the blood are regulated by the hypothalamic-thyroid-pituitary-adrenal (HPTA axis), while tissue thyroid hormone levels are regulated by the thyroid hormone cell transporters and deiodinase enzymes. This means that the T4 and T3 levels in your blood may not reflect tissue or cellular levels of T4 and T3. TSH is a much better reflection of T4 and

T3 in the blood than it is of tissue levels of T4 or T3. Why doesn't TSH truly reflect the tissue levels of thyroid hormones? Because tissue and cellular availability is a complex dance involving several possibilities. The level of hormone available may be the result of

- an interplay between the supply of thyroid hormone—that is, how much is made by the thyroid gland—and the amount available in the blood;
- thyroid hormone transport into the cells and tissues, which is dependent on cellular energy and thyroid hormone transporters; or
- activation versus deactivation of thyroid hormones, which is based on cellular stress and deiodinase activity.

No matter what your doctor tells you, TSH on its own cannot determine your cellular or tissue thyroid hormone status throughout your body. The complexity of all the reactions occurring in your various cells and tissues can alter TSH, causing blood and tissue levels of thyroid hormone to be regulated independently of each other. For this reason, deiodinase-mediated thyroid hormone activation and deactivation controls metabolism. The following quote emphasizes this point. "Individual cells outside of the central nervous system (CNS) are also actively involved in the regulation/modulation of TH (thyroid hormone) signaling through deiodinase expression and activity. This can create a local tissue-specific state of hypothyroidism or thyrotoxicosis even in the setting of systemic euthyroidism.[164]

What the author is expressing here is that your thyroid gland can be working properly, and your TSH and T4 can be normal, but cells of individual tissues (in this case, the cells outside of the central nervous system) can still increase thyroid hormone activation or deactivation locally in that tissue only to cause a hypothyroid or hyperthyroid state locally within that tissue. This allows the body to regulate multiple systems differently at the same time. If individual tissues of the body could not self-regulate, we could never have evolved.

To look at this another way, consider the power in your house. You have a main breaker that turns power to the house on or off. But you have multiple levels of site-specific control as well. For example, each room can be individually controlled by a switch or multiple switches. If you didn't have this type of control in your home, you would have to turn off the main breaker every time you wanted to turn off the kitchen lights. As a result, all power in the house would go off. Nothing else would work—fridge, heater, or lights.

To allow for individual tissue and cell control of metabolism, the body has mechanisms for local control of thyroid hormones independent of the thyroid gland. Think of the thyroid gland as being more like the main breaker.

TSH may be a relatively reliable marker of thyroid hormone levels in the blood in a homeostatic (nonstressed) state, but nonstressed people are usually not the people struggling with chronic hypothyroid symptoms. If you are struggling with chronic hypothyroid symptoms, you likely are not in a homeostatic state. How could you be? You aren't getting eight hours of quality sleep every night. And that is just one stressor that can cause cellular hypothyroidism.

The number-one problem affecting most people and resulting in life-long health problems is chronic, low-grade inflammation. The inflammation is secondary to some level of chronic stress—the same stress that triggers a cell danger response. (See chapter 6.) Chronic inflammation and cellular stress trigger the release of inflammatory chemicals called "cytokines." One of those cytokines, IL6, can cause cellular and tissue hypothyroidism without a rise in TSH.

An increase in IL6 increases D3 activity, causing the deactivation of thyroid hormones in the peripheral cells to increase. This leads to reduced levels of fT3 reaching the thyroid receptors in the cells, causing hypothyroid symptoms. You might expect that would cause a rise in TSH. However, IL6 can suppress the pituitary gland's ability to make TSH, making blood levels of thyroid hormones appear to be within their reference ranges or lower.

If TSH and blood levels of T4 and T3 do not necessarily reflect what is happening inside your cells and tissues, how can your doctor determine what is happening in them or whether or not you have cellular hypothyroidism? And how can your doctor detect cellular hypothyroidism if he or she is testing for only TSH and maybe T4?

First, your allopathic doctor's intention is not to evaluate what is happening in your cells and tissues. According to the medical guidelines of hypothyroid care, intervention starts when the thyroid gland becomes 90 percent dysfunctional.[165] Unfortunately, there is no strategy in place to address the cellular and tissue aspects of hypothyroidism.

There is, however, a blood test that can evaluate whether your cells are favoring activation or deactivation of thyroid hormone. That test is to measure rT3. When your cells favor the deactivation of thyroid hormone with a rise in deiodinase 3 activity, your rT3 levels rise. The other way to evaluate whether your cells are favoring deactivation is to look at the ratios of T3 to rT3 and free T3 (fT3) to rT3. When T3:rT3 is low, your cells are favoring deactivation, especially if you have hypothyroid symptoms.

If you dig into the research, you will find that researchers test T3 and rT3 levels and utilize T3:rT3 and fT3:rT3 ratios to determine cellular hypothyroidism. Therefore, I believe that these tests must be included in every blood test panel a doctor orders for a person with hypothyroid symptoms.

I will further discuss the evaluation of the thyroid blood test panel in chapter 13. But now, know that there are tests to determine whether or not the hypothyroid symptoms you are struggling with are due to cellular hypothyroidism.

WHAT INFLUENCES DEIODINASE ACTIVITY?

Simply put, everything happening in the body influences deiodinase activity. There is constant fine-tuning of thyroid hormone within the cells and tissues. Each tissue—heart, lung, gastrointestinal tract, and so forth—must regulate its cells' thyroid physiology based on the demands being put on the body.

When you eat, the gastrointestinal tract's metabolism must be upregulated to deal with the digestion and absorption of food and excretion of waste. The body does not need to increase every cell and tissue's metabolism, just the ones required for optimal gastrointestinal physiology. The body is constantly reorganizing thyroid hormone resources. The hypothalamus-pituitary-thyroid axis ensures enough, but not too much, bulk production of thyroid hormones. At the same time, individual tissues and cells control thyroid hormones' fine-tuning based on their needs.

Various stressors can alter the deiodinase activity in your cells and tissues, resulting in increased activation or deactivation of thyroid hormone within a specific tissue type. This happens all the time in relation to acute, short-term stressors. Therefore, even if you are in optimal health, you can experience both hypothyroid and hyperthyroid symptoms at times, and sometimes at the same time, as a result of some stress on your body. Why? Because in a given situation, one tissue may need its cells to downregulate thyroid physiology while it is upregulated in another tissue.

While it is normal for thyroid physiology to fluctuate and adapt to acute stressors, research shows that when some of those short-term stressors become chronic, prolonged adaptations in thyroid physiology occur, leading to cellular hypothyroidism and hypothyroid and hyperthyroid symptoms.[166]

Based on my review of the research, it is my assertion that the body's attempt to adapt to chronic stress drives hypothyroid symptoms and cellular hypothyroidism, ultimately causing thyroid gland destruction and a diagnosis of primary hypothyroidism.

So what is influencing your deiodinases? As I said, nearly everything. I cover some specific examples of chronic stressors that downregulate tissue and cellular thyroid physiology in the following chapters.

In summary, let me simplify what impacts deiodinase activity to induce and favor a state of cellular and tissue hypothyroidism in the presence or absence of primary hypothyroidism. Some form of physical, chemical, emotional, or microbial stress, or a combination thereof, causes a cell to perceive danger. When danger is perceived, the cell's physiology changes from growth and development to defense. This shift in physiology results in symptoms. If the stressors are acute and short-term, the symptoms are temporary. If the stressors become chronic, chronic cellular and tissue hypothyroidism and chronic hypothyroid symptoms develop.

THYROID-HORMONE NUCLEAR RECEPTORS

The last piece of the puzzle influencing cellular thyroid hormone status is the thyroid hormone receptor. When thyroid hormones (T4 and T3) enter your cells, the T4 converts to T3, and all the resulting T3 exerts its actions by binding to thyroid hormone receptors in your cells.

Figure 3: T3 binding to thyroid receptor in the nucleus.

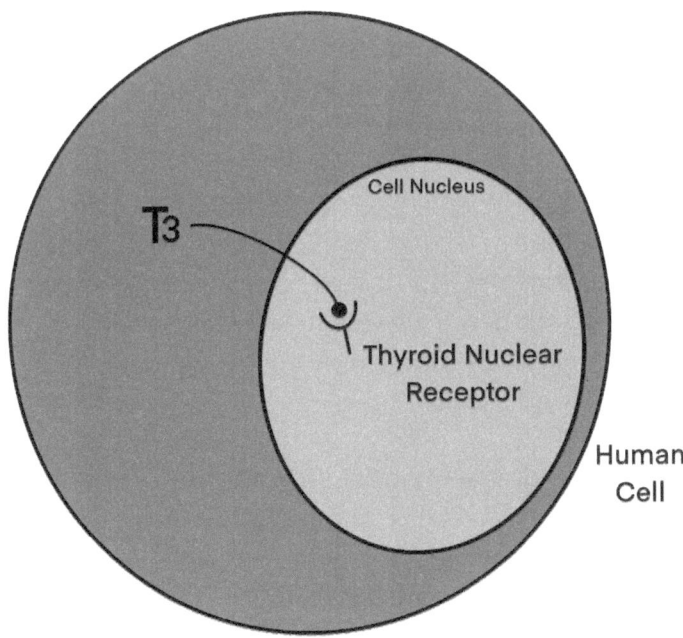

Those actions could inhibit or stimulate the cell, depending on the cell and tissue type. There is more than one type of thyroid hormone receptor. Each type responds a bit differently to thyroid hormones, and the type of receptor present varies among tissue types. Again, this means that thyroid hormone physiology varies among tissue types, especially in times of cellular stress.

The primary types of thyroid hormone nuclear receptors are alpha receptors and beta receptors. (The word "nuclear" will become important in a moment.) Today scientists believe that when thyroid hormone (primarily T3) binds to receptors in the cell, it prompts specific actions on specific genes. This phenomenon is called genomic action.

Currently, there are four known thyroid nuclear receptors: alpha 1, alpha 2, beta 1, and beta 2. The different receptors have patterns of activity that vary by tissue and by the stage of the body's development.

There is a level of complexity to thyroid hormone receptors that goes beyond this book's scope, but here is one example that illustrates what may occur. Thyroid receptor beta has two forms (called isoforms): TRB1 and TRB2. TRB2 is found primarily in the central nervous system (CNS), hypothalamus, and pituitary gland. TRB1 is found primarily in peripheral tissues.

Very few people seem to understand that all thyroid receptors do *not* have the same sensitivity to thyroid hormone. Even though thyroid receptors beta 1 and beta 2 are very similar, their sensitivity to thyroid hormone is significantly different. For instance, beta 2 is ten times more sensitive to T3 than beta 1.

This is likely a protective mechanism. When the central nervous system, hypothalamus, and pituitary gland register an influx of T3 and T4, they shut down further thyroid hormone production before there is an excessive amount in circulation. However, because beta 2 receptors in these areas are so sensitive, they may become satisfied and shut down thyroid hormone production well before peripheral tissues are satisfied, causing peripheral cellular hypothyroidism.

But what if you are on thyroid hormone replacement therapy?

If thyroid hormone replacement is given and the central nervous system, hypothalamus, and pituitary gland are satisfied with a minimal dose of thyroid hormone, TSH blood levels will drop and not necessarily reflect the status of T3 in the peripheral tissues.

The action of T3-binding to the nuclear receptor can be stimulating or inhibiting, depending on the receptor and the cell and tissue type. Just as the thyroid hormone transporters and deiodinases, many forces can affect thyroid receptor function and activity.

THYROID HORMONE NON-NUCLEAR RECEPTORS

Advances in understanding thyroid hormone function continue to unravel the complexities of thyroid physiology. The classic pathway is one in which thyroid hormones enter the cell and bind to receptors. However, recent research has uncovered a "nonclassical" pathway in which some forms of thyroid hormones bind to receptors on the surfaces of cells.

Figure 4: Classical and nonclassical binding of thyroid hormone.

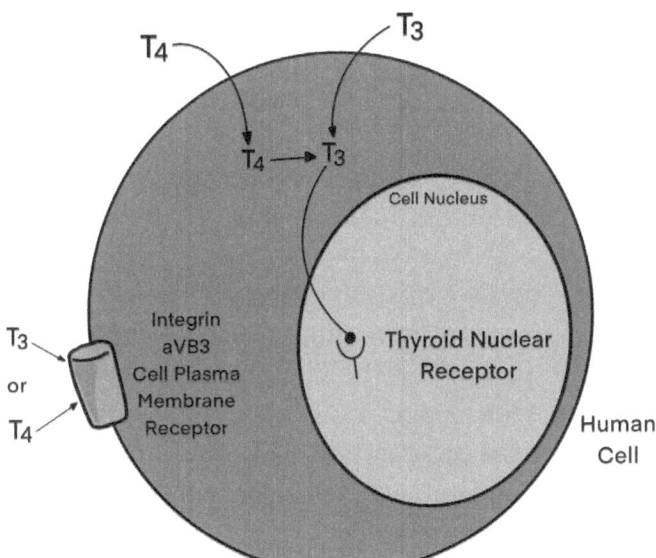

Receptors on the outer surfaces of cells are called integrin receptors, specifically integrin αvβ3 (alpha-v beta-3). The complexity of integrin activation and its full impact on cell physiology has yet to be fully elucidated. Still, researchers think that it allows the thyroid hormones to contribute to a cell's structure and basal metabolic rate and even regulate the proliferation of cells. In addition, when thyroid hormones bind to nonnuclear receptors, many forms of thyroid hormone, not just T3, can influence cell and tissue physiology.

That last part is what is most concerning. In Dr. Kelly's and my opinion, chronic cell danger or cellular stress initiates the global downregulation of thyroid physiology, which can damage the thyroid gland and lead to a diagnosis of primary hypothyroidism. In these situations, it seems the body's protective mechanism is trying to reduce thyroid hormone production and action. Cells are actively reducing thyroid hormone transport and favoring thyroid hormone deactivation globally. Thus, cells, tissues, and the immune system are actively attempting to reduce thyroid hormone production as a protective mechanism.

If thyroid hormone medication floods the body with T4 while the cells are trying to downregulate cell metabolism, growth, and replication, could there be a risk of increasing abnormal cell growth and metabolism? Is there a risk of increasing the proliferation of cancer cells? Some of the most recent literature raises this concern: T4 and possibly rT3 may be able to support cancer cell growth by binding to the integrin αvβ3 receptors on cancer cells.

This concept is extremely important because it questions how cautious doctors should be about providing thyroid hormone replacement therapy. If doctors flood patients' bodies with thyroid hormones, they may increase the binding of T4 to integrin receptors, which risks increasing cancer cell proliferation. However, much more research is needed to fully understand the implications of thyroid hormone actions via integrin receptors.[167,168,169]

CHAPTER 9

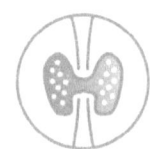

THE EVOLUTION OF A HYPOTHYROID CONDITION

Up to this point, Dr. Kelly and I have asked you to consider that hypothyroidism (at least when it begins) is not the problem but is the body's adaptation to excessive cellular stress. It is the body's attempt to slow metabolism and address the stress or threats putting your cells and tissues in danger.

The stressors that induce cell stress and prompt the cell danger response are often one or more of the following:

- unhealthy food choices
- poor sleep
- overbreathing and mouth-breathing
- environmental exposures to toxins
- lifestyle factors
- negative mindset
- infection

The hypothesis that excessive cell stress is at the root of all things that ail you is not a new concept. The problem has been that there is so much variation in how different stressors impact each individual. Your tolerance for cell stress is unique to you.

Allopathic medicine has few tools to detect excessive cell stress early and address it. Rather, it flourishes when a consistent pattern leads to a specific disease, which allows for a consistent diagnosis and treatment. That is why allopathic medicine does so well in acute care, symptom suppression, and disease management. There is a playbook or algorithm to follow. One symptom, one remedy. One sign, one remedy. One disease, one treatment protocol. In a health crisis, this makes sense. When you are in crisis, you want and need immediate relief.

Most allopathic doctors have ten to fifteen minutes to assess their patients and prescribe treatments. There is not a lot of time spent looking at root-cause issues. I don't think the doctors are bad; I think it's the industry. How many people who have high cholesterol are worked up to determine why it's elevated? Not many. It's assumed to be due to a lousy diet or genetics. The patient gets a mini-lecture to eat right and exercise, along with a prescription for a statin. Do you think most medical doctors would say, "Hmmm ... maybe there is a tissue hypothyroid condition occurring in the liver"? I don't think so.

Allopathic medicine focuses on what it can more easily detect and manage, which is the outcome of excessive cell stress, not the cause. Judging by the nature of the types of tests allopathic doctors order, the reference ranges of blood tests, and the tools they use to treat signs and symptoms, it seems they see the end stage of excessive cell stress, not the beginning. Since allopathic medicine treats the aftermath of persistent excessive cell stress, it doesn't address its original cause or the evolution of a problem.

In contrast, identifying and addressing the cause of signs, symptoms, dysfunction, and disease is difficult, inconsistent, and messy. Why?

The same diagnosis in twenty people could have different root causes in each case. Therefore, doctors either need to identify each person's root cause or causes and treat them as an individual or default to treating the signs, symptoms, and diagnosis.

The solutions of allostatic medicine keep us alive and functioning despite chronic insults on our cells and tissues. Don't think for an instant that we could survive with the onslaught put upon our cells and tissues without medical intervention. But managing the outcome is not the same as addressing the root issues. Medical treatment is not the same as identifying and removing or reducing excessive cellular stress. Scientists call the damage resulting from that excessive cell stress "allostatic overload." Disease results from excessive cell stress that pushes you into sustained allostatic regulation and eventually leads to allostatic overload or disease.

When you are constantly being bombarded by cellular stress, your physiology changes; every system in your body must change how it functions and regulates. The concept of how the body responds to excessive cellular stress has been beautifully discussed in a research paper in the journal *Mitochondrion* by one of the brilliant minds of our time, Robert Naviaux, MD, PhD, titled, "Metabolic Features of the Cell Danger Response."

THE CELL DANGER RESPONSE

The cell danger response is a complex innate defense response by individual cells to a threat.[170] At a basic level, the human body is a complex organism made up of individual cells. The cells work together as small communities to form tissues and organs. Each cell is itself a complex working organism. Within the cells are many components. Among the most important are the mitochondria.[171]

Mitochondria are the power plants of cells. They produce energy from the food you eat to power your cells, tissues, and organs. The mitochondria have two other important roles: They are energy sensors within the cells and agents of cell defense.[172]

Figure 1: Mitochondria, the power plants of the cell.

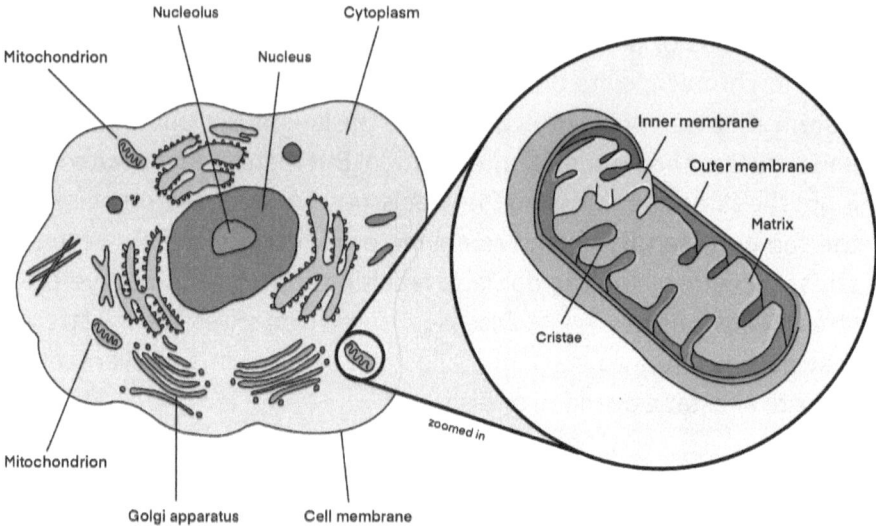

Cells must maintain a certain level of energy to maintain homeostasis. Put another way, a minimum level of energy is required to maintain cells' day-to-day functions. Homeostasis means that energy demands meet energy availability. The mitochondria are constantly monitoring cellular energy levels to keep the energy available within a set range. When the energy available starts to drop, the cellular machinery kicks in to increase energy production. When the energy level reaches maximal need, energy production lessens.

If the cell energy level drops below a specific threshold, the mitochondria sense the decrease as a threat. Something is "stealing" energy from the cell. The mitochondria then activate a cell danger response and change their primary function from energy production (power plant function) to cell defense.

This "energy steal" reaction sets off an almost instantaneous series of events designed to protect the cell, warn surrounding cells, and neutralize the threat. When danger is detected, the mitochondria alter cells' metabolisms to help shield them from further injury. The cell membranes stiffen, which alters the transmission and transport of substances in and out of cells. The cell danger response involves activating the production of inflammatory cytokines and unruly oxygen molecules called reactive oxygen species (ROS) to kill or otherwise address the threat. (I explain reactive oxygen species later in this chapter.)

The cell danger response involves changes in many physiological pathways involved in cell metabolism to limit pathogen replication and the spread of the source of danger. These alterations in cell metabolism lead to changes in cellular physiology to cause inflammation and activate innate and adaptive immunity, much of which you experience as symptoms and, eventually, autoimmunity and disease.

Damage to tissue triggers inflammation. The inflammatory response is a defense mechanism that evolved in higher organisms to protect them from infection and injury. Its purpose is to localize and eliminate the injurious agent and to remove damaged tissue components so that the body can begin to heal. The inflammatory response consists of changes in blood flow and increased blood vessel permeability so fluid, proteins, and white blood cells (leukocytes) can migrate from the circulation to the site of tissue damage. An inflammatory response that lasts only a few days is called acute inflammation, while a response of long duration is referred to as chronic inflammation.

> The immune system is typically divided into two categories—innate and adaptive—although these distinctions are not mutually exclusive.
>
> - "Innate immunity" refers to nonspecific defense mechanisms that come into play immediately or within hours of an antigen's appearance in the body. (An antigen is any substance—chemical, bacterial, viral, and so forth—that causes your immune system to produce antibodies against it.) These mechanisms include physical barriers, such as skin; chemicals in the blood; and immune system cells that attack foreign cells in the body. The chemical properties of the antigen activate the innate immune response.
> - "Adaptive immunity" refers to an antigen-specific immune response. The adaptive immune response is more complex than the innate response. The antigen first must be processed and recognized. Then the adaptive immune system creates an army of immune cells specifically designed to attack that antigen. Adaptive immunity also includes a "memory" that makes future responses against a specific antigen more efficient.

REINTERPRETING SYMPTOMS

Many common symptoms, such as fever, fatigue, and depression, are not disorders or diseases themselves but "normal" consequences of the cell danger response. In fact, the cell danger response is initially a healthy response. The problem occurs when it becomes chronic. The adaptive changes eventually cause allostatic overload, dysfunction, and disease.

We believe that in many, if not most, cases, many of our diagnosed disorders and diseases—such as cardiovascular disease, neurodegenerative diseases, and, yes, hypothyroidism—are the result of an unrelenting cell danger response.

Even the inflammation that is at the root of most acute and chronic health problems is a "normal" consequence of cellular stress. Too often, doctors attempt to suppress the signs and symptoms their patients experience when the inflammation and the reactive oxygen species cells generate are for the body's self-defense. Unknowingly, the treatments suppress the adaptive cell danger response, so the thing or things inducing the response take hold. For example, when a person with an immune condition is given steroid medication to prevent his or her immune system from damaging tissue, the unintended consequence may be that the steroid prevents the immune system from fighting an infection, should one be present or occur. As a result, the person may develop a chronic infection.

Physicians and their patients often mistake the symptoms for the illness, when in most cases, the symptoms result from the cells' response to a threat. Intervening and suppressing natural innate defense mechanisms often contribute to a lingering or chronic illness and perpetuate the cell danger response.

But could excessive stress and activation of the cell danger response cause hypothyroidism? Much of what you have been taught or told is that hypothyroidism starts in the thyroid gland and that the primary cause of hypothyroidism in most developed countries is an autoimmune disorder where your immune system loses control and attacks you and destroys your thyroid tissue. (Autoimmunity is a type of immunity wherein the immune response is directed against one's own body, attacking its tissues, cells, or cell components.) I don't believe these concepts are true in most people. Both Dr. Kelly and I think that something less sinister is going on. Your immune system is not attacking your thyroid gland by mistake but is trying to protect you. After decades of helping people with hypothyroidism, we propose that hypothyroidism starts in the peripheral cells as a response to excessive cellular stress. Hashimoto's thyroiditis is often not the initial root cause of hypothyroidism but the effect of excessive cellular stress and a prolonged cell danger response. Thus, we look at hypothyroidism as a spectrum disorder rather than as a single disease.

Much of what I explain in the next section flies in the face of what the current dogma would have us believe. Allopathic medicine teaches that many of the symptoms are "the problem" or "the disorder." Doctors learn that the body is breaking down and that these signs and symptoms need to be suppressed. But many of the symptoms you experience are not the result of broken physiology. Instead they are the "normal" cell response to excessive cell stress. Many hypothyroidism symptoms are induced by the cell danger response, not as a result of malfunction of thyroid physiology but as an adaptation to support cell defense. When the cells are under stress, the cell danger response is activated. Thyroid physiology often adapts to support the shift from growth and development to cell defense.

The problem occurs when the cell danger response is chronic. Then the adaptive changes eventually cause allostatic overload, dysfunction, and disease. The prescribed treatment may then suppress the adaptive protective response, resulting in the thing or things inducing the cell danger response to take hold. For example, a person with an immune condition may be prescribed a steroid to prevent his or her immune system from damaging tissue. Unfortunately, the immune suppression caused by the steroid does not allow the immune system to fight infection, and the person develops a chronic infection.

WHEN CELLS FIGHT BACK

Thyroid hormone transport into the cells is an energy-dependent system. (See chapter 6.) One thing that triggers the cell danger response is a drop in cellular energy. If the energy within the cell drops, there is less energy to transport thyroid hormone into the cell. In the old paradigm of thyroid physiology, it was believed that thyroid hormones simply diffused from the blood into the cells.

The current science shows that thyroid hormone transport into the cells occurs by transport molecules like MCT8, MCT10, OATP, and LAT. Nearly all of these transport proteins require cellular energy. If the cell is under stress and energy is reduced, thyroid hormone transport into the cell will diminish.[173] If less thyroid hormone (T4 or T3) enters the cell, less thyroid hormone is available to reach the thyroid receptor, resulting in hypothyroid symptoms.

When the cell danger response is activated, inflammatory chemicals are released, resulting in increased deactivation of T4 and T3 within the impacted cells. If higher levels of T4 and T3 are deactivated, less thyroid hormone (T3) is available to reach the thyroid receptors, resulting in hypothyroid symptoms.

When cells trigger the cell danger response, they also release signaling molecules called "damage-associated molecular patterns" (DAMPs) and "pathogen-associated molecular patterns" (PAMPs) into the bloodstream to alert the immune system that the cells need help fighting the threat. The immune system then ramps up to kill or address the threat[174], which could be an organism, a heavy metal, or a toxin.

> DAMPs are materials released from damaged cells that alert the immune system to damage and injury.
>
> PAMPs are materials released from organisms that initiate and perpetuate the infectious, pathogen-induced inflammatory response.

What is extremely interesting is that the cells of the thyroid gland are uniquely sensitive to DAMPs and PAMPs. When the cells of the thyroid gland (called thyrocytes) sense DAMPs or PAMPs, they essentially initiate self-destruction of the thyroid gland.[175] "We show that thyroid cells express functional sensors for exogenous and endogenous dangers and that they are capable of launching innate immune responses without the assistance of immune cells. Such responses may relate to the development of thyroiditis, which in turn may trigger autoimmune reactions."[176]

In other words, when the thyroid cells sense the DAMPs and PAMPs, they activate an inflammatory response called "thyroiditis." Thyroiditis leads to thyroid cell damage and loss of thyroid hormone production. In time, that damage may cause the immune system to participate in even more thyroid cell damage, a condition called "thyroid autoimmunity." (I have a different theory on thyroid autoimmunity that I describe ahead.)

The thyroid sensing of DAMPs and PAMPS is huge because it may mean that when the thyroid cells detect danger signals from surrounding thyroid cells or from peripheral cells, they can induce a self-destruct response. Thyroid cell damage and thyroiditis may not be mistakes by the immune system but part of a natural process to reduce cell metabolism throughout the body. So when there is an active cell danger response, the body reduces thyroid hormone physiology in one or more of the following ways:

- reduced production by the thyroid gland
- reduced free hormone available to enter the cell
- reduced transport into the cell
- reduced conversion and increased deconversion of thyroid hormone
- increased metabolism or deactivation of thyroid hormone

When cells perceive a threat, one of the key objectives is to slow metabolism in some tissues and increase metabolism in other tissues. As a result, some aspects of physiology in threatened cells are upregulated, and others are downregulated. Tissues in a cell danger response want to temporarily reduce their cells' metabolism to limit fuel resources for the perceived threat. Initially the reduced cellular energy limits transport of thyroid hormone into the cells. Next there is an increase in the deactivation of some of the thyroid hormones that enter the cells to lower cellular metabolism.

Thyroid hormone that isn't being deactivated increases the production of reactive oxygen species to kill the threat. However, the same reactive oxygen species also damage cell membranes, making them less permeable to oxygen. Thus, the reduction in cellular oxygen is another tool for cell defense.

With reduced active thyroid hormone within the peripheral cells, glucose transport into the cells lessens, limiting the glucose available for the perceived attacker to use as fuel. As a result, there is an upregulation of a process called "autophagy," which means "self-eating." When a cell is in danger mode and glucose transport decreases, the cell initiates autophagy to use old or damaged cellular material as fuel.[177] Intracellular organisms can also be consumed and destroyed as part of autophagy.[178] Several processes occur within the cell that focus on reducing the cellular threat, including stiffening cell membranes, increasing inflammatory cytokines, and reducing cell replication.

> Autophagy is a unique process employed by eukaryotic cells to recycle some of their components, including macromolecules, such as proteins and organelles. It is triggered in the event of starvation or when cellular components are damaged.

Any form of excessive cellular stress can activate the cell danger response to wall off and then eliminate the threat. In most cases, viruses, bacteria, parasites, fungi, toxins, exposure to an electromagnetic field (EMF), or emotional stressors trigger short-term or acute cellular stress. Once the threat is identified and eliminated, the cell danger response subsides, and the cell healing response kicks in to restore the cell physiology to homeostasis.

Figure 2: The vicious cycle of the cell danger response.

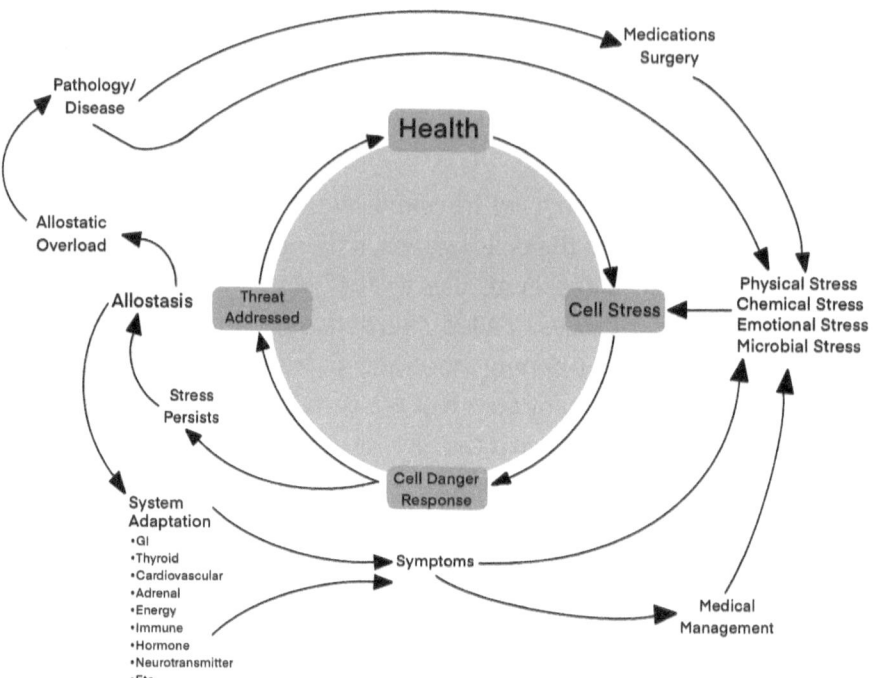

But what if excessive cell stress becomes chronic? What if the cell danger response becomes chronic? What if the shift from homeostasis to allostasis becomes chronic? In any of these situations, cells and tissues never get a chance to recover. Signs and symptoms that persist require medical intervention. While those medical interventions are sometimes necessary, they may add to cellular stress, causing more symptoms, autoimmunity, and pathology, and requiring more medications and procedures that ultimately lead to a downward spiral.

Dr. Kelly and I believe that excessive cell stress and an unrelenting cell danger response are at the crux of hypothyroidism and nearly every chronic disease. Whether real or perceived, excessive stress is at the root of all health problems. Stress is not just emotional; it's physical, chemical, and microbial.

STOPPING DAMAGE AT THE SOURCE

If the stress or threat is chronic, the best way to slow metabolism throughout the body is to shut it off at the source and not to spend excessive resources within each cell to do so. If you wanted to change the nozzle on your garden hose while the water pressure was on, you could simply pinch the hose to stop the flow of water, take off the old nozzle, and screw the new one on. This is similar to your cells deactivating thyroid hormone locally. If there is a short-term threat, the cells deactivate thyroid hormone locally to slow metabolism. As a result, you may have short-term hypothyroid symptoms, which are the typical symptoms of illness. The cellular danger response addresses the threat, and eventually metabolism returns to normal. Thyroid hormone deactivation in the cell diminishes.

If the threat is persistent, the cells undergoing the cell danger response release DAMPs and PAMPs to alert the immune system that backup is needed. The thyroid gland also senses the DAMPs and PAMPs and lessens thyroid hormone production.[179]

Multiple papers discuss how the release of DAMPs and PAMPs by damaged cells contributes to thyroiditis and autoimmunity.[180,181,182,183] When the thyroid gland is shut down with an immune attack, it produces less thyroid hormone. With less thyroid hormone, there is less for individual cells to deactivate.

Think of the garden hose analogy. If I have the new nozzle in hand, I may just pinch the hose quickly and make the change. But if I don't have the nozzle I need, I will not stand there and pinch the hose forever to control the water. Instead I shut off the water at the source, the spigot. This frees me up to go to the hardware store to buy a new nozzle.

To review, when the cells and tissues are under persistent attack and the cell danger response is chronic, the damaged cells continually release DAMPs and PAMPs to activate the immune system. When receptors in thyroid gland cells receive these dangerous signaling molecules, they instigate an inflammatory and immune process within the thyroid gland. Thus, the thyroid cells themselves activate a self-destruct mode. This self-destruction is called an "autoimmune attack," and it can destroy the thyroid gland. This autoimmune destruction is not an accident, not a mistake by the immune system, but a properly regulated immune response to one or more threats. When the cell danger response resolves, the thyroid gland may be able to recover.

I know this is not what you were told or taught. This science is fairly new, and to be fair, researchers are still trying to figure out thyroiditis and thyroid autoimmunity. However, science seems to be reasonably sure that the incidence of hypothyroidism and Hashimoto's thyroiditis is not slowing down.

HOW HYPOTHYROIDISM DEVELOPS

The current medical hypothesis is that two possible mechanisms cause thyroid disease: iodine deficiency, which is the most common cause in underdeveloped countries, and autoimmunity, the most common cause in developed countries. Destruction or disease of the thyroid gland diminishes thyroid hormone production. This leads to insufficient thyroid hormones in your blood, so less is available to enter your cells and attach to hormone receptors. The net result is hypothyroid symptoms.

According to this line of thinking, the solution is to put more thyroid hormone into the body. Since allopathic doctors believe hypothyroidism starts in the thyroid gland and the damage is beyond repair, they think the only option is to replace what the thyroid gland can no longer make. This remedy brings your TSH blood level back into its reference range and creates a biochemical euthyroidism. According to allopathic medicine, once TSH returns to the normal range (biochemical euthyroidism), your thyroid condition has been fixed.

Here are the problems with this line of thinking:

1. It assumes that every aspect of thyroid physiology beyond the thyroid gland is working.
2. It assumes that normalizing TSH in the blood indicates thyroid physiology is restored in all tissues. The allopathic model focuses on restoring TSH, which for many people does not improve their symptoms, function, or quality of life.
3. It assumes that thyroid physiology regulates the same in homeostasis as it does in allostasis.
4. It assumes that no cellular stress persists.
5. It assumes that hypothyroidism starts in the thyroid gland via autoimmunity or iodine deficiency, the two assumed primary causes of hypothyroidism. Unfortunately, very few people are evaluated for iodine deficiency, and rarely, if ever, does the allopathic doctor try to identify the cause of thyroid autoimmunity.
6. The allopathic model puts no effort into identifying the cause of your hypothyroidism, which is why you are never done with taking thyroid hormone. If you never address the real problem, lifelong medical management becomes the only solution.

After twenty years of helping patients recover from chronic hypothyroidism and combing through the scientific research, it is our opinion that most hypothyroid conditions do not start in the thyroid gland. Instead, for most people, hypothyroid symptoms start long before the thyroid gland becomes dysfunctional. And it begins well before a diagnosis of primary hypothyroidism or intervention occurs.

Instead of hypothyroidism starting in the gland, Dr. Kelly and I believe hypothyroidism begins in the peripheral tissues, away from the thyroid gland. We consider hypothyroidism as a continuum or spectrum disorder. By the time you have been diagnosed with primary hypothyroidism, you may have been struggling with cellular hypothyroidism for decades. You are probably thinking, "If allopathic medicine is looking at hypothyroidism from the wrong end, what is really going on? How does a thyroid physiology problem develop?" I'm glad you asked.

CHAPTER 10

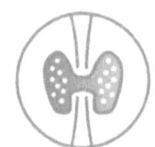

HYPOTHYROIDISM IS A SPECTRUM DISORDER

A major problem with the allopathic approach to hypothyroidism is the assumption that hypothyroidism is a single disorder that begins when the thyroid gland can no longer produce sufficient thyroid hormone. Nor is there a uniform reduction in thyroid physiology in all tissues when the production of thyroid hormones decreases. That's because the effects of hypothyroidism on the body's metabolism depend on several factors:

- the underlying cause of the cell danger response
- the phase of hypothyroidism
- the extent to which thyroid hormone levels have decreased
- the tissues impacted

Another major problem with the allopathic model of thyroid care is the idea that hypothyroidism is caused by a mistake of the immune system. Dr. Kelly and I do not believe that to be the case in most instances; it is more likely a defense mechanism. Thyroid hormones regulate the cells' adaptations to danger by protecting energy storage in times of stress. In addition, research shows that thyroid hormones regulate the shift from cell growth to cell defense.

Lastly, in the allopathic model, treatable hypothyroidism starts when TSH is elevated and T4 is low. Also, when TSH is normal, there is little discussion regarding tissue thyroid physiology. Dr. Kelly and I believe that hypothyroidism begins in the cells and tissues due to diminished amounts of T3 reaching thyroid receptors. This occurs long before an allopathic doctor diagnoses thyroid gland dysfunction and primary hypothyroidism. For these reasons, we redefine hypothyroidism not as a thyroid gland disease but as a spectrum disorder that begins in the peripheral cells.

PHASES OF DYSFUNCTION

I could spend two days explaining the intricacies of the development of a thyroid condition, but for now, I am simplifying it to three primary phases:

- phase 1: cellular hypothyroidism
- phase 2: thyroid gland destruction
- phase 3: thyroid gland exhaustion, or primary hypothyroidism

Allopathic medicine focuses mainly on identifying and intervening when someone is in phase 3. Functional medicine traditionally focuses on phase 2 and tries to identify thyroid gland dysfunction early by looking at more complex thyroid blood test panels and specifically testing for thyroid antibodies.

In the Strategic Thyroid Solution, Dr. Kelly and I go one step further to identify and address hypothyroidism at its site of origin—that is, at the cellular level. While identifying and supporting a hypothyroid condition can significantly benefit someone regardless of the phase he or she is in, identifying cellular hypothyroidism at the earliest point possible allows for the best outcome.

Phase 1: Cellular Hypothyroidism

Allopathic and functional medicine practitioners agree that hypothyroidism occurs when a less-than-optimal amount of T3 reaches the receptors in cells and tissues. However, allopathic medicine assumes that this happens only when the gland is diseased to the point where TSH is high and T4 is low. Research shows, and functional medicine considers, that cell receptors receive less than optimal T3 for many reasons apart from thyroid gland production. Cellular hypothyroidism can begin in any tissue in the body, but it may not occur in all tissues simultaneously or with the same intensity.

When the cells of any tissue, such as in muscle, the GI tract, liver, or thyroid gland, perceive danger, physiology changes. The cells switch from normal growth, repair, and regeneration mode to cell protection mode. Thyroid hormone's role within the cell changes from supporting growth, repair, and energy production to supporting cell defense.

I explain some aspects of this process in chapter 9, but here are more details about the ebb and flow of energy within your cells. Cells contain mitochondria, which play three significant roles in cellular health. They are as follows:

- a "thermostat" of energy flow.
- a power plant to generate energy
- a critical component in the launching of cell defenses

Mitochondria are constantly making energy molecules or fuel called adenosine triphosphate (ATP). In the process of creating and utilizing ATP, there is an "exhaust" called reactive oxygen species (ROS). This is similar to what happens in a car. As the car uses fuel to power your car, it releases exhaust.

> Oxidative stress is an imbalance of free radicals and antioxidants in the body, leading to cell and tissue damage.

The mitochondria are constantly monitoring the energy flux within cells. When cellular energy use increases and energy levels start to drop, signals are sent to the mitochondria, the other parts of the cells, and the brain to increase ATP production. To increase ATP production, cells need more T3 to reach hormone receptors in the cells.

When energy levels exceed what the cells need, they scale back energy production. They decrease the amount of T3 that reaches the hormone receptors in the cell by reducing the amount of thyroid hormone transported into the cells and by deactivating the thyroid hormones in the cells.

There is a general range of energy ebb and flow that the cells sense as normal and appropriate. If the energy flow drops significantly out of the healthy or homeostatic range, alarms go off in the cell.

Think about your refrigerator. The thermostat senses the temperature inside your fridge. The goal is to maintain a specific temperature range. Every time you open the refrigerator, the temperature changes. The thermostat senses the rise in temperature and kicks in the cooling system to drop the temperature. It's part of the ebb and flow of maintaining the temperature. When the door is closed for extended periods, the temperature is easy to maintain, and there is less need for the cooling system to kick in. But suppose you leave the door ajar for a long time. In that case, the temperature rises dramatically out of the established normal range, and newer models emit a beeping alarm to alert you to close the door.

The mitochondria in your cells work in a similar fashion. As long as the energy flow remains within what the cells have established as the healthy range, no alarms sound. But if energy flow drops significantly, the mitochondria have to determine whether the change results from an increase in demand or a threat—that is, something robbing the cell of energy.

If the mitochondria sense that more energy is needed, thyroid physiology ramps up to meet the demand. However, this may cause some cells, tissues, and body processes to slow until the mitochondria meet the energy demand. Think about it like food. If you have enough food in your house to feed five people, but twenty people show up for dinner, you might ration how much food you serve everyone until you can prepare more.

If the mitochondria sense that something is robbing or stealing energy from their cell, they change their role from energy production to cell defense. They shut down energy production in favor of making ROS and inflammatory chemicals to kill the threat. The cell also deactivates some thyroid hormone to slow energy production. Without sufficient levels of thyroid hormone, the major ATP-generating system of the mitochondria and the electron transport chain (ETC) cannot generate energy. Instead, as the ETC is disrupted, more defense products, more inflammatory chemicals, and even more ROS are created. The cellular defense strategy called autophagy also kicks in to scour the cell for the perceived threat.

In a healthy person, the ebb and flow of energy within cells doesn't elicit a cell danger response and doesn't last long enough to create a problem. Occasionally, though, even when you are in relatively good health, the cell danger response occurs. When it does, you feel its effects. You may feel tired, exhausted, feverish, and depressed. These signs and symptoms are not the problem. They are the result of your body's natural defense response to a threat or excessive cellular stress. When the stress is significant enough to induce the cell danger response, thyroid hormone physiology in the cell downregulates to reduce cell metabolism. The cell danger response is a protective mechanism.

If bacteria, a virus, a heavy metal, or a toxin enters your cells, the mitochondria activate the cell danger response, and cellular chemistry shifts to protect the cells. There are two primary changes in cellular thyroid physiology during the cell danger response that cause cellular hypothyroidism and hypothyroid symptoms. The first is the reduction in thyroid hormone transport into the cell.

The second is the deactivation of thyroid hormones at or within the cell. These two mechanisms result in less T3 reaching the thyroid receptors in your cells.

The goal of the cell danger response is to reduce cell metabolism to prevent the bacteria, virus, or other invaders from multiplying, limit the spread of the threat to other cells, and make the cell toxic to the invader. If cell metabolism slows, the organism can't multiply. Once your cells eradicate the threat, metabolism is turned back up, and cell defense is turned down. The amount of available thyroid hormone in the cell, specifically T3, plays a significant role in the cell danger response.

Any factor that reduces cellular energy (electron flow) or increases cellular stress to the point that activates the cell danger response can cause cellular hypothyroidism and initiate the hypothyroid spectrum. Some of the factors that can reduce thyroid hormones in the cell even when the thyroid gland and TSH, T4, and T3 blood levels remain normal are

- heavy metal toxicity[184];
- hypoxia, or low oxygen[185];
- inflammation[186];
- medications[187];
- infection with a microorganism[188];
- nutrient depletion or deficiency[189];
- organic chemical exposure[190];
- oxidative stress[191];
- toxin exposure[192];

The cell danger response to a stressor like one of those listed above is meant to be a short-term acute response. So you may feel lousy for a few days. But even when the cell danger response persists, thyroid hormones in the cell don't completely deactivate. Nevertheless, thyroid physiology changes significantly enough to cause chronic symptoms of altered metabolism. So the symptoms you experience are real even though your TSH and T4 blood levels are normal and the condition isn't detected.

Having a chronic cell danger response with some of the thyroid hormones in your cells being deactivated is like running your home on a generator after a storm knocks out the power. The generator can supply some energy but not enough to power the whole house, so you plug in only the most important things. Likewise, when energy production in your cells diminishes, there is still enough energy to support the most critical cellular processes that keep your cells alive and able to defend themselves.

Deactivating thyroid hormone has another vital role. When a cell deactivates thyroid hormone, it pulls iodine off the thyroid hormone molecule. Iodine is one of the most potent natural antimicrobial agents. Isn't it interesting that the cells increase free iodine in the presence of a threat? Dr. Kelly and I don't think this is a coincidence. We believe it is the innate intelligence of the cells doing what they are supposed to do.

Understanding phase 1 is crucial because thyroid physiology first changes within the cells and tissues. When your cells perceive danger, the role of thyroid hormone changes. Think of the thyroid hormone in your cells as employees in a factory. When times are good, they are busy working, but when alarms start going off at the factory (signaling cell danger), the nonessential employees are evacuated (thyroid hormone deactivates), and some employees alter their roles to try to identify what is triggering the alarms and fix the problem.

If your allopathic doctor orders TSH and T4 tests during phase 1, your TSH blood level will be normal. If you see a functional medicine practitioner who orders a comprehensive thyroid panel, all the blood levels are likely to be within the reference ranges except reverse T3 (rT3), which is likely to be above the reference range.

However, if the stressors robbing your cells of energy become unrelenting, the thyroid hormone deactivation in the cells and the cell danger response become chronic. And when that happens, which may take weeks to decades, the hypothyroid symptoms become chronic too. So now, phase 2, thyroid gland damage, kicks in.

Phase 2: Thyroid Gland Damage

There is a tipping point when a chronic cell danger response begins to impact cells away from those actually in danger. The peripheral cells experiencing the cell danger response release products, such as cytokines, that affect the hypothalamic-pituitary-thyroid axis.

Figure 1: The impact of the CDR on thyroid regulation.

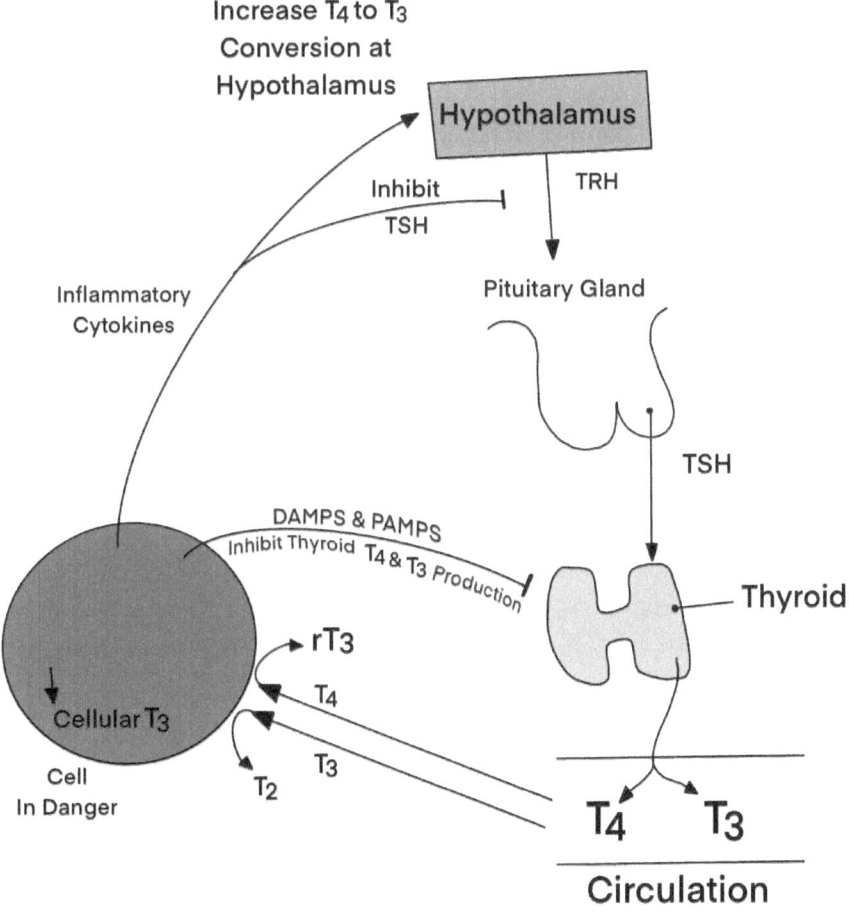

Inflammatory cytokines increase the conversion of T4 to T3 in the hypothalamus, resulting in a drop in thyrotropin-releasing hormone (TRH). With less TRH, there is less stimulation of the pituitary gland to make thyroid-stimulating hormone (TSH). Therefore, your TSH blood levels may be normal or low on your blood test, but your thyroid gland will make less T4 and T3—a change that is detectable with the appropriate blood tests.

The cellular danger response also releases DAMPS and PAMPS, which are used to stimulate the immune system to defend the cell. (See chapter 9.) DAMPS and PAMPS stimulate both the innate (fast-acting) immune system and the adaptive (slow-acting, antibody-producing) immune system. Activation of the innate and adaptive immune systems produces inflammatory chemicals, such as cytokines and antibodies, to aid in cell defense in the moment and the near future.

Nonimmune cells can also detect DAMPS and PAMPS in the circulation, and among the tissues that respond to circulating DAMPS and PAMPS are those of the thyroid gland.[193,194] Circulating DAMPS and PAMPS bind to specific receptors on thyroid gland cells and convert them into active, immune-like thyroid cells. Activated thyroid cells produce and release inflammatory cytokines, which inhibit thyroid function, reducing thyroid hormone production. Cytokines also send a danger signal to the immune system so it becomes active. In addition, activated thyroid cells release chemical signals into the bloodstream to attract special immune cells called lymphocytes to the thyroid gland.

The combination of inflammatory cytokines and infiltrating lymphocytes damages thyroid cells and disrupts thyroid hormone production. This process can cause slow and progressive or rapid and aggressive damage to thyroid gland cells.

It is still unknown whether thyroid cell destruction results from an out-of-control immune system or is an innate response to excessive cell danger. Still, Dr. Kelly and I believe that destruction of the thyroid gland is part of a defensive strategy rather than a mistake of the immune system. If part of the cell danger response is to slow down metabolism to starve invading organisms, what better way to slow down metabolism than to shut it off at the source, the thyroid gland.

The damage to thyroid cells results in more inflammation and DAMPS released. The immune system then uses DAMPS to create antibodies to find and clean up the cellular debris. The two most common antibodies produced in response to thyroid cell damage are TPO antibodies and TG antibodies.

TPO is one of the crucial enzymes in thyroid hormone production. TPO antibodies bind to TPO and mark it for destruction and removal. The thyroid gland uses the protein matrix of thyroglobulin to make thyroid hormones. Thyroglobulin antibodies bind to and eliminate free-floating thyroglobulin. These antibodies are rarely present unless there is thyroid gland damage.

A big misunderstanding is that thyroid antibodies are responsible for most damage to the thyroid gland. This does not appear to be the case. Thyroglobulin antibodies do not appear to damage the thyroid gland, but TPO antibodies do have destructive potential. However, the damage TPO antibodies cause pales compared to that done by activated thyroid cells themselves and invading lymphocytes.[195]

This concept that the activated thyroid cells themselves and the immune cells they invite or attract cause most of the damage to the thyroid gland seems to validate our belief that thyroid gland destruction is likely a defensive mechanism and not an immune mistake.

Depending on whether you are in early, middle, or late phase 2, the levels of your thyroid hormones and antibodies may vary in the following ways:

- TSH could be low, normal, or elevated.
- T4 and fT4 are likely to be normal.
- T3 and fT3 are likely to be lower than the optimal or healthiest range.

- rT3 will be functionally high if not higher than the reference range.
- Thyroid antibodies may be negative or positive.

Your allopathic doctor will say you are euthyroid if your TSH is normal or that you have subclinical hypothyroidism if your TSH blood level is higher than the reference range but your fT4 blood level is normal. In both of these situations, it is unlikely that they will prescribe any treatment. The guidelines are pretty clear that thyroid hormone replacement therapy is not recommended. Even if your doctor diagnoses subclinical hypothyroidism, it is usually a "wait and see what happens" process.

One of two things is likely to happen if you have subclinical hypothyroidism. The first is that the excessive cellular stress diminishes, the cellular danger response subsides, and your thyroid physiology returns to normal. The other possibility is that excessive cell stress leads to thyroiditis, which continues to damage the thyroid gland, leading to excessive destruction and progression into phase 3, thyroid gland exhaustion.

Phase 3: Thyroid Gland Exhaustion

During phase 3, the excessive cell stress that triggered thyroiditis persists and becomes chronic, leading to such excessive thyroid cell damage that thyroid hormone production drops enough to raise your TSH blood level above the reference range and lowers your T4 blood level below the reference range. By the time this finally happens, more than 90 percent of your thyroid gland function is lost.

Now it's likely that you are at the point where your doctor prescribes thyroid hormone replacement therapy. This is the beginning of hypothyroidism, as allopathic medicine defines it. In other words, thyroid destruction is so severe that it warrants medical treatment. However, Dr. Kelly and I believe that this is the late stage of a thyroid condition, not the beginning.

In phase 3, your allopathic doctors' guidelines recommend providing enough thyroid hormone replacement therapy to restore your TSH blood level to the reference range or below it. There is much debate about what the TSH should be for those on thyroid hormone replacement therapy, but that is a discussion for another day.

When TSH is within the reference range, allopathic medicine concludes that biochemical euthyroidism is achieved. In other words, your thyroid physiology is restored. But is it? Maybe. Some people do well on thyroid hormone replacement therapy. Their hypothyroid symptoms go away, and they return to an optimal state of health.

But far too many patients continue to complain of hypothyroid symptoms despite biochemical euthyroidism. Some will be told their chronic complaints are not the result of a thyroid condition because treatment has restored their TSH blood levels to normal. Their doctors often prescribe medications to suppress or manage symptoms or refer patients to other medical specialists for help with their other, newly diagnosed, conditions.

Your doctor may try switching to another type of thyroid hormone replacement therapy. He or she may try increasing or decreasing the dose to improve symptoms. But for many people, nothing the doctor does works to eradicate hypothyroid signs and symptoms.

Some doctors realize that their patients are still struggling with chronic hypothyroid symptoms despite normal TSH blood levels. So to help them, the doctors prescribe higher doses of T4, driving down TSH to almost unmeasurable levels. Those patients then experience a brief honeymoon period during which they feel better. But just like honeymoons, bliss doesn't last. In a short time, the symptoms return, including weight gain. At this point, everyone is frustrated.

Why does this happen? It happens because adding thyroid hormone to a body experiencing excessive stress, a cell danger response, and in thyroid allostasis will not restore thyroid physiology. It can restore a normal TSH blood level but not thyroid physiology. To improve thyroid physiology, your doctor must identify the stress or stressors that drove you into the hypothyroid spectrum in the first place.

Unfortunately, too few people find functional medicine early in phases 1 or 2. Instead they get stuck in the downward spiral of allopathic medicine. That is, once biochemical euthyroidism has been achieved, doctors may tell you that the signs and symptoms that persist are due to another condition, resulting in additional diagnoses and more medication.

People are told that their signs, symptoms, and disorders are unrelated to each other or their thyroid condition. In reality, this couldn't be further from the truth. All the signs, symptoms, and conditions result from excessive cell stress and the cell danger response to the excessive cell stress. So you don't have five, ten, or twenty unrelated issues. Instead you have excessive cell stress, which activates a cell danger response, resulting in adapted allostatic physiology and a multisystem adaptive disorder.

Multisystem Adaptive Disorder

You've likely never heard this term before reading *The Thyroid Debacle*. "Multisystem adaptive disorder (MSAD)" is a term Dr. Kelly and I coined to explain the changes we see in our patients struggling with excessive cell stress, the cell danger response, and cellular hypothyroidism.

Figure 2: Multisystem adaptive disorder.

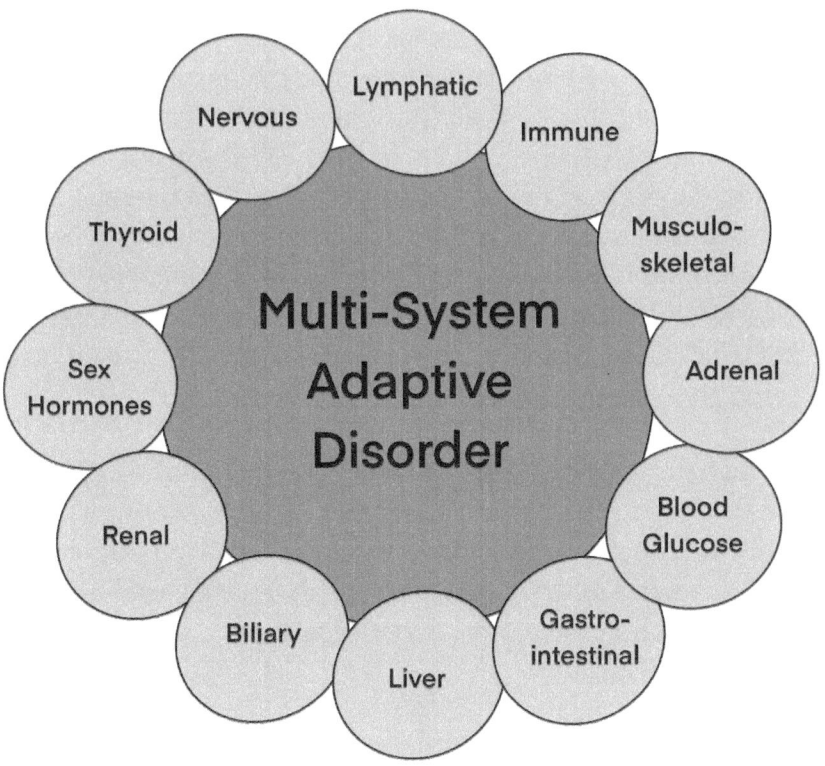

What Is Multisystem Adaptive Disorder (MSAD)?

MSAD is the adaptation of multiple tissue systems to chronic cell danger response, during which thyroid physiology in various tissues, organs, and systems changes, compromising numerous organ systems. Someone with chronic cell danger response and cellular hypothyroidism might develop blood sugar dysregulation or insulin resistance or GI tract, adrenal, hormone, or neurotransmitter disorders. Instead of looking at all of the signs, symptoms, and disorders separately, consider them all together as the allostatic overload of chronic cellular stress and a chronic cell danger response. This may occur in phase 1, 2 or 3.

When your body's cells are in a state of cell danger response, cell physiology shifts energy toward cell defense and away from functions that are not critical to cell survival. In chapter 9, I explain how the physiology of the cells and tissues of the body shifts from homeostatic to allostatic regulation. In allostatic regulation, multiple systems operate at less than their optimal function. They are adapting their operations to support the cell danger response. This can cause many of the body's tissues and organs to demonstrate signs and symptoms of dysfunction in the absence of disease. Your doctor may say you have a functional disorder, such as depression, anxiety, adrenal fatigue, irritable bowel syndrome, chronic fatigue syndrome, or high blood pressure, just to name a few.

In allopathic medicine, these disorders are unrelated. They aren't. They are the result of multiple systems adapting to excessive cellular stress. They are the result of allostatic regulation. In the absence of a disease to treat, allopathic medicine suppresses or manages the signs and symptoms. Eventually, allostatic regulation results in allostatic overload and disease.

Dr. Kelly and I tell people that the multiple conditions they are told they have are not likely to be separate and unrelated health problems but signs and symptoms of multiple body systems struggling to adapt to excessive stress, a cell danger response, and cellular hypothyroidism. So they are struggling not with ten unrelated conditions but one multisystem adaptive disorder.

Figure 3: The downward spiral from danger to death.

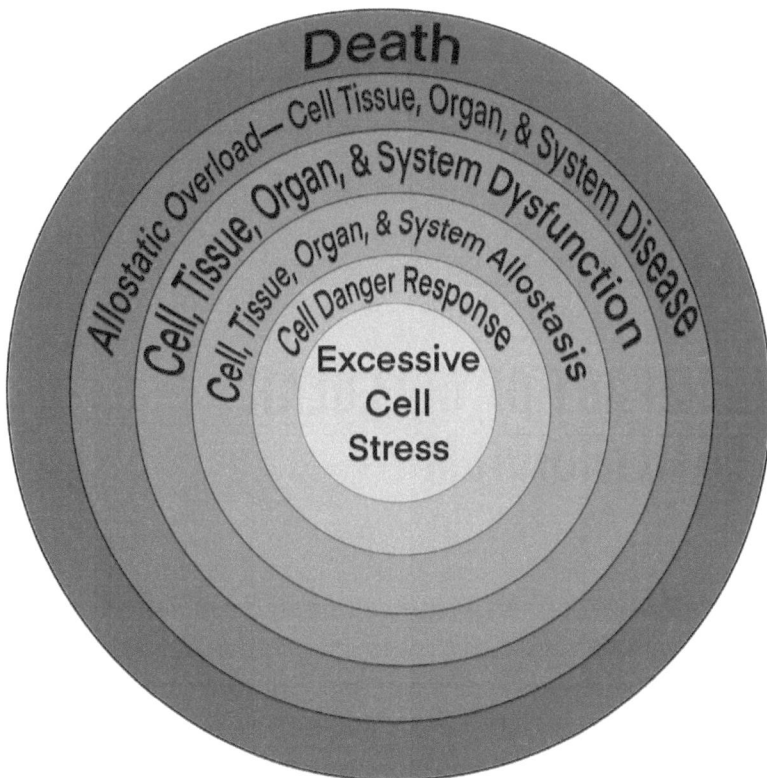

The challenge is that everyone with excessive cell stress, a persistent cell danger response, and cellular hypothyroidism does not experience the same symptoms. MSAD appears differently in everyone. The signs and symptoms you experience, which systems of your body become dysregulated, and the disorders and diseases you develop are due to your unique life experiences, genetics, epigenetics, diet, lifestyle, environment, and interventions. This creates a serious hurdle for health care because, unless doctors are willing to put the work into identifying each person's unique "why" for his or her excessive stress, medicine can do no more than attempt to manage signs, symptoms, disorders, and diseases.

CHAPTER 11

THE IMPACT OF CELLULAR HYPOTHYROIDISM

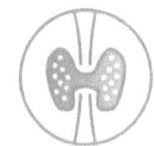

In the previous two chapters, I explained the progression of a hypothyroid condition and described it as a spectrum disorder. At least in the early phase of the hypothyroid spectrum, much of what you experience as signs and symptoms results from adaptive changes thyroid physiology makes in response to excessive cellular stress. Your complaints are the consequences of a shift from a homeostatic regulation of thyroid hormones to an allostatic regulation. Dr. Kelly and I contend that early aspects of the hypothyroid spectrum don't represent a mistake of physiology but are an intentional, adaptive change.

The longer you are in an allostatic state—that is, the longer your thyroid physiology is under allostatic regulation, the more likely it is that the function of some systems of your body will begin to break down and become dysfunctional or diseased. This is allostatic overload. (See chapter 9.)

Extended periods of cell danger and thyroid allostasis lead to signs and symptoms in many tissues and organ systems away from the thyroid gland. Indeed it's likely that thyroid allostasis and cellular hypothyroidism play a critical role in many chronic disorders and diseases. However, it is no surprise that neither you nor your doctor considers that cellular hypothyroidism is playing a role in your hyperlipidemia, cardiovascular disease, diabetes, and GI disorders. And yet cellular hypothyroidism can impact a number of systems in your body and lead to multiple symptoms, disorders, and diseases.

CELLULAR HYPOTHYROIDISM AND THE GI TRACT

Alterations in cellular thyroid physiology can impact every aspect of GI function, including saliva, acid, and enzyme production, as well as bowel motility and integrity.[196]

Saliva Production

Thyroid hormone can directly impact the GI tract, beginning in the oral cavity with the salivary glands. As a result, people with either hypothyroidism or hyperthyroidism often have dry mouth, or xerostomia, meaning they produce little or no saliva.[197] While dry mouth is a symptom of many diseases, it's most often the result of an autoimmune disorder called Sjögren's syndrome.

Like most autoimmune disorders, Sjögren's syndrome results from various factors, including genetic susceptibility and a microbial or environmental trigger. However, at the root of Sjögren's syndrome is the cell danger response. In one study, researchers found that people with Sjögren's syndrome were 3.3 times more likely to develop thyroid disease than those who didn't have the disorder.[198] In another study, more than half of people with xerostomia exhibited some form of thyroid disease.

Why is there such a correlation? While this hasn't been identified conclusively, Dr. Kelly and I assume that at least part of the reason is that damage to salivary gland cells releases DAMPs and PAMPs (see chapter 9), which thyroid gland cells detect, causing them to initiate thyroid gland self-destruction.

Thyroid hormone also plays a role in saliva production. When the salivary gland cells are under excessive stress, cellular thyroid allostasis and cellular hypothyroidism occurs. There is a drop in thyroid hormone within the cells of the saliva glands, which decreases vasoactive intestinal peptide (VIP) production. Less VIP reduces saliva production. Even if cell stress doesn't directly impact the salivary glands, a person with hypothyroidism may develop a dry mouth due to insufficient circulating thyroid hormones.[199] Many other things can negatively influence saliva production, but cellular thyroid allostasis and cellular hypothyroidism clearly plays a role.

Esophagus and Stomach

Your esophagus is the tube that connects your throat with your stomach. In cases of cellular stress and cellular thyroid allostasis, low levels of cellular thyroid hormone disturb the function of the esophagus, causing difficulty swallowing (dysphasia) and inflammation (esophagitis); bloating, stomach discomfort, nausea, and burping (dyspepsia); and low or no stomach acid production (hypochlorhydria and achlorhydria). Low cellular levels of thyroid hormone can impair every aspect of stomach and esophagus function and physiology.[200]

Intestine and Colon

Cellular hypothyroidism's impact on the intestines and colon occurs via multiple factors, including altering gastrointestinal hormone production, smooth muscle function, and motility. In addition, thyroid hormones play a role in the contractile movement of the GI tract, called the migrating motor complex.[201]

Cellular hypothyroidism in the GI tract leads to common symptoms like constipation, diarrhea, bloating, and excessive bowel gas. It also contributes to conditions like irritable bowel syndrome (IBS)[202], small intestinal bowel overgrowth (SIBO)[203], and inflammatory bowel disease (IBD).[204]

Glandular hypothyroidism may also impact the GI tract because a drop in the production of thyroid hormones reduces the production of a hormone called motilin. Motilin is primarily produced in the GI tract and drives the contractile movement of the GI tract. But the thyroid gland also produces motilin, which contributes to stimulation of the migrating motor complex of the GI tract. When the thyroid gland has been removed, destroyed, or damaged by radiation therapy or certain medication, or is subject to autoimmune attack, motilin production drops or stops entirely. The reduction or elimination of thyroid-produced motilin results in a dysfunction of the migrating motor complex, leading to constipation and other GI symptoms and disorders, such as SIBO.[205]

Without sufficient thyroid hormone in the cells of the GI tract or sufficient motilin, GI motility slows, causing constipation. Food moving too slowly through the GI tract allows for increased bacterial overgrowth and fermentation and putrefaction of food, resulting in symptoms like bloating, gas, abdominal pain, and inflammation. Many other factors impact gastrointestinal function and motility, but as you see, thyroid physiology plays a significant role.

Your cellular hypothyroidism may have led your doctor to diagnose your bowel complaints as IBS. IBS is a functional disorder of the GI tract in which the bowels move too slowly, causing constipation (IBS-C); too fast, resulting in loose stools (IBS-D); or a combination of periods of constipation and diarrhea (IBS-M). Regardless of your GI symptoms or diagnosis, you can bet that cellular thyroid allostasis and cellular hypothyroidism are part of the problem.

Any disruption of normal GI physiology also creates cellular stress, leading to cellular hypothyroidism, Hashimoto's thyroiditis, or primary hypothyroidism. Your oral cavity and GI tract house trillions of organisms. The balance of quantity and quality of these microbes impacts the health and function of your GI tract and other tissues. An imbalance of microbes of the GI tract, called dysbiosis, can result in inflammation and damage in the GI tract. When microbes or their toxins escape the GI tract because of tissue damage, they trigger cellular stress in other body tissues, cellular hypothyroidism, and Hashimoto's thyroiditis.[206]

HYPOTHYROIDISM AND BILE PHYSIOLOGY

It's not unusual for patients struggling with chronic hypothyroid symptoms to have a history of gallbladder dysfunction or gallstones, or to have previously had their gallbladder removed by a cholecystectomy procedure. There is a connection between cellular thyroid allostasis, cellular hypothyroidism, and bile physiology. Cellular hypothyroidism can cause bile and gallbladder dysfunction via multiple mechanisms.

First, cellular hypothyroidism raises cholesterol levels. A large percent of people with hypothyroidism have elevated cholesterol.[207,208,209] High blood cholesterol results in supersaturation of bile, making it thick, sluggish, and slow-moving.

Second, cellular hypothyroidism can reduce the ability of your liver cells to release bile into your bile ducts.[210]

Third, cellular hypothyroidism reduces bile flow from your bile ducts into your duodenum, the upper part of your small intestine. After you eat, the movement of your stomach contents into your duodenum stimulates the production and release of bile and pancreatic enzymes. The enzymes move from their respective tissues into tubes that join to form one larger tube called the ampulla of Vater. The ampulla of Vater then releases the bile and pancreatic enzymes into the duodenum. Separating the ampulla of Vater from the duodenum is a valve, or sphincter muscle, called the sphincter of Oddi. That sphincter can be influenced by many factors but requires optimal levels of T3 binding to receptors to relax it enough to allow bile and pancreatic enzymes to flow through it into the intestines.[211]

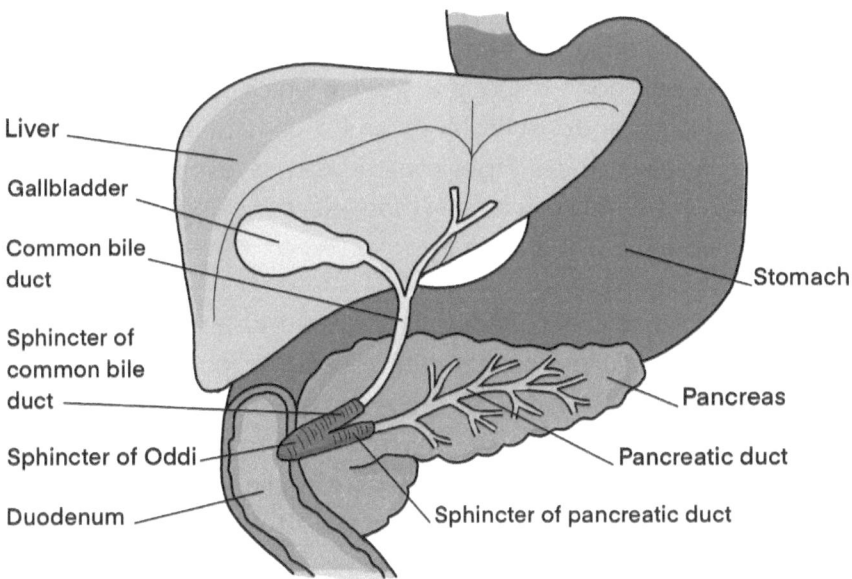

Figure 1: Liver, gallbladder, pancreas, and the sphincter of Oddi.

The significance of this can't be understated. Proper bile quality, quantity, flow, and release are critical to detoxification, absorption of fat and fat-soluble vitamins, microbial control in the GI tract, maintenance of intestinal cell tight junctions, and hormone signaling in the body. Leaky gut syndrome is a common disorder often manifesting from excessive GI cellular stress and cellular hypothyroidism. Optimal cellular thyroid physiology enables proper bile function, and less-than-optimal bile physiology can disrupt it. Too much or too little bile resorption in the GI tract impacts cellular levels of T3. Circulating bile salts can increase the activity of deiodinase 2 in various tissues in the body, influencing cellular and blood levels of thyroid hormones.[212]

HYPOTHYROIDISM AND LIVER FUNCTION

A drop in cellular thyroid hormone levels in the liver compromises liver function and detoxification. (There is a link between hypothyroidism and a condition called "nonalcoholic fatty liver disease [NAFLD]" or "nonalcoholic steatohepatitis [NASH].") When cellular stress initiates the cell danger response in liver cells and cellular thyroid allostasis develops, resulting in cellular hypothyroidism, the cells of many tissues in the body, including the liver, have a reduced ability to transport glucose. The cells don't respond to insulin, which causes an increase in blood glucose and insulin levels and a condition called insulin resistance. As glucose levels rise, insulin levels rise to force the glucose into tissues, ultimately resulting in more glucose being stored as fat, especially around the abdomen.

When your liver cells become insulin resistant as a result of cellular hypothyroidism, glucose can't get in. Your fat (adipose) cells release fatty acids (triglycerides) and send them to the liver. The liver converts those fatty acids to acetyl-CoA, which converts to glucose, which the liver cells use for energy. If the liver cells are insulin resistant, however, the glucose the liver makes from the fatty acids converts back to fat, which is then stored in the liver. Essentially, fat is moved from your fat cells to your liver. Your adipose tissue is supposed to store excess glucose as fat; your liver isn't. The cycle continues until the liver is so saturated with fat that it becomes dysfunctional and diseased. This is NAFLD or NASH.[213]

As the liver becomes more compromised and less functional, glucose from your diet is stored as fat. The increase in your body's fat storage prompts the release of inflammatory molecules from your adipose cells. This fat-driven inflammation causes increased

- conversion of 25OHD to 1,25OHD, which are types of vitamin D, making you appear to be vitamin D deficient;
- systemic inflammation, resulting in aches and pains;
- production of deiodinase 3, which causes T4 and T3 deactivation, lower T4 and T3 blood levels, and increased rT3 blood levels, which worsens cellular hypothyroidism; and
- insulin resistance.

This scenario eventually results in high blood levels of lipids, such as triglycerides, total cholesterol, low-density lipoprotein (LDL) cholesterol, very-low-density lipoprotein (VLDL) cholesterol, and conditions such as diabetes and a fatty liver. As liver physiology becomes compromised, it is less able to support healthy T3 blood levels. Remember that 90 percent of the thyroid hormone that the thyroid gland makes is T4, and only 10 percent is T3, yet T3 is the active hormone. Also keep in mind that your body fights to defend T3 blood levels at the expense of hormone levels in your peripheral tissues.

If liver conversion of T4 to T3 diminishes, your peripheral cells will divert the T3 they need for critical functions to your bloodstream. If the peripheral cells are healthy and not in a cell danger response, the "steal" of T3 from them may not cause cellular hypothyroidism and hypothyroid symptoms. But if the cell danger response with cellular hypothyroidism is underway, stealing more T3 from within the peripheral cells to support the T3 blood level exacerbates your cellular hypothyroid state.

The cells of most tissues have the ability to convert T4 to T3, depending on their need. However, some tissue cells cannot make that conversion. Therefore, they rely on the T4-to-T3 conversion in other cells and tissues to maintain a healthy T3 blood level to sustain their metabolism.

If the liver cells become less functional, their ability to convert T4 to T3 suffers, resulting in a lower T3 blood level. Defending T3 blood levels within the reference range is a biologic priority, so if the liver cells fail to do their job, peripheral tissues will supply T3 at their own expense.[214]

Cellular hypothyroidism in the liver can significantly impact cholesterol and LDL levels, too. High blood cholesterol and LDL are often blamed on diet or genetics, but research shows that a primary cause of elevated cholesterol and LDL is the result of cellular hypothyroidism.[215,216,217] T3 is needed for liver LDL receptors to work correctly.

When liver T3 levels are low, LDL cannot bind to the LDL receptors and release cholesterol into the liver. This results in more cholesterol and LDL in the blood. Since hypothyroidism is often the cause of elevated cholesterol and LDL, everyone should be evaluated for glandular and cellular hypothyroidism before being put on a statin. An interesting statistic estimates that 12 percent of the US population has a cholesterol level greater than 240 mg/dL. That is pretty close to the estimate of people with primary hypothyroidism.

HYPOTHYROIDISM AND GLUCOSE REGULATION

Glucose must get into the cells to be useful. In fact, high glucose levels in the blood are not just unhelpful to your cells and tissues; they can be highly toxic.

In a state of low stress and optimal thyroid physiology, your body converts the food you eat to glucose, and the glucose enters your cells and tissues to support their needs. The mitochondria, the power plants of cells, can efficiently use one glucose molecule to make thirty-six molecules of ATP.

When there is enough glucose to satisfy the muscle, liver, and other tissues' cell requirements, the excess glucose goes into storage as glycogen and fat. Your fat cells release a hormone called leptin to signal to your brain that you are satisfied and should stop eating. Those same leptin signals let your brain know that your metabolism needs to increase to burn off the excess caloric load.

Leptin signals the hypothalamus to trigger TRH production, which is sent to your pituitary gland to stimulate TSH production. TSH signals the thyroid gland to increase T4 and T3 production and release them into the blood. Once in the blood, the T4 and T3 are circulated through the blood to support needy tissues with thyroid hormone and boost metabolism. But remember: it's up to the individual tissues to decide how that thyroid hormone is used.

In times of cellular stress, however, glucose regulation changes. The cell danger response involves an increase in inflammation, which curtails T4-to-T3 conversion in the cells and creates a state of cellular hypothyroidism. It is more difficult for glucose to get into the cells with low thyroid hormone levels.

Glucose is transported into your cells by glucose transport molecules, or GLUTs. There are four primary GLUT transporters—GLUT1, GLUT2, GLUT3, and GLUT4—and all four require T3 inside the cells for optimal function. The glucose transporters are found in varying levels in the various tissue types of the body. Therefore, a drop in T3 levels in the cells under cellular stress hinders glucose transport into most of your cells, except for your fat cells.

When you are not eating and your cells need glucose, they use GLUTs 1–3 to move glucose into the cells. If T3 is low in the cells, less glucose can be transported into them, raising fasting glucose levels in the blood. After a meal, when large amounts of glucose enter the blood, the pancreas releases the hormone insulin to move large quantities of glucose into tissues. Insulin-induced glucose transport utilizes GLUT4. If there is low T3 inside your cells, the cells can become insulin resistant. As cells become more resistant to insulin and glucose, the pancreas has to work harder to make insulin to force glucose into cells. The cells least impacted by low levels of T3 for glucose transport are white adipose cells. An increase in glucose storage in those white adipose cells leads to obesity.

Cellular stress and cellular hypothyroidism are likely a more significant cause of obesity and diabetes than too many calories taken in versus not enough calories burned. When you have cellular hypothyroidism, you can gain weight even on a lower-calorie diet. This is because the cellular hypothyroid state results in more fat storage and reduced calories burned.

Remember: deactivation of thyroid hormone is occurring in the cells initially. So all this is happening, at least in the early stages, with a normally functioning thyroid gland and normal levels of thyroid hormones—or at least TSH and T4—in the blood. Because your TSH is normal, your doctor will likely not realize your weight gain results from a hypothyroid condition.

As cells and tissues become resistant to glucose and insulin, your body starts to manufacture glucose from stored fat and protein catabolism. This ultimately results in a rise in blood triglyceride levels and the development of fatty liver, as I described earlier in this chapter.

Cellular glucose resistance is more of a protective mechanism than a dysfunction. In times of cellular stress, your cells reduce the transport of glucose into cells in an effort to reduce fuel for the "threat." Instead of bringing glucose in, the cells increase autophagy and mitophagy. Autophagy and mitophagy result in phagosomes within the cells engulfing damaged tissue, debris, and organisms; breaking them down for energy; and recycling them for rebuilding. Thus, autophagy and mitophagy serve multiple purposes; they provide fuel, clean up the cell, and eliminate organisms that may threaten the cell.

HYPOTHYROIDISM AND ADRENAL HORMONES

Thyroid and adrenal hormones affect each other in cells, tissues, and their respective organs. In times of homeostasis, your adrenal glands—small but powerful glands resting on top of your kidneys—produce a hormone called cortisol. Cortisol is essential for the optimal functioning of your physiology. Regardless of what you may have heard or read about cortisol, it's not good or bad. Cellular stress gives rise to either cortisol elevations or deficiencies.

The amount of cortisol the adrenal glands produce depends on two primary regulatory systems. One is the circadian rhythm of your body. In the wee hours of the morning, sometime after 3:00 a.m., the adrenal glands begin ramping up cortisol production and releasing it into the bloodstream to get your body ready for the day ahead.

This rise in the cortisol level in your blood increases glucose production to prepare you for awakening. You need glucose to power your brain, muscles, and other tissues so that you are ready to hit the ground running on awakening. Throughout the day and into the evening, your cortisol level slowly declines, setting the stage for sleep. Your cortisol blood level should be at its lowest point around 3:00 a.m.

You might wonder why your cortisol level drops throughout the day if it helps support your blood glucose level. Once you are up and moving, you are likely to be eating, too. When you eat and digest food, your body absorbs glucose and other nutrients. With glucose in your bloodstream and available for use, cortisol is not needed to increase blood glucose levels.

Now, this scenario applies to individuals who have little or no stress. However, if you have cellular stress, regardless of the cause—microbes, a family conflict, a physical injury, lack of sleep, or lack of food—your body will adapt by increasing cortisol. Why?

When your cells and tissues sense danger, they change their physiology. They know that something is wrong, something is threatening, and they are in for a fight. But, unfortunately, your cells and tissues have no way of knowing how long the fight will last, so they make tactical moves.

For instance, as stress and cortisol levels rise, global thyroid physiology lowers. If you are stressed, you want your overall metabolism to slow down so your body can use glucose for its most essential needs. For example, if you were starving, your body would slow your tissues' metabolism to minimize energy use. If you were running from a tiger, your body would slow metabolism in some tissues, such as those involved in growth (think hair and skin) and functions such as digestion, sleep, and reproduction. None of these functions are critical to the primary mission of survival. Cortisol is upregulated under stressful conditions to help slow metabolism and increase cell defense.

This works great when the stress is short-term. For example, if you are fasting or lost in the woods for a few days, the rise in cortisol is beneficial. But that is not the kind of stress that most people are dealing with. Instead what is driving up your cortisol might be night after night of short, disrupted sleep. It might be night after night of mouth-breathing, snoring, and hypoxia. It might be emotional stress at work or with family. It might be physical stress caused by a food reaction or a microbial imbalance in your GI tract. It might be chemical stress from medication or toxins in your food, water, and environment.

The type of stress that induces hypothyroidism is typically neither short-term nor arises from a single stressor. Instead it's chronic, cumulative, and usually low-grade stress, at least in the beginning. As a result, you may not even recognize the stress or realize its effects on you. Or maybe you acknowledge a stressor or two and wear them like badges of honor.

Stress and the rise in cortisol significantly impact cellular thyroid hormone levels and the thyroid hormone production by the thyroid gland. A rise in cortisol reduces the amount of thyroid hormones in your blood and tissue, and even in a healthy thyroid gland. An allopathic physician might tell you that you don't have a thyroid problem because your TSH is normal, but that is flat-out wrong. If you experience a rise in cortisol, it will reduce TSH production, potentially hiding your thyroid gland's hypothyroid state. Or, worse yet, cortisol will suppress your TSH so much that your doctor might tell you that you are hyperthyroid, meaning the symptoms you are complaining of couldn't be the result of hypothyroidism. Or your doctor might suggest that your symptoms are coming from depression, anxiety, overeating, or too little exercise.

How does cortisol shut down thyroid physiology? Let us count the ways. As cortisol rises above normal homeostatic levels, it triggers the release of inflammatory cytokines, which directly inhibit TSH production. This makes sense from a survival standpoint: If the body is under stress, slowing metabolism is a great way to prevent the cellular threat from multiplying. Inflammatory cytokines also increase activation of deiodinase 3, the enzyme that boosts the deactivation of T4 and T3. Cortisol-induced inflammation can also be a driver of chronic joint or muscle pain. Chronic stress, cortisol, inflammation, and cellular hypothyroidism are often the drivers behind fibromyalgia, chronic pain syndromes, and chronic fatigue.

Thyroid hormone also affects cortisol physiology. The liver is the major site of the metabolization of cortisol. Cellular hypothyroidism reduces your body's ability to metabolize cortisol, which can lead to elevated levels of circulating cortisol, contributing to high blood glucose, inflammation, and further thyroid hormone dysregulation. Cellular hypothyroidism can also impact cortisol production. Low adrenal T3 results in reduced cortisol production.

Cellular stress should be short-term, and therefore the stress response should be short-lived. The problem is that for many of us, stress becomes chronic. Over time, the sustained levels of high cortisol and slow metabolism can result in the hypothalamus-pituitary-adrenal axis no longer responding to the stimuli. Essentially, the hypothalamus ignores the stress signals because they have become so constant that it no longer initiates the chemical signals to the adrenal glands. When cortisol production drops, a condition called "adrenal insufficiency"—or, in its more severe form, "Addison's disease"—occurs.

HYPOTHYROIDISM AND THE IMMUNE SYSTEM

You can be certain that cellular stress, cellular thyroid allostasis, and cellular hypothyroidism involve your immune system somehow. Hashimoto's thyroiditis most certainly involves your immune system.

You are probably getting the gist that thyroid physiology affects every cell, tissue, and system in your body and that every system impacts thyroid physiology. The immune system is no different. What is essential to know is that if you have primary hypothyroidism, it probably stems from immune system damage to the gland.

Dr. Kelly and I think this is a big misunderstanding in most cases of hypothyroidism. The idea that your immune system is attacking your own body for no good reason makes little sense. The more sensible way to look at thyroid autoimmunity or any other autoimmune condition is from a different perspective. Some form of cellular stress triggers an immune system response to cell damage and destruction.

The scientific literature is pretty clear that the immune system has a role in the thyroid gland damage that leads to glandular hypothyroidism. Doctors often assume that since a person's own immune system is attacking tissues, his or her immune system is out of control. However, what Dr. Kelly and I consider, especially in the context of the thyroid gland and other tissues, is that something is causing the immune cells to infiltrate the thyroid gland and damage it.

The concept that the autoimmune condition *is* the problem is born out of a lack of understanding of cell physiology. Blaming the body's response to excessive cellular stress and cell damage as the cause of health problems must stop. Firefighters aren't blamed for causing fires just because they are always around fires. Firefighters are there to put out the fires. Likewise, your immune system is the firefighter of your body, and it is called to action because there are fires to be fought. Your immune system gets a call to action because of damage from toxins and organisms.

It seems crazy to think that the solution to an autoimmune condition is to suppress the immune system to gain control of it. To some degree, this line of thinking makes sense, at least in the short run. Suppressing the immune system lessens inflammation, pain, and possibly tissue damage. But unless the root cause of your cellular stress is addressed, that stress or stressors will persist. If the immune system is suppressed with medical intervention, the excessive stress activating the cell danger response will continue to cause damage and destruction. If the stressor is an organism, which it often is, that organism will flourish.

Treatment with immune suppressants can make you feel better, at least temporarily. Ultimately, however, immune suppression has devastating effects on long-term health and function for at least three reasons:

1. The cause of the cellular stress is ongoing, leading to more damage.
2. Because your immune system is suppressed, you are vulnerable to new threats.
3. Immunosuppressive therapy has the potential to cause significant side effects. Furthermore, when you come off the therapy, the rebound response of the immune system can be horrific.

What is the relationship between the immune system and thyroid physiology? Does an out-of-control immune system cause immune system-induced hypothyroidism (Hashimoto's thyroiditis)? Or is something complex and centered around a protective mechanism more to blame than an incompetent immune system?

If you've gotten this far in *The Thyroid Debacle*, you are probably open to the idea that cellular stress is at the root of your thyroid challenges. What I describe next may solidify that thought for you.

Most of us are taught that TSH is made in the pituitary gland and is responsible for T4 and T3 production. But what if we told you that this isn't always the case? It turns out that nonpituitary cells make TSH, too.[218] They do not make large amounts of it, but the fact that cells other than those of the pituitary gland can produce small quantities of TSH may be significant, considering that cellular stress is the initiator of cellular thyroid allostasis, cellular hypothyroidism, and Hashimoto's thyroiditis.

Active microbes may be one factor at the root of cellular stress, inflammation, and cellular hypothyroidism. British biochemist Douglas

Kell, PhD, does a brilliant job of laying out how chronic low-grade infections caused by active organisms are at the root of most common health conditions.[219] What he doesn't do is tie in how that affects thyroid physiology. That's what I am about to do.

Your cells and tissues are exposed to microbes that enter your body through your mouth, lungs, or GI tract at various times in your life. If there is sufficient available iron and other resources to feed the microbes, they may make you sick. If there is insufficient iron or other resources, the microbes either die or go dormant.

Excessive cellular stress and cell damage release free iron, which reactivates dormant microbes. The damaged cells release inflammatory chemicals, affecting thyroid physiology. Short-term, limited tissue damage isn't typically a big deal and would not induce sustained disruption of cellular thyroid physiology. But if that tissue damage and subsequent inflammation becomes chronic or reactivates organisms, cellular stress and the cell danger response launch a whole new level of urgency. There is a cellular and systemic alteration in thyroid physiology and a substantial shift toward cell defense. Cellular actions that are not critical for cell defense downregulate. There is a net deactivation of thyroid hormones within the cells. This is the beginning of events that cause your hypothyroid symptoms.

Now, with less glucose entering your cells, you become insulin resistant, and the glucose is stored as fat instead of being used for energy. Cellular energy production decreases in favor of increased oxidative stress and inflammatory chemicals. Autophagy is upregulated to use cellular debris for energy. Mitochondrial function and biogenesis (growth) decrease in an effort to adapt to the limited resources available. It's like taking the engine out of a race car and replacing it with the engine from a lawnmower. The race car will still go, but not as it did when it had its high-performance engine. The result? Chronic fatigue.

Local cell defense seeks out and identifies reactivated microbes and releases more inflammation to kill the threat and activate the immune system. As a result, inflammatory chemicals and fragments from damaged microbes (PAMPs) enter your circulation. PAMPs and inflammatory cytokines in your hypothalamus increase conversion of T4 to T3, so TRH production decreases, preventing the pituitary gland from increasing TSH production.

These defensive activities occur while cellular stress continues, so the body's natural response is to slow metabolism.

Remember that the body accomplishes this by deactivating thyroid hormone in individual cells and tissues. If the cell danger response becomes chronic, the next step is to reduce thyroid hormone production by the thyroid gland.

Your TSH, T4, and T3 in this situation may look normal or functionally low. You may have hypothyroid symptoms despite normal blood test results. Your thyroid physiology is being suppressed in both your brain and your cells. So your TSH blood level is not a valid indicator of your thyroid physiology. If your doctor orders only TSH and T4 tests, it's likely he or she will conclude that nothing is wrong with your thyroid gland.

Low or normal TSH results in reduced conversion of T4 to T3 in your peripheral tissues. This is good for your cells but not great for your symptoms. (When T4 doesn't convert to T3 in your cells, this can and often does result in hypothyroid symptoms.) The global metabolic activity drop and the shift to cell defense allow your immune system to restore control of free iron and put the microbes back into dormancy, allowing the restoration of thyroid physiology and cell repair and regeneration.

The cycle of chronic excessive stress continues endlessly for some of us due to our diets, lifestyles, sleep habits, emotional stressors, and more. There continues to be ongoing cell damage, release of free iron, and reactivation of dormant organisms.

The cell danger response becomes chronic, the inflammatory response becomes chronic, cellular hypothyroidism becomes chronic, and the release of DAMPs and PAMPS becomes chronic. (Chapter 9 explains how the thyroid gland can respond directly to DAMPs and PAMPs, initiating thyroid cell destruction and Hashimoto's thyroiditis.) Over time, the thyroid gland becomes so compromised that it doesn't make enough thyroid hormones to support critical cell functions, including cell defense. That is primary hypothyroidism, but it is far from primary. It's far from the beginning of a thyroid problem.

Here is a quick review of how the immune system works to reduce thyroid physiology in the presence of excessive cellular stress. The immune system

- plays a role in deactivating cellular thyroid hormones;
- shuts down TSH production, preventing the thyroid gland from producing more thyroid hormones; and
- launches an autoimmune attack to destroy the thyroid gland.

The immune attack on the thyroid gland and the global suppression of thyroid physiology are often not mistakes or the result of an immune system gone haywire. Instead the immune system is orchestrating a mission to slow metabolism and prevent the spread of microbes while it works to regain control. There are currently at least ten theories as to the mechanisms of autoimmunity, and all of them involve the immune system losing control. But maybe the immune system has not lost control and is simply doing its job, at least initially. Perhaps the real problem is that the cause of cellular stress is still present. And for this reason, the immune system is still trying to slow your metabolism. Maybe the immune system is still attempting to address the threat.

So what is the significance of nonpituitary cells being able to produce TSH? Once the immune system regains control of the cell danger response, it may reactivate the thyroid gland to produce more T4 and T3 to support repair, regrowth, and regeneration. This concept is laid out in a research article, "The Immune System as a Regulator of Thyroid Hormone Activity," published in the journal *Experimental Biology and Medicine* in 2016.

> During acute infection, inflammatory mediators released into the circulation would stimulate the conversion of T4 to T3 in tanycytes of the third ventricle. This in turn would hold TSH in check, lowering thyroid hormone output. Physiologically, this would initiate and sustain an overall condition of curtailed metabolic activity. Low metabolic activity would encourage energy conservation by the host and discourage attempts to over-exert during the period of infection—a time when rest would be important. Once the infection is under control through the generation of innate and adaptive immune responses, the immune system would provide the initial signal (through intrathyroidal TSH synthesis by CD11b+ cells from the bone marrow and possibly also from the peripheral immune system) that would lead to an adjustment in thyroid hormone activity with concomitant recovery in metabolic activity. This system offers the added advantage, particularly during times of acute infection, of drawing upon the inherent power of the immune system into the process of metabolic regulation in ways that could not be accomplished solely through classical HPT circuitry.[220]

In other words, the immune system initiates the shutdown of the thyroid gland in reaction to a cell danger response and initiates the restoration of thyroid function and thyroid physiology once the cellular stress is eliminated. Thus, when you reduce or remove your cellular stressors and the cell danger response shifts to a cell healing response, restoration of thyroid physiology at the cellular level and potentially in the thyroid gland occurs. The challenge for many people is that they never address their stressors, and therefore the cell danger response never entirely ceases. For this reason, many people never recover from hypothyroidism and require lifelong thyroid hormone medication.

HYPOTHYROIDISM AND SEX HORMONES

Hypothyroidism can compromise androgen and estrogen physiology and vice versa—that is, sex hormones can be a factor in causing hypothyroidism. Elevations in primary and secondary estrogens are notorious for causing hypothyroidism at both the glandular and cellular levels. Therefore, if your primary or secondary estrogen levels rise, you can experience both hyperthyroid and hypothyroid symptoms.

High estrogen levels hinder your body's ability to transport iodide into your thyroid gland. Without sufficient iodide, the thyroid gland can't make adequate thyroid hormones. The result is low thyroid hormone production and enlargement or swelling of the thyroid gland, often referred to as a goiter.[221]

Many women gain weight after they begin taking birth control pills. The reason is that the estrogen in the contraceptive reduces the amount of iodide moving into their thyroid cells, resulting in less thyroid hormone production.

Elevated estrogen levels can also increase the levels of sex hormone–binding globulins (SHBGs) and thyroid-binding globulins (TBGs). SHBGs are the proteins that transport androgens and estrogens in the blood. When estrogen increases TBG levels, more thyroid hormone may be bound, so less is free to enter cells and tissues, causing cellular hypothyroidism. Lastly, elevated estrogen increases the expression of deiodinase 3, the deactivating enzyme. (See chapter 7.)[222]

Understanding the effects of elevated estrogen on thyroid physiology is extremely important for women on hormonal birth control or receiving hormone replacement therapy (HRT). For example, suppose you complain of irregular menstrual cycles or low libido in menopause and your doctor puts you on birth control or HRT. In that case, your thyroid physiology may become stunted, and you could develop hypothyroid symptoms. (These problems are likely the result of cellular hypothyroidism and reduced liver metabolism.)

The tissues impacted by cellular hypothyroidism and the state of the hypothyroid spectrum you are in may determine to what degree your sex hormones are affected. Hypothyroidism often causes low estrogen and androgen production, but elevations often occur as well owing to poor metabolism when cellular hypothyroidism impacts the liver. In times of cellular stress and limited cellular energy, the body views estrogen and androgen production as less critical than the physiology that supports your sympathetic nervous system or fight-or-flight systems, so production of the sex hormones are often downregulated. Hypothyroidism has been linked to multiple hormone disorders, including

- disturbances in the ovarian cycle and ovulation,[223]
- dysmenorrhea,[224]
- polycystic ovarian syndrome,[225]
- infertility,[226]
- miscarriage,[227]
- prostate disorders,[228]
- erectile dysfunction[229], and
- sexual dysfunction[230].

HYPOTHYROIDISM AND NEUROTRANSMITTERS

A neurotransmitter is a chemical one nerve releases to communicate with another. There are many neurotransmitters, and hypothyroidism may affect them all. Optimal thyroid hormone physiology is critical to brain and neurotransmitter function.[231] Small fluctuations in brain and neuronal thyroid hormone levels can significantly impact mood, temperament, focus, and memory.

An important neurotransmitter that is affected by cellular stress is serotonin, which affects sleep, bowel motility, mood, and motivation.

Cellular stress can cause serotonin production by the brain and GI tract to decrease.

An increase in cellular stress can result in higher levels of another neurotransmitter, dopamine, as well as toxic dopamine metabolites, norepinephrine, and epinephrine. As dopamine, norepinephrine, and epinephrine levels rise, more of their component, tyrosine, is required. Therefore, tyrosine may be taken from the thyroid gland, decreasing thyroid hormone production. In addition, elevated dopamine has been associated with suppressing TSH production and lowering fT4. Both situations can result in less thyroid hormone reaching the cells, causing cellular hypothyroidism.[232]

It is likely that in the early phase of cellular stress and activation of the cell danger response, overall thyroid physiology in the brain is upregulated. Serotonin production is downregulated along with serotonin signaling pathways, while dopamine, norepinephrine, and epinephrine are upregulated. As acute cellular stress and the cell danger response become chronic, global thyroid production starts to decline. As it does, a systemic state of hypothyroidism occurs, along with a potential decline in nerve and neurotransmitter functions.

Cellular or glandular hypothyroidism impacts many systems of the body, including the ones this chapter describes. As you understand these interactions, you will better understand how optimal thyroid physiology is critically important to your overall health. Almost any condition you experience may reflect some level of altered thyroid physiology.

CHAPTER 12

INTERPRETING THYROID LAB TESTS

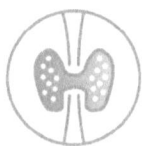

This chapter is not meant to make you a master at understanding and interpreting thyroid blood test results. Instead the purpose is to give you a sense of how to interpret them and, more importantly, to help you understand why you need more than TSH and T4 blood tests. I hope it becomes clear that interpreting blood test results involves more than just looking for *H* for high or *L* for low on your lab report. A thyroid panel of blood tests on its own is simply not enough to explain the complexity of your thyroid physiology problems.

READING VERSUS INTERPRETING

People often assume that lab tests are easy to interpret, but interpretation can be a complex process. Blood test results are easy to read if all you are trying to do is identify whether lab values are out of their reference ranges. In the allopathic model, the results are often reviewed for values that fall above or below the reference range. If the lab value is within the reference range, it is normal. An abnormal result is a value above or below the reference range. This is when an allopathic physician often prescribes medication to bring the value into the reference range. Doing that isn't interpreting a test result; it's reading a number. Your blood test results are not the problem; they are a reference for what is happening in your body. They are signs of health or signs of a problem.

Interpreting blood test results is a bit of an art, and how well a doctor interprets them is based on his or her skill set and knowledge base. Interpretation involves looking at every lab value in conjunction with a person's history, signs and symptoms, medications, supplements, and other tests. First, a doctor must consider whether the lab value is normal or abnormal, appropriate or inappropriate for each patient. The next step is to identify why the lab value is what it is. Lastly, the doctor determines the best way to address the cause of the abnormal result.

You don't need an ounce of biochemistry training to read a lab report. The average doctor can read your report and prescribe a drug or supplement that might bring a lab value back into the lab reference range. If there are no abnormal high or low values, your test results are considered normal. You are told that everything is normal and that you are healthy. It takes an exceptional doctor to interpret your lab values, determine strategies to address the root cause of abnormal ones, and restore your health and quality of life using as few medications or supplements as possible.

Functional medicine practitioners, whose goal is to identify and address root-cause issues, must do more than look for high or low lab values. We must interpret patients' test results. If not, we aren't doing our job.

Replacing Medications with Supplements Isn't the Answer

Both functional medicine practitioners and people looking for a functional medicine approach must understand that a supplement for every symptom or a supplement to restore a lab value without addressing the root-cause issues is not functional medicine. If you are trading five medications for twenty supplements that you will take for years, you are still working within the allopathic model. For me, functional medicine should not be replacing medication with supplements. Instead the goal is to use supplements strategically to restore your physiology while addressing the root causes of your compromised health.

Some practitioners tell their patients that functional medicine is better because it uses "natural" supplements to help the body. That is not my perspective. The shutdown of thyroid physiology is often not the "problem" but a protective response. (See Chapter 9.)

When it comes to thyroid physiology, allopathic medicine considers thyroid replacement—T4 therapy with levothyroxine—the only solution. The general philosophy regarding T3 therapy was that there was no need for it. However, more integrative doctors now use T3 when patients don't get well on T4 only.

Many functional medicine practitioners seem to believe that T4/T3 combined is best because both are closer to what the body makes. Others feel T3 is the only way to go because it bypasses the need for the body to convert T4 to T3 in those with chronic symptoms despite T4 therapy. It is assumed these patients have a conversion problem.

It is our opinion that in many cases, the type of thyroid medication isn't to blame for a patient's lack of significant improvement. Rather, the thyroid hormone is being deactivated at the cell and tissue level for many people. A person may feel a temporary improvement with a change of medication. Still, in time, if the cell danger response continues, the person's cells deactivate the thyroid hormone, resulting in ongoing symptoms. The solution isn't the type of thyroid medication—T4 or T3 or some secret combination of both. The key to improving the effectiveness of thyroid hormone medications is to reduce the cell danger response and support the return of thyroid homeostasis in the tissue. When that happens, the medication improves blood levels of TSH, T4, and T3, and signs and symptoms of hypothyroidism improve or resolve. As a result, we often see a need to reduce the dose of thyroid hormone medication, if not eliminating the drug entirely.

Dr. Kelly and I cover the following points in earlier chapters, but a few are worth reiterating:

- **Standard lab reference ranges are not health ranges.** This is what you see on a traditional lab report. Its reference range is not a "health" range but a "treatment consideration" range and may be based on the results of the population being tested in that particular lab. Having values above or below the lab reference range is like getting an F in high school. Optimal ranges are the standard when the focus is on assessing, restoring, or improving health. (See chart below.)
- **Lab values are just snapshots.** Some blood test results vary widely depending on whether you are fasting, drinking a lot of fluids, exercising, or experiencing any significant stressors prior to testing. Also, supplements and medications may influence your results, making them appear normal or abnormal when they truly are not.
- **A single test result rarely tells the whole story.** Again, TSH is a great example. Your blood level of TSH can be influenced by multiple factors, including the number-one problem people struggle with: chronic, low-grade inflammation. Chronic, low-grade inflammation suppresses TSH production. Therefore, without evaluating your inflammatory state, your doctor cannot make a sound, clinical decision about what your TSH value means. Instead he or she must consider all values and look for patterns. For example, your TSH may be normal, but if rT3, insulin, cholesterol, and c-reactive protein (CRP) tests show elevated levels, you probably have cellular hypothyroidism.

- When doctors look at test results, they must consider the context.
- **What gets measured gets managed.** If your doctor runs a limited panel of blood tests, he or she can only evaluate those few results. If you have hypothyroidism, a broad panel of blood tests gives the doctor some clues as to why you have it. Confirming a diagnosis to convince a patient that he or she has a disease or to get the insurance company the information it needs to pay the bill is fine, but properly evaluated lab tests can provide a skilled doctor with a great deal of insight into what is showing compromise or dysfunction long before disease occurs. A broad panel of blood tests helps identify root causes of cellular stress and see the adaptation happening, possibly long before signs, symptoms, and disease are recognized.

Blood Test Result Ranges

Hormone	Optimal Range	Reference Range
TSH (uIU/mL)	1.0-2.0	.45-4.5
T4 (ug/dL)	6.0-12.0	4.5-12.0
T3 (ng/dL)	100.0-180.0	71.0-180.0
FTI	1.2-4.9	1.2-4.9
T3U (%)	28.0-38.0	24.0-39.0
fT4 (ng/dL)	1.0-1.5	.82-1.77
fT3 (pg/mL)	3.0-4.0	2.0-4.4
rT3 (ng/dL)	9.2-18.0	9.2-24.1

Figure 1: Common optimal and lab reference ranges of thyroid hormone tests

THE SEVEN-STEP PROCESS

First let me say that Dr. Kelly and I rarely run a thyroid panel of blood tests alone. Why? Because, as we have stated throughout this book, a thyroid panel needs to be assessed in context with other things, especially other blood tests. A patient's thyroid values may appear normal, but a comprehensive metabolic panel of blood tests often reveals key indicators of cellular hypothyroidism.

Rejuvagen Requested Comprehensive Labs List:

Chemistry Profile:

Albumin	TIBC	CRP-hs
Globulin	Ferritin	BUN
A/G Ratio	Magnesium	Creatinine
Protein	LDH	BUN/Creatinine Ratio
AST	Glucose	Cholesterol
ALT	HA1C	Triglycerides
Alkaline Phosphatase	Uric Acid	LDL
Total Bilirubin	Calcium	HDL
Vitamin D (25-OH and 1,25OH)	Sodium	VLDL
	Potassium	Cholesterol/HDL Ratio
Homocysteine	Phosphorus	GGT
Fibrinogen	Chloride	RBC Magnesium
Iron	CO2	Insulin

CBC w/ Differential:

WBC	RDW
RBC	Neutrophils
HGB	Lymphocytes
HCT	Monocytes
MCV	Eosinophils
MCH	Basophils
MCHC	Platelets

Thyroid Panel:

TSH	TPO AB
T4	TBG AB
T3 Uptake	T3
FTI	fT3
Reverse T3	fT4

Figure 2: Comprehensive metabolic panel tests

Recommended Comprehensive Metabolic Panel

Let's start by breaking down the metabolic panel of blood tests that Dr. Kelly and I order in an initial office visit. With a patient's list of medications and supplements in front of us, we evaluate and interpret the results of the tests using a seven-step process:

1. Determine whether the lab values are normal or abnormal based on optimal ranges and reference ranges.
2. Determine whether the values are appropriate or inappropriate based on medications and supplements the patient is taking.
3. Evaluate for cellular hypothyroidism based on rT3, T3/rT3, fT3/rT3, and fT3/fT4 ratios.
4. Assess the progression of the patient's thyroid disorder: from cellular hypothyroidism to thyroid autoimmunity to primary hypothyroidism.
5. Look for signs of the cell danger response: inflammation, oxidative stress, and tissue damage.
6. Look for signs of multisystem adaptive disorder caused by cellular hypothyroidism.
7. Summarize the findings.

Step 1

If a test result is out of the functional or reference range, Dr. Kelly and I jot down the possible reasons. We also want to ensure that the patient's thyroid hormone production isn't creating a crisis. If TSH is greater than 6 mIU/L with T4, T3, and rT3 below the reference range, we will probably recommend thyroid medication to support the failing thyroid gland. In this case, the thyroid gland has become so dysfunctional that prescribing proper medication is a priority. By the time TSH and T4 are out of the reference range, and it's clear the patient has primary hypothyroidism, more than 90 percent of the thyroid gland is destroyed.[233]

That last statement may be disheartening. You may be thinking, "If my thyroid gland has sustained that much damage, why should I bother reading the rest of this book?" You might think you are a lost cause. On the contrary, we urge you to keep reading for two reasons. First, we see many patients' thyroid gland function improve when the cell danger response and root cause issues are addressed. Second, even if the thyroid gland has been removed or there is severe damage because of an autoimmune attack, radiation, or medication, it's still essential to improve thyroid physiology within your cells.

If TSH is normal or high with normal values of T4, fT4, T3, and fT3, thyroid hormone medication is not likely to be helpful, especially if rT3 is elevated or ratios of T3/rT3 and fT3/rT3 indicate cellular hypothyroidism.

Step 2

We want to determine whether a value is normal or abnormal as a result of the influence of medications or supplements. Also, as we list the reasons a particular value is out of range, we start building a picture of whether or not there are patterns of problems.

Step 3

We look for cellular hypothyroidism. The clearest indicator would be an rT3 value above the reference range, which is typically 24 ng/dL (nanograms per deciliter). Often, rT3 is higher than normal in people undergoing LT4 therapy. In many cases, especially for those not on LT4 therapy, the pattern of cellular hypothyroidism may be less obvious. For this reason, we prefer to use an upper limit of 18 ng/dL for rT3. If your rT3 is above 18 ng/dL, you have a reasonable probability of having cellular hypothyroidism.

Like all lab tests, however, rT3 values can be influenced by other factors, so even a value of less than 18ng/dL does not rule out cellular hypothyroidism. Why? Because to make rT3, you must have sufficient levels of T4. If T4 or fT4 is low, rT3 levels are often within the normal range. That is because there isn't sufficient T4 to deactivate to rT3.

Along with rT3, we look at some other indicators that the cells and tissues favor the deactivation of thyroid hormone. T3/rT3 and fT3/Rt3 ratios of less than 10 and 0.2, respectively, are indicators of cellular hypothyroidism. We can also look at proxies for cellular hypothyroidism. (See step 6.) For example, do we see signs of insulin resistance, elevated glucose, hemoglobin A1c (HbA1c), or insulin? High cholesterol is another common sign of cellular hypothyroidism.

To summarize step 3, we want to identify whether the patient has cellular hypothyroidism by answering the following questions:

- Is rT3 > 18 ng/dL?
- If rT3 is < 18 ng/dL, is T4, fT4, T3, or fT3 lower than the reference range or functionally low? If so, rT3 may be normal only because of low T4 in the blood.
- Is the T3/rT3 ratio < 10?
- Is the fT3/rT3 ratio < 0.2?

Step 4

We determine whether or not cellular hypothyroidism has progressed to an immune attack on the thyroid gland by looking at thyroid antibody levels. If thyroid antibodies TPO and/or TGA are above the reference range, the diagnosis is thyroid autoimmunity, or Hashimoto's thyroiditis.

Even if thyroid antibodies are negative, Hashimoto's thyroiditis or an immune attack on the gland cannot be ruled out. Why? Because Hashimoto's thyroiditis is often a TH1-dominant disorder ("TH" stands for "T-helper cell"). There are two key types of T cells that influence thyroid antibody production: TH1 and TH2 cells. If you are TH1 dominant, your TH2 immune system may be suppressed, and you might not make sufficient antibodies in your current state for the thyroid antibody tests to be positive. As a result, they will be falsely normal.

We also must determine whether anything could be increasing TH1 levels and suppressing TH2. The most common suppressor of thyroid antibodies and TH2 is a high level of 1,25(OH)D (an active form of vitamin D) because of chronic cellular stress and vitamin D supplementation.

Vitamin D Testing

Evaluation and interpretation of vitamin D status and vitamin D supplementation is an area that is poorly understood. Yet there are endless research papers and blog posts regarding vitamin D deficiency as a primary cause of impaired health and its association with a lack of sufficient sun exposure, the latitude of residence, dark skin color, and broad-spectrum sunblock.

Dr. Kelly and I go against the tide on what most allopathic and functional medical practitioners say about vitamin D. We believe that the vast majority of people are not vitamin D deficient. The problem is that what gets measured gets managed.

Vitamin D testing most often measures 25-hydroxy vitamin D [25(OH)D]. Much like T4, 25(OH)D is a prohormone. To be effective, it must be converted to 1,25(OH)D, the active form of vitamin D. Measuring only 25(OH)D does not tell the whole story. If your 25(OH)D is low, we do not know whether it's low because you have insufficient vitamin D production through your skin or because you are not eating sufficient vitamin D foods in your diet. It does not tell us whether you are magnesium deficient and cannot convert vitamin D to 25(OH)D. Nor does it tell us whether 25(OH)D is being deactivated as part of the cell danger response or whether it's being overconverted to 1,25(OH)D.

Why is all this important? Because most people undergo a blood test only for 25(OH)D and are told that they are deficient. Consequently, most of them are getting vitamin D supplementation, yet they still have chronically low 25(OH)D. If their doctors also looked at their 1,25(OH)D, they would see that their patients have an overconversion of 25(OH)D to 1,25(OH)D, resulting in a high 1,25(OH)D as well as a low 25(OH)D.

For now, you need to know a few points regarding vitamin D testing and evaluation:[1]

---

[1] M. Mangin, R. Sinha, and K. Fincher, "Inflammation and Vitamin D: the Infection Connection," Inflammation Research 63, no. 10 (2014): 803–19, doi:10.1007/s00011-014-0755-z

1. Appropriate evaluation of vitamin D status requires at least three tests: red blood cells (RBC) magnesium, 25(OH)D, and 1,25(OH)D.
2. If all three values are functionally low, supplementation with magnesium and sun exposure should be the initial treatment. To convert vitamin D (made in the skin from sunlight or from diet or supplements), you must have optimal magnesium levels in your cells.
3. If your RBC magnesium is normal and 25(OH)D and 1,25(OH)D are functionally low, you should take a vitamin D supplement.
4. If 1,25(OH)D is greater than 25(OH)D, you should not take a vitamin D supplement.
5. Elevated levels of 1,25(OH)D suppress the conversion of vitamin D to 25(OH)D.[21,32]
6. Sustained 1,25(OH)D levels greater than 42ng/mL have been associated with osteopenia and osteoporosis.
7. In homeostasis, 25(OH)D should be 1.3 times 1,25(OH)D. Over time, having higher levels of 1,25(OH)D than 25(OH)D will suppress the adaptive TH2 immune response, artificially lowering thyroid antibody production and increasing the innate immune response.

If your thyroid antibodies are normal but you have elevated 1,25(OH)D or your 1,25(OH)D is greater than your 25(OH)D, the high 1,25(OH)D may be suppressing thyroid antibody production and hiding the immune attack on the thyroid gland.

---

[1] Bell NH, Shaw S, Turner RT. Evidence that 1,25-dihydroxyvitamin D3 inhibits the hepatic production of 25-hydroxyvitamin D in man. J Clin Invest. 1984;74(4):1540–1544. doi:10.1172/JCI111568

[2] Kell DB, Pretorius E. No effects without causes: the Iron Dysregulation and Dormant Microbes hypothesis for chronic, inflammatory diseases. Biol Rev Camb Philos Soc. 2018;93(3):1518–1557. doi:10.1111/brv.12407

Step 5

We evaluate the rest of your metabolic panel for inflammation, oxidative stress, and tissue damage markers. These things confirm whether or not the cell danger response has begun, leading to cellular hypothyroidism, hypothyroid symptoms, Hashimoto's thyroiditis, and primary hypothyroidism.

Some of the key indicators on our comprehensive metabolic panel include

- elevated uric acid,
- ferritin levels of greater than 25,
- elevated CRP,
- elevated homocysteine,
- low or elevated bilirubin,
- elevated fibrinogen, and
- 1,25(OH)D greater than 25(OH)D.

Step 6

If we see inflammation, oxidative stress, and tissue damage indicators, we attempt to identify the cause or causes of cellular stress and the cell danger response. This involves identifying systems that likely have become compromised because of cellular stress, activation of the cell danger response, inflammation, and cellular hypothyroidism—a condition we call "multisystem adaptive disorder." Key areas include the following:

- blood glucose regulation with blood tests, such as glucose, insulin, HbA1c, cholesterol, triglycerides, lactate dehydrogenase (LDH), aspartate aminotransferase (AST), alanine transaminase (ALT), and gamma-glutamyl transferase (GGT)
- gastrointestinal physiology
- liver and bile physiology

- renal physiology
- immune system function
- indicators of infection
- hormone physiology

Step 7

Now to summarize the findings and initiate a plan of action. First we consider the rest of the patient's history, health timeline, and assessments. Then, when Dr. Kelly and I understand what each test result means both on its own and in context with other lab tests, your symptoms, and your medications and supplements, we have a better grasp of why you have specific symptoms and what follow-up tests are going to be the most helpful in identifying your root-cause issues.

Our plan of action for helping every person improve his or her symptoms, function, health, and quality of life involves five key principles. Our Strategic Thyroid Solution Protocol involves the following steps:

1. Identify the stressors inducing a patient's cellular stress, cell danger response, and cellular hypothyroidism.
2. Identify which systems are compromised resulting in their multisystem adaptive disorder.
3. Remove or reduce as many of their stressors as possible by addressing their fitness factors. (See part 3.)
4. Support the cell healing response and the return of adapted systems to homeostasis by implementing supplemental support protocols and improving fitness factors.
5. Monitor health and fitness factors with functional lab testing of blood, stool, and urine, as well as assessments.

THE FACES OF HYPOTHYROIDISM

Let's look at a few case studies to get a better understanding of the Strategic Thyroid Solution.

Pam Has Hashimoto's Thyroiditis

Pam is a thirty-four-year-old female who has been diagnosed with Hashimoto's thyroiditis and primary hypothyroidism. She is struggling with chronic hypothyroid symptoms. Her current medications and supplements include 10 mcg of T3 twice a day and 65 mg of Nature-Throid, iodine, and 5,000 IU of vitamin D3 daily.

Here are her comprehensive thyroid panel results:

- TSH: 5.32 uIU/ml (high)
- T4: 4.80 ug/dL (functionally low)
- T3: 187 ng/dL (high)
- FTI: 1.30 (normal)
- T3U: 28.0% (normal)
- fT4: 0.67 ng/dL (low)
- fT3: 4.60 pg/mL (high)
- rT3: 12.40 ng/dL (normal)
- TPO Ab: 146 (high)
- Tg Ab: < 1.0 (normal)

Step 1: We've documented the lab values above, noting whether they are in or out of the reference range.

Step 2: Pam's TSH is high, which is inappropriate for a person taking thyroid hormone medication. This tells us that the thyroid hormone is not sufficiently supporting her hypothalamus. Her T4 is functionally low, which is appropriate considering that she has damage to her thyroid gland and takes T3 medication. Her T3 is high but appropriate, given that she is taking T3 medication. Her T3U is normal and, based on the information we had at the time, appropriate. Her fT4 is low, which is appropriate given that her total T4 is low. Her fT3 is high, which is appropriate for someone on T3 therapy and struggling with chronic hypothyroid symptoms. Her rT3 is normal and appropriate, given that she has low T4 to convert to rT3. It would likely be elevated if her T4 were normal.

Step 3: We want to identify whether Pam has cellular hypothyroidism. Her rT3 is within the reference range, but because she has low T4 and fT4, she has reduced levels of T4 to convert to rT3, possibly making the rT3 value normal only because of the low T4. Next we look at the other indicators of cellular hypothyroidism. Finally, we can consider the ratios of T3/rT3 and fT3/rT3. Unfortunately, because she is taking T3 medication, the ratios will not be helpful.

Step 4: We look for signs of autoimmunity and Pam's hypothyroid condition progression. She has elevated TPO antibodies, indicating that an immune attack on her thyroid gland is underway. She has already been diagnosed with primary hypothyroidism.

Step 5: We look at the metabolic panel for signs of inflammation, oxidative stress, and tissue damage, and we find them. Her metabolic panel of tests shows a high ferritin level of 45 ng/ml, and 1,25(OH)D is greater than 25(OH)D.

Step 6: We look for other indicators of multisystem adaptive disorder (MSAD) caused by cellular hypothyroidism in the rest of her comprehensive metabolic panel. Her tests show signs of hypochlorhydria, a condition of low stomach acid production that can be caused by cellular hypothyroidism. Her lab panel also demonstrates nutrient malabsorption, an indicator of GI dysfunction.

Step 7: Our summary of Pam's case is as follows:

1. The patient is on two types of thyroid hormone medication, but they are not sufficiently supporting her brain and peripheral tissues.
2. She has all phases of hypothyroidism: cellular, Hashimoto's thyroiditis, and primary hypothyroidism.
3. Her therapy is not working as intended based on her symptoms and blood test results. The medications have not addressed her root-cause issues, which likely stem from GI dysfunction, but there may be other issues, too.

What can we do for Pam? First, we need to identify and address her cellular stressors. Second, her prescribing doctor needs to reduce the T3 medication and possibly switch to T4 medication only. Pam's endocrinologist originally prescribed LT4 therapy. Then he switched to Nature-Throid and T3 for two reasons: Pam wasn't feeling well, and her rT3 values jumped when she was taking LT4. He wanted to lower her rT3 by placing her on T3 therapy, which we often see physicians do. Some doctors believe that rT3 blocks T3 from binding to receptors within the cells. There is no evidence that this happens and a great deal of evidence that it doesn't.

We need to discontinue the vitamin D supplements based on Pam's vitamin D ratios. Also, she should stop taking supplemental iodine, which can worsen TPO antibody levels. We also need to perform functional testing on her GI tract.

Susan's Missed Diagnosis

Susan is a seventy-two-year-old female. Her symptoms include weight gain, fatigue, sleep disruption, bloating, diarrhea, excessive smelly gas, dry skin and hair, hair thinning, sugar and salt cravings, sweating episodes, depression, lack of motivation, headaches and migraines, and low libido. However, she has been told that she does not have a hypothyroid condition and is not taking any medications.

Here are her comprehensive thyroid panel results:

- TSH: 2.23 uIU/ml (functionally high)
- T4: 6.9 ug/dL (normal)
- T3: 99 ng/dL (functionally low)
- FTI: 1.90 (normal)
- T3U: 28% (normal)
- fT4: 1.3 ng/dL (normal)
- fT3: 3.2 pg/mL (normal)
- rT3: 19.6 ng/dL (functionally high)

- TPO <10 (normal)
- TG Ab: < 1.0 (normal)

On the surface, I can see why she was told that she does not have a hypothyroid problem. Both TSH and T4 are within the reference range. If those two test results are within the reference range in allopathic medicine, an allopathic doctor would conclude Susan has normal thyroid physiology. But when I ordered a thorough thyroid panel of blood tests and interpreted the results—not just reading it looking for H and L—her results told a different story.

Step 1: All lab values are within normal lab range, but TSH, T3, and rT3 are out of optimal range.

Step 2: We determine whether the blood tests are appropriate given the patient's medications and supplements. Susan is not taking any medications that would influence her lab values.

Step 3: Susan's rT3 is 19.6 ng/dL. This is above the optimal range and an indicator of cellular hypothyroidism. It suggests that her cells favor T4 deactivation. When we look at her T3/rT3 and fT3/rT3 ratios, we see that both are below the optimal range.

Step 4: We look for progression of thyroid adaptation. Currently Susan does not have thyroid antibodies. In addition, her TSH is not high, and her T4 and fT3 appear normal, indicating that she does not have glandular dysfunction or primary hypothyroidism.

Step 5: We look for signs of inflammation, oxidative stress, and tissue damage. Susan had seven tests to identify these factors, and all seven were out of the optimal range. Some were out of the reference range as well, indicating inflammation, including uric acid, alkaline phosphatase, ferritin, RDW, homocysteine, CRP, and a 25OHD:1,25OHD ratio of less than 1:3.

Step 6: We look for signs of multisystem adaptive disorder caused by cellular hypothyroidism. Susan does have insulin resistance and prediabetes, hyperlipidemia, and hypochlorhydria.

Step 7: Susan's TSH is functionally high but may be suppressed as a result of inflammation. Her blood levels of T4 and T3 are normal; this is potentially due to reduced thyroid transport into her tissues. However, her T3 is functionally low, and rT3 is functionally high, indicating cellular hypothyroidism. A finding of cellular hypothyroidism is appropriate given Susan's test results and symptoms. She may or may not have Hashimoto's thyroiditis at this point, but we can't tell with certainty because her elevated 1,25(OH)D may be suppressing an appropriate antibody response.

In this case, Susan's primary care doctor was correct: she does not have primary hypothyroidism. However, her doctor considered only her TSH and did not evaluate her for cellular hypothyroidism, which is typical for allopathic doctors. Consequently, her doctor was not aware of her cellular hypothyroid condition.

Cheryl's Weight Issue

Cheryl is a sixty-two-year-old female. She is obese and has been diagnosed with type 2 diabetes, high blood pressure, hypothyroidism, hyperlipidemia, and arthritis. Her primary complaints are joint pain, inability to lose weight, and depression. Cheryl's medications include Levemir, Metformin, and Victoza for diabetes; Rosuvastatin for high cholesterol; Losartan and Metoprolol for high blood pressure; Synthroid for hypothyroidism, and aspirin for pain.

Her most significant concern is that she cannot lose weight. Her doctors told her that because her "thyroid numbers" had been medicated into the reference range, her weight problems resulted from overeating and exercising too little. As a result, she eats one meal a day and works out with a personal trainer three times a week.

Here are her comprehensive thyroid panel results:

- TSH: 2.89 uIU/mL (normal)
- T4: 10 ug/dL (normal)
- T3: 122 ng/dL (normal)
- FTI: 2.6 (normal)
- T3U: 26% (functionally low)
- fT4: 1.55 (functionally high)
- fT3: 3.1 ng/dL (normal)
- rT3: 44.6pg/mL (lab high)
- TPO: < 34
- TG Ab: < 1.0

Step 1: Her lab values are listed above. By her primary care doctor's and endocrinologist's standards, she is euthyroid with the help of medication.

Step 2: Her TSH, T4, and T3 are all within normal range. However, she is morbidly obese. She does not appear to be a person who is euthyroid with a normally functioning thyroid hormone. Three of her medications suppress TSH, potentially hiding a hypothyroid state. Her T4 is within the lab reference range because she is taking levothyroxine. Her T3U is functionally low, indicating that much of her thyroid hormone is bound to circulating carrier proteins. These are typical results for someone taking multiple medications to force lab values into reference ranges.

Step 3: Her rT3 is elevated to almost twice the upper limit of the reference range, indicating that her cells are deactivating her thyroid hormone support. It's a clear case of cellular hypothyroidism. Her T3/rT3 ratio and fT3/rT3 ratio are 2.74 and 0.07 respectively. Both indicate cellular hypothyroidism.

Step 4: We know that this patient has cellular hypothyroidism. Her thyroid antibodies are negative, but her 1,25(OH)D is three times higher than her 25(OH)D, which suppresses her immune system's ability to make antibodies. We know that she has primary hypothyroidism from her previous diagnosis.

Step 5: Multiple tests in the comprehensive metabolic panel of blood tests indicate inflammation, oxidative stress, and tissue damage. Those outside of the optimal range include alkaline phosphatase (ALP), AST, ALT, ferritin, red cell distribution width (RDW), fibrinogen, 25(OH)D:1,25(OH)D ratio, homocysteine, and c-reactive protein (CRP).

Step 6: Signs of multisystem adaptive disorder include diabetes, hyperlipidemia, fatty liver, GI dysfunction, and hypochlorhydria.

Step 7: This woman is the poster child for what is wrong with allopathic thyroid care. Her doctors have her on multiple medications to force her lab values into range. Her TSH and T4 are within normal range, but clearly her metabolism is not working properly. Despite her medications, she still has high blood pressure, and her lipids are above the reference range. Her HbA1C is above 10 mmol/mol with elevated insulin, which means despite diabetes medications, she is still struggling with blood glucose dysregulation. Her doctors are failing to normalize her blood levels and failing to improve her health. Out of frustration, they blame the patient, maintaining that she must be doing something wrong. She, however, is following their advice—eating less, working out daily, taking her medications—yet she is getting worse, and her doctors keep prescribing more medications and browbeating her.

You will be happy to know that all three women improved significantly after following our prescribed protocols. However, it's important to understand that each woman needed a different set of recommendations. This is because while many people are diagnosed with hypothyroidism, what causes each person's hypothyroid condition is different.

In allopathic medicine, the model is one diagnosis, one treatment. In functional medicine, the diagnosis is less important. What matters more is addressing the cause of cellular hypothyroidism and all of the diseases and disorders that come after it so that health can be restored.

PART 3

THE STRATEGIC THYROID SOLUTION

We have been helping people recover from chronic health conditions for over two decades. We understand that people struggling with these problems want a simple, quick solution for their chronic health challenges. In our experience, though, a simple, quick solution doesn't exist for most people. If it did, you wouldn't be struggling with a chronic thyroid condition, and it's unlikely that you would be reading *The Thyroid Debacle.* That's not to say that improving your thyroid physiology is impossible—far from it. But recovery does require a different journey for each person.

We often find that people hope one drug or one supplement will be the fix. While taking a pill a day works for some people, it is the exception, not the norm. Instead we know that some concepts, habits, and behaviors need to change for most people to improve their health and quality of life. We incorporate this knowledge into our practices and our personal lives.

Part 3 lays out the concepts, habits, and behaviors that are the foundation of the Strategic Thyroid Solution. You can start applying these strategies right now. The Strategic Thyroid Solution has improved the thyroid physiology, symptoms, health, and quality of life for hundreds of our patients.

What's great about the Strategic Thyroid Solution is that much of what we describe in part 3 are things you can do for yourself. In most cases, you can incorporate most of these concepts and strategies into your life without a doctor's help. The strategies are time-tested and are simple to do. This does not mean that implementing some of them is easy. Changing your diet, lifestyle, habits, mindset, and behavior is a challenge. If the changes were easy to make, you would be doing them already. Without addressing and putting into action all the diet and lifestyle concepts we describe, the success you experience is likely to be short-lived, if you see any success at all.

Very little of what we discuss in part 3 will be new concepts. You may read a chapter and say to yourself, "I know I should be doing this or that, but I don't think it's related to my thyroid issues or health problems." We urge you not to blow off these strategies and concepts. They may seem too insignificant to cause your thyroid problem, but we beg to differ. The lack of doing the right things consistently undermines health and leads to multisystem adaptive disorder, a web of physiological dysfunction, hypothyroidism, and other diseases.

If you were one of our patients, we would ask you to bring the strategies covered in part 3 into your life to reduce your cellular stress. Many of our patients improve by just following the recommendations in the Strategic Thyroid Solution. For some, it may be the only support they need to improve their health. For others, guided professional help is essential to help them address the results of years of chronic cellular stress and dysfunction. This is where your doctor's input becomes critical. Still, the sooner you use these concepts before reaching out to a functional medicine practitioner, the better. By starting now, you will be ahead of the game and save yourself time and money.

WHAT IS THE STRATEGIC THYROID SOLUTION?

We developed the Strategic Thyroid Solution to be straightforward suggestions that our patients could use to improve their chronic hypothyroid symptoms, thyroid disorder, and nearly any chronic health condition. The following strategies require that you

- identify the root cause issues of your cellular stress;
- identify your dysfunctional organ systems;
- reduce or remove as many cellular stressors as possible;
- support cell, tissue, and system repair and regeneration by improving your health Fitness Factors and supplemental support;
- monitor and manage health, not disease, with functional medicine testing and achieve optimal health reference ranges for thyroid hormones circulating in your bloodstream.

You will notice that we don't offer much in the way of nutritional supplement strategies. The reason for this is that the supplements beneficial for you, and their dosages, depend on your personal health history, signs and symptoms, and the results of your blood tests.

It is true that many health-care professionals provide broad suggestions or protocols to "treat" your thyroid, IBS, reflux, allergies, and multiple signs, symptoms, and diagnoses. In our practices, though, we see that these generalized recommendations lead people to try to "treat" their conditions with supplements in place of prescribed medications. This leads people away from improving their diets and lifestyles. Relying on supplements can cause people to believe that those pills and capsules fix the problem, though they really are just a tool, not *the* tool. It is not unusual for someone who has read multiple books or blogs on "healing the thyroid" to show up with shopping bags of supplements he or she takes on a daily basis. So far, the record for us is one patient who was taking 106 capsules per day from 35 individual supplement bottles.

When I asked the patient why he was taking so many supplements, the patient said they were a combination of recommendations from multiple practitioners plus his own additions based on books and blogs he reads. To be clear, taking thirty-five different supplements a day is not the solution. It is not functional medicine. So instead, we want you to focus first on the Fitness Factors we describe in the following chapters. We want you to take these suggestions and recommendations to heart and implement them in your life.

In chapter 13, we break down some common terms used in health care and medicine to make sure we are thinking from the same mindset. Then we will discuss the health continuum and the ten health categories of the Wellness Wheel. Finally, we will describe how your fitness level in each category determines your overall state of health, wellness, and well-being and where you are on the Illness–Wellness Continuum.

Next we describe each of the ten health categories, or Fitness Factors. Then we explain some simple strategies you can use to evaluate your fitness level and provide recommendations and strategies for improving your fitness in each category. As you improve, your physical, chemical, emotional, and microbial stress will decrease, and your health will start to improve.

(As your level of fitness in one or more of these categories goes down, your physical, chemical, emotional, and microbial stresses go up.)

Figure 1: Wellness Wheel

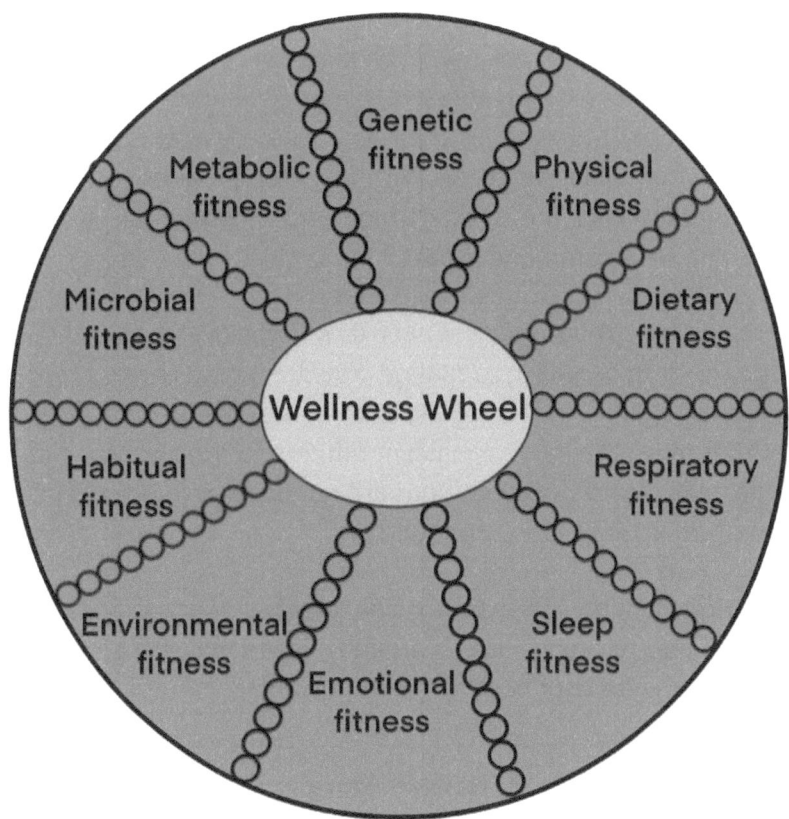

You can improve in many of these health categories without much professional help. However, the last two—metabolic and genetic—are likely to require the skills and expertise of a functional medicine practitioner.

There are many things you are doing that are likely good or even great for your health. But other things aren't. Be humble. Be coachable. Be willing to make some changes that may seem difficult, if not nearly impossible. Just give our recommendations a chance.

Nothing we discuss in this part of the book is voodoo or some foreign idea that came to us in a dream. Instead these strategies are based on science, thousands of patient experiences, and plain common sense.

YOU CAN DO THIS

Before you think it, we will say it. Change can be challenging. Doing anything new is often hard at first. So when patients tell us that eating healthy is tough, turning off their electronic devices is difficult, or fasting is impossible, we agree. With the wrong mindset, everything is difficult. But with the right attitude and willpower, anything and everything we recommend in part 3 is possible.

You can do this. You can. We've seen it over and over in our practices. You just have to be willing to change. You don't have to make massive changes all at once. In fact, small, incremental changes are often the ones that make the most significant difference. Vincent Van Gogh is credited with saying, "Great things are not done by impulse, but by a series of small things brought together."

Small things done consistently can resolve your chronic health problems and turn your health around. That's why the choices you make in caring for your body are so important.

> ### Nancy's Story
>
> Nancy was fifty-five years old when she came to the office. She struggled with dozens of chronic symptoms. She was taking eleven prescriptions (three for blood pressure, one for her thyroid, a statin for cholesterol, two for diabetes, one for reflux, two for allergies, and one for depression) and ten nutritional supplements in an attempt to manage her symptoms, disorders, and diseases. In addition, she was nearly sixty-five pounds overweight. She was totally frustrated and not living the life she had anticipated. The cost of doctors' visits, prescriptions, and supplements was having a massive impact on her finances. The combination of the financial burden and lack of health was crippling her quality of life. In a last-ditch effort to improve her situation, she turned to Dr. Eric and functional medicine.

After reviewing her history, I explained my plan. It caught her off guard. She came to me hoping I would recommend more supplements to add to what she was already taking to fix her problems. I told her that no supplement would cure her. Instead I told her my job was to help her identify her cellular stressors and remove or reduce them as much as possible with functional medicine tests and interpretation. I would help her address each of the Fitness Factors in the Strategic Thyroid Solution by modifying her diet and her lifestyle, as well as by implementing strategic supplemental protocols based on my interpretation of her signs, symptoms, and lab test results. I explained that it would be a challenging process initially but would be worth the effort in time. She would one day wonder how it could have been so simple.

Over the following six months, I addressed each fitness factor. She modified her diet and improved her sleep quality and quantity. I addressed her breathing issues. She took steps to improve her emotional state, habits, and physical fitness. I ordered a comprehensive metabolic blood panel of blood tests and functional testing of her GI tract function. I identified stressors and dysfunctional systems and prescribed specific supplements to address her stressors and support the repair and generation of compromised organ systems.

It was a challenge at times for Nancy to make some of the changes. A few of the recommendations contradicted what her medical doctors were advising, but she followed them. After six months, she was a new woman. She had lost forty-two pounds and eight inches from both her waist and hips. She had energy and vitality. Of the twenty-five symptoms she had started with, all had improved, and 80 percent of them were no longer an issue. With the help of her medical doctors, she was able to eliminate all but one of her medications.

Nancy's story is Nancy's story. You will have your own. The road to recovery will not be easy, but much of what needs to be done for you to improve your health are simple strategies that most people are either not aware of, ignore, or believe won't have an impact. We believe that the strategies we describe in the following chapters will improve your health and quality of life; in fact, without implementing them, you may find it impossible to improve your health and quality of life.

We've seen the powerful impact of these strategies in our patients and our own lives. Every small positive change you make creates a ripple effect on your physiology, your health, your quality of life, and the lives of your circle of influence. You've got nothing to lose and so much to gain.

CHAPTER 13

THE DICHOTOMY OF HEALTH

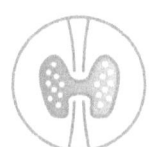

This chapter lays the foundation for part 3. Before discussing the Fitness Factors, which are key to improving your cell danger response, hypothyroidism, and every aspect of your health, we need to define some common terms. When we ask people what health is, very few can provide a clear, concise definition. Most doctors will throw out the World Health Organization definition from 1948. It defines health as "a state of complete physical, mental, and social well-being and not merely the absence of disease." If that "state" has to be "complete," there may not be a person on the planet in a state of health! We have no tools to define a complete state of health, so how could anyone be "healthy?"

Webster's dictionary defines health as "freedom from physical disease or pain." Are we really considered "healthy" if we don't have any formal medical diagnoses, take no medication, or have no pain? Couldn't we still have pain and be healthy? If a man stubs a toe or gets a splinter, he may be in pain. Does that mean he is no longer healthy? Doctors are able to identify patterns that predate formal diagnoses like diabetes and will address and reverse them. But if we never look for those patterns and simply define health as "no diagnosis, no pain," then we are doomed.

What if you have a tumor too small to detect but that will eventually grow and be diagnosed as cancer? Or a blood vessel in your brain on the verge of bursting and becoming a brain aneurysm is seen on a CT scan or an MRI? Or your angiogram reveals clogged coronary arteries. You don't have chest pain, but a heart attack may be in your future. Are you genuinely healthy until the minute you are given a diagnosis? After all, at this point, you have no physical disease or pain. Do you remember the former host of *Meet the Press*, Tim Russert? He was given a "clean bill of health" just days before his sudden death from a massive heart attack.

We often see patients whose doctors say they are healthy. But their health history includes multiple diagnoses, and they are taking numerous medications. Are you healthy if you have various conditions, disorders, or diseases? Are you healthy if you require one or more medications? If you say yes, what would you be if you had no conditions, disorders, or diseases and took no medications?

We can't tell you how many people we see who tell us, "I am really healthy. I just have a thyroid disorder." And often we see people struggling with chronic signs and symptoms of hypothyroidism but who have been told that since their TSH levels are normal, they don't have thyroid problems. Their doctors say they are healthy and suggest they may be depressed.

Are people wrong? Are doctors wrong? Or is it that the definitions we use don't accurately define health in a specific manner? Have the definitions of words such as "fit," "fitness," "health," "healthy," "well," "wellness," and "well-being" become so distorted that they have lost their meaning? The crazy thing is that you can't find a definition for any of these terms that does not use at least one of the other terms. We think it is time to clarify some of these terms.

It is time to redefine the word "health" and look beyond our limited way of assessing it. No definition is perfect, but the definition we offer at least gets us closer to a more realistic definition of health.

Our definition of "health" is "a state of physiological function and adaptability within the environment." Our interpretation of a "state of health" has a different meaning for someone living in polar regions than for someone living near the equator. For example, extra body fat is an adaptation and supports health in an arctic area, but it might infer disease in an equatorial region. This is one reason why the diet of one culture or region does not always benefit people of a different culture or in another area of the world.

Health is personal. Each of us has our own perception of what health is based on the context of our preconceived notions, biases, and environment. Health is not a static state. It can improve or regress based on our actions, habits, and behaviors. Health is measured on a continuum from illness to wellness.

Figure 1: Simplistic interpretation of the Illness–Wellness Continuum.

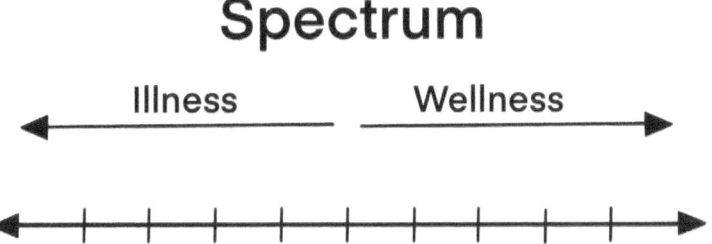

THE HEALTH CONTINUUM

Multiple variations of the health continuum have been proposed. Our interpretation is slightly different than other models. That does not make it right, but it works for our beliefs and bias.

You are entitled to your personal perception of health, but we are going to explain our criteria. We grade health on a continuum from zero to ten. Zero is terrible or critically ill health or fitness, and ten is excellent or exceptional health or wellness. Average or fair health is the midpoint. When most people look at their health, they typically consider where they are as compared to others in their environment. Therefore, there must be some context by which you judge yourself.

Figure 2: Complex version of the Illness–Wellness Continuum

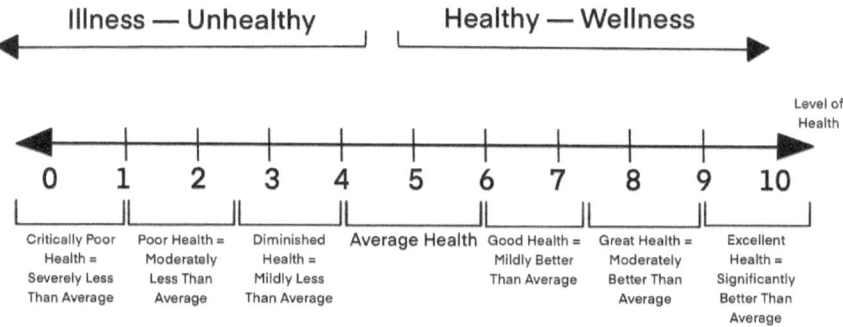

When you have less-than-average health, you are favoring a state of illness. When you have above-average health, you are favoring a state of wellness. "Illness" is another term that has many definitions. For our purposes, illness is a state of less-than-average health. When you are moving down the health continuum, you are losing function, adaptability, resilience, strength, and the ability to self-manage. As signs and symptoms become chronic, you begin to accumulate diagnoses of conditions, disorders, and diseases like yellow jackets at a fall picnic. You start to rely on medical care for treatments to manage symptoms that arise as you continue to decline.

It is easy to move down the continuum. The dichotomy, however, is that the further you move down the continuum and deeper into illness, the more difficult everyday life becomes. But conversely, when you move up the continuum into a higher state of wellness, you improve your function, adaptability, resilience, and strength, and everyday life becomes more manageable.

When you participate in activities that improve and maximize your fitness and potential in all of the Fitness Factors, moving up the continuum is often difficult. It sometimes takes effort that you do not want to invest. The dichotomy here is that as you do the difficult things—the hard tasks, work, and training necessary to move up the continuum—the easier day-to-day life becomes.

HEALTHY VS. UNHEALTHY

"Healthy" and "unhealthy" are adjectives that describe a person, place, or thing. If someone is said to be healthy, he or she should have above-average health. If someone has below-average health, he or she is unhealthy. If some food, drink, or action is to be considered healthy, it should promote a higher state of health. It should make you more adaptable and more resilient, and it should improve your ability to manage without medications. It should move you up the health continuum.

Our society tends to look at a person's diet, lifestyle, or behaviors and then make a value judgment on whether the person is healthy. Not everyone who has a healthy diet, lifestyle, and habits is healthy. However, everyone who is healthy has a healthy diet, lifestyle, and habits. This is an important distinction to make. Just because someone who is obese and has cardiovascular disease and diabetes is running or lifting weights at the gym, that does not make him or her healthy. Just because someone takes multiple medications to manage his or her high blood pressure, TSH, diabetes, or cholesterol does not mean the person is healthy. An unhealthy person can have a healthy diet and behaviors and still be unhealthy or ill. A healthy person can engage in unhealthy behaviors and still be healthy.

As we previously stated, the definition of health is your state of physiological function and your adaptability to your environment. For you to have average or baseline health—the midpoint of the continuum—you must have functional physiology that can adapt to your environment, and you need to be able to self-manage. Being healthy should not require ongoing treatment with medications.

You can and should absolutely engage in activities that we deem healthy because they help improve your physiological function and adaptability. Therefore, we consider specific actions or behaviors as healthy even though the person isn't. At least not yet.

WELL-BEING VS. ILL-BEING

For us, "well-being" and "ill-being" are about your mindset. They are about how you act, think, and behave. They are about how you are functioning, given your situation, environment, and state of health. You could be unhealthy; you could be in poor health and still project well-being. Well-being is your outlook. It is having a state of inner peace, happiness, contentment, and satisfaction. What we call "Ill-being" and "being in illness" occurs when your life is one of inner turmoil, unhappiness, and lack of contentment and satisfaction. Well-being and Ill-being can swap fairly quickly. We often see people in illness who are angry, irritable, and unhappy suddenly come to grips with their situations. We see their emotions, energy, and spirits change. Almost in an instant, they flip the switch.

FIT AND FITNESS

"Fit" is an adjective. When we say someone is fit, we often think of it in physical and athletic terms. We may infer that the fit person is in great shape. But being fit applies to all of the Fitness Factors. To us, being fit means that one can adapt, self-manage, survive, and thrive in one's environment. "Fitness" is a noun that reflects your level of being fit. It is your level of strength, stamina, stability, and adaptability. The more fit you are or the higher your fitness level in the Fitness Factors is what determines your level of health.

THE TRUE MEANING OF HEALTH

Health includes normal blood test values, CT scans, and MRIs, but it is not limited to them. Health also includes positive states of mind, such as feelings of happiness, contentment, and belonging, but it is not limited to those either. Health implies physical fitness, strength, and flexibility, but it is not limited to those qualities. Health is only perfectly defined when you lose it, but it is not simply the absence of disease. We should not diagnose someone as healthy if he or she requires medications that "normalize" lab values by manipulating them into a reference range based on 97 percent of the population—a population that is overweight, chronically ill, and overmedicated. Two examples are how statins are used to lower blood cholesterol or how blood pressure medication maintains normal blood pressure. Those are false and dangerous assumptions that leave the body's physiology on a pathological path that leads, most likely, to a formal diagnosis of one of the top killers—heart disease, cancer, and stroke.

Health cannot be defined by a simple yes or no. It is a dynamic, ever-changing, complicated process in which a trillion cellular events happen within your body every second of every day. You can't control them and are not even aware of them. Therefore, the myopic label of being in a "state of health" is obsolete.

Health is best defined by what we do every day to maintain it, not by what it is not or the way we chemically manipulate it. Health is all the choices we make hour by hour each and every day. It is what we feed our bodies, what toxins we ingest or absorb, how we move, how we treat each other, how we react to stress, how we manage life's curveballs, and how we support our physiology with vitamins and minerals.

CHAPTER 14

DIETARY FITNESS

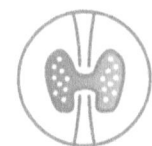

When we bring up the idea of dietary fitness, what we are really getting at is the health of your diet. What is the quality of the food you are putting into your body? Do you eat more whole foods than processed foods? Are you eating more burgers and fries than fish, fruits, and veggies? Quality and quantity of food are essential to optimal health but so are the frequency of your meals, your mindset about eating, and your emotional state when you eat.

If you're struggling with chronic hypothyroid symptoms, improving your dietary fitness can have a massive impact on reducing your cellular stress and enhancing your thyroid physiology.

Hundreds, if not thousands, of books have been written about diet and nutrition. The question then becomes one of which dietary advice to follow. Should you be eating low-carb, no-carb, vegetarian, vegan, paleo, autoimmune paleo, autoimmune protocol (AIP), ketogenic, ketotarian, carnivore, low-fermentable carbs (FODMAP), low-histamine, gluten-free, or Mediterranean? All of these eating styles have some benefits and some drawbacks. Every diet will work a bit differently based on your current state of health, physiology, metabolism, and goals. But just because a woman on Instagram who follows the carnivore diet looks great does not mean it's the proper diet for you.

Based on the current state of your GI physiology, you may find that one of these diets works for you better than another. There is no perfect diet for everyone, even when you begin to recover your health. We typically have people start with the autoimmune protocol, or AIP, diet. It's a great place to start evaluating what works best for you. But, depending on your health history or response to the AIP diet, you may need to opt for a variation of AIP or one of the other dietary protocols.

Chad's Story

Chad was a fifty-year-old physician when we first met to discuss his situation. He was sixty pounds overweight and taking medications for his high blood pressure, high cholesterol, and diabetes, and his doctors were considering putting him on insulin to control his diabetes.

He had heard me on a podcast discussing the concept of the cell danger response, cellular hypothyroidism, and the hypothyroid spectrum. He wondered whether he had cellular hypothyroidism and whether that was why, despite following autoimmune protocol (AIP), vegetarian, and keto diets, nothing was working to improve his weight and chronic health challenges.

After reviewing his lab test results and history and assessment forms, I confirmed he had a cellular hypothyroid condition. After agreeing to work together to improve his health, one of the first things we did was discuss his current diet and make a change that to him, a cardiologist, sounded like blasphemy.

> His signs, symptoms, and struggles with previous diets led me to suggest a trial of the carnivore diet, a meat-only diet. No plants. He was stunned that I would suggest he eat only meat and asked whether I realized what he did for a living. I explained I fully realized what his profession was and how what I was asking him to do flew in the face of the advice he gave to his patients.
>
> I pointed out that he had failed with what were considered "healthy" diets and that continuing to do the same thing was likely not to start working miraculously. Finally, I explained the premise of the carnivore diet and why it seemed to be helping so many people. At that point, Chad was at his wits' end and decided that not much could go wrong with a one-week trial.
>
> After a week, he checked in. Not only had nothing gone wrong, but a lot had also actually gone right. Within that short week, he had noticed a change in his signs and symptoms. In addition, he lost a couple of pounds. He was now curious about how this meat-only diet could make him feel better when the current wisdom was that red meat was unhealthy.
>
> Chad decided to try another week, and again he lost weight and felt better. We agreed to commit to thirty days of the carnivore diet while we started working on his many health problems. At thirty days, we had seen so much improvement that he had no interest in stopping the diet. To make a long story a bit shorter, with the help of the carnivore diet and following the Strategic Thyroid Solution recommendations, Chad was able to eliminate all his medications and lose sixty-five pounds.
>
> I continue to work with Chad to monitor his health. He continues to follow a primarily carnivore diet with limited integration of plant-based foods.

Also, the best diet for *improving* your health may not be the best diet for sustaining it. Many of our patients experience amazing benefits when they switch from the current standard American diet to one of the restrictive diets. That's because all the diets we mention above remove some of the most toxic foods. The challenge, however, is that many of these restrictive diets can result in nutritional deficiencies and reduced health if not performed precisely.

All of these diets are great starting points, but very few of them are meant to be long-term strategies. Instead they share a common goal: to remove poor-quality food as well as potentially healthier foods that cause unhealthy reactions in your body. Each of these diets has a slightly different focus. All of them can work to aid in someone's recovery. But which one is best for you? That I don't know. This is where a functional medicine doctor can be beneficial. You can try any one of the diets and see how you tolerate it. Or you could simply start removing toxic, low-quality foods from your current diet and adding more high-quality, healthy foods. This is the strategy we think works best if you are working on your own.

FIND YOUR STARTING POINT BY KEEPING A FOOD LOG

The first step to improving your dietary fitness is to be aware of your starting point. What are you eating now? How many meals per day do you eat? How many snacks? What is the quality of the food you eat?

We often ask our patients to provide a list of three days' worth of eating and drinking. We want to know what they eat and drink from the time they get up until they go to bed. We want to know the times of the day they are eating, how often they are eating, and why they are eating. We want to know everything—even the little snacks they grab between meals.

This is where you should start as well. Do you have to write it all down? Yes! We tend to have a skewed vision of how and what we eat. For example, patients tell us all the time that they eat a good diet. Yet when we see their three-day logs, they are dominated by processed foods, with whole foods and vegetables being almost nonexistent.

As you track what you eat for a few days, you might notice that your diet is not nearly as good as you thought it was. The only way to truly fix a problem is to identify it. So the first step before you change anything about what you eat and drink is to understand better what your current diet looks like. Once you've recorded three days of eating and drinking, you want to take an objective look at what you've written down.

- How many meals per day are you eating—one, two, three, four?
- Are you eating multiple snacks between meals?
- Are you constantly snacking throughout the day?
- Do you have dessert most nights?
- Is winning the lottery a more likely scenario for you than eating five to six servings of vegetables per day?
- Is most of the food you eat processed?
- Do you seem to eat mostly when you are stressed or on the run?
- What are you drinking?
- How much are you drinking?

These are questions that can easily be answered once you have completed your three-day eating log.

HOW TO EAT FOR BETTER HEALTH

Now let's discuss what we consider the foundation for dietary fitness. In the Strategic Thyroid Solutions program, we recommend starting with four foundational dietary principles. Don't worry about keto, vegetarian, carnivore, or Paleo for now. Just start with the following four principles.

1. Eat more whole, real foods, and less processed foods.

The diets we previously mentioned have one thing in common: They focus on eating more whole, real food, and less processed food. So, for now, let's set aside all the nonsense about which diet is best and focus on the one principle that all of these diets can agree on: eating more whole, real food.

Food Choices Made Simple

Whole food: Whole food is any minimally processed food that is free of additives and other artificial substances. Whole foods are often one-ingredient foods.

Real food: Real food is single-ingredient food that is free of additives and minimally processed.

Organic food: Organic food is produced without the use of most conventional pesticides, fertilizers containing synthetic ingredients or sewage sludge, bioengineering, and ionizing radiation.

Non-organic (inorganic) food: Non-organic food is produced using conventional pesticides, fertilizers containing synthetic ingredients or sewage sludge, bioengineering, and ionizing radiation. Additionally, this includes inorganic foods modified at a molecular or genetic level.

Processed food: Processed food is any food that undergoes a series of mechanical or chemical operations to change or preserve it. Processed foods typically come in a box or bag and contain more than one ingredient.

The goal is to eat more food in a state as close to how it was found in nature—how it walked the earth, swam in the water, came out of the ground, or came off the plant. For example, choose the roast over the processed beef patty. Choose fresh fish over the fish sticks or imitation crab meat. Pick the potato over the potato chips. Pick the orange over the orange juice.

Is it hard to eat whole food all the time? No. But is it easier to eat processed foods? Yes, absolutely. It is often more difficult to find whole, unprocessed foods than processed foods, especially when you haven't planned ahead. Will there be times when you have to choose something that has been processed? Absolutely. But always opt for food as close to its natural state as possible.

When buying processed foods, keep these simple tips in mind:

- Choose foods with the fewest ingredients.
- Avoid foods with added sugar.
- If you can't pronounce the name of an ingredient or don't know what an ingredient is, don't buy it.
- Remember that just because something is gluten-free, sugar-free, or low fat doesn't mean it's healthy.

When you eat out, choose a restaurant that serves locally raised organic foods. If you are in a pinch and need to pick up something quickly, select one of the many healthier fast-food options. If you are going to a friend's home for dinner, don't freak out. You don't have to be perfect; you just need to be better.

If you know you have a food allergy or sensitivity, you obviously want to avoid those foods that cause you to react. But for now, you do not need to focus on gluten-free or dairy-free. Instead try first to simply shift from processed Frankenfoods to more whole, real foods. You will notice that as you make this shift, it is easy to become naturally gluten-free. That's because gluten-containing foods tend to be the processed foods that you eliminate anyway.

2. Eat mindfully.

Every time you put food into your body, it's a good idea to ask yourself these key questions:

- What am I eating?
- Why am I eating?
- When am I eating?
- How does what I eat make me feel?

What am I eating?

If you don't know what you are eating and your goal is to improve your health, you probably shouldn't be eating it. Sure, some processed foods taste awesome, but that doesn't mean they are healthy. Those foods don't necessarily have any redeeming value in your body. Check the labels next time you are at the store. How many ingredients are in a food? Does it contain more than six ingredients? Can you pronounce the names of the ingredients? Do you know what those ingredients are?

When you eat real, whole foods versus processed foods, you tend to be less hungry. You feel satisfied for much longer. Processed foods are designed to get you to consume more of them. You wind up eating more food because you don't feel satisfied, and in the long run, you spend just as much, if not more, money on your food.

Why am I eating?

Are you eating because you are hungry? Because you're bored? Because it's breakfast, lunch, or dinnertime? Because you're depressed? Because you're nervous? Because you are with friends? Because you are watching TV or a movie? Because the bowl of peanut M&Ms is right next to you?

Most people eat or drink for many reasons other than hunger or thirst. For example, you may be eating first thing in the morning because you were told that breakfast is the most important meal of the day.

Or maybe you were told that you need to eat at least three meals and three snacks per day to manage your blood sugar. Unfortunately, most of the dietary advice we've been given is bogus. It is based on assumptions, flawed science, and outright lies.

If you are overweight, your main challenge is that your body is storing too many calories as body fat. It's not able to burn the calorie load you are putting into your body. Because of your hypothyroidism, your metabolism is slow and you are less able to burn calories. Continuing to put calories into your body that cannot use them results in those calories being stored as fat. The fat you have on your body is the excess calories your cells can't burn.

Your challenge is to get your cells and tissues to burn those stored calories. If you have cellular hypothyroidism, are gaining weight easily, and have excess body fat, you may feel hungry at times, but you aren't starving. There is little chance that your body will burn your excess body fat if you are constantly eating. That's why it is important to ask, "Why am I eating?"

When am I eating?

The simplest advice we give people to improve their health is to eat less often. Most of us eat too often. Some of us eat too much. And some of us eat too much too often—the worst-case scenario.

While medical and health experts say we should eat every two to three hours to maintain blood sugar, that advice leads us to consume more food, store excess calories in body fat, become obese, and develop diabetes at alarming rates. When you eat frequently, you are always giving your cells and tissues access to a quick-burning fuel, or glucose. Your cells and tissues prefer using glucose for fuel. When glucose is available, there is less need to burn other food sources, such as fat.

> **Burn Fat, Not Carbs**
>
> When the body does not have enough carbohydrates to convert into glucose, the liver breaks down fat into an organic compound called a ketone, which can be used for energy. What most people want their cells to burn is excess body fat. Unfortunately, as long as you are putting food (especially carbohydrate-based food) into your body every couple of hours, there is little chance that your body will ever burn fat efficiently.

Before you have your next meal or snack, ask yourself *why* you are eating. If you can't say that you are truly hungry, don't eat. If you are having low blood sugar symptoms, such as feeling dizzy, light-headed, or shaky, you should eat. But if you are eating out of boredom, because it is a specific time of day, or because you are stressed, find something else to do. Your brain may be telling you that you're hungry, but if you have extra belly and body fat, you have plenty of food resources on board. You will not starve. Skipping a meal, two meals, or even a whole day or two of eating will not hurt you. There are many religions whose followers fast for days at a time.

When you have cellular hypothyroidism, your body burns calories less efficiently, while its efficiency at storing fat increases. You may still get the urge to eat, but unless you are super active, frequent meals and snacks make it even harder to lose body fat.

If you can resist the temptation to snack constantly, your body will be forced to burn excess body fat. But if you are snacking every time you get the urge, your body will never dip into your fat stores. You don't need to eat just because it's breakfast time or lunchtime or dinnertime. You just don't. You should eat when you are truly hungry, not because of the time of day. If you have excess body fat, you have plenty of stored calories. The only way to get your body to use those calories is to not bring in more calories in food.

Yes, we are fully aware that you have probably already tried a low-calorie diet. We are not instructing you to eat a low-calorie diet. What we are suggesting is that you eat less frequently. Time-restricted eating is a concept that is taking hold in clinical research, cancer therapy, and the treatment of diabetes, obesity, and gastrointestinal disorders. The idea behind time-restricted eating is to shorten your eating window to six to ten hours per day. It is important to start slowly and work up to what you can tolerate in terms of your personal eating window.

People often use the terms "time-restricted eating (TRE)" and "intermittent fasting (IF)" interchangeably. Technically, they are not the same thing. With TRE, you are reducing your eating window to somewhere around eight hours. For the remaining sixteen hours, you don't eat. With IF, you choose not to eat for a set period; the time frame ranges from a few hours to days.

Many people eat from the time they get up until just before bed. For example, if you start eating at 6:00 a.m. and your last meal or snack of the day is at 8:00 p.m., your eating window is fourteen hours and your fasting window is ten hours. During that time frame, you may be eating every couple of hours. You may have only one or two meals, but snacks and sugary drinks count as well. Remember what we said: as long as you are putting food into your body fairly regularly, your body will use what is coming in for its needs and will store the rest as fat. Your body will not burn stored fat as long as there is a constant supply of food.

Constantly eating, snacking, or grazing on food and calorie-laden drinks can create a series of problems. One is that you train your body not to burn stored fat. If you are constantly feeding your body when your blood sugar starts to drop, your fat-burning system rarely gets used. As a result, your body becomes inefficient at burning fat but really good at storing it. This creates a real problem at night because your body is expecting food every couple of hours. When you are sleeping and aren't burning fat efficiently, your fight-or-flight nervous system may need to kick in to make more glucose to satisfy your cellular needs. When your fight-or-flight system kicks in to release more blood sugar, it disrupts your quality of sleep, creating cellular stress.

If you struggle to stay asleep at night, this may be the reason. During the day, you are training your body to expect food every two to three hours. At night, when that two-to-three-hour time frame hits and there is no glucose ready for use from a new intake of food, your fight-or-flight system kicks in to make sugar from your tissues. Unfortunately, it also pulls you out of restorative sleep. To manage cellular energy better at night, you must train your body to be more efficient at fat-burning during the day. The best way to do that is to fast for extended periods.

The simplest way to perform time-restricted eating is to skip either breakfast or dinner. Most people find that they are busy and not super hungry in the morning, and breakfast is the easiest meal to skip. You should do what works best for your lifestyle. If dinnertime is the one time of the day when you get together with others, that is probably not the meal to skip. There is something positive about eating and celebrating with others. If, however, you are a morning person, love to eat in the morning, and find it easier to skip dinner, then that is the meal to skip.

How do you start? Try scaling back so that you are eating within a ten- to twelve-hour time frame. Then scale back further with a goal of six to ten hours. You can eat one, two, or three meals during that window. You shouldn't consume anything but water, black coffee, or tea during the fasting period. Make the transition gradually so you don't shock your system. If you are one of those people who isn't hungry in the morning, the transition may be pretty easy. If you are usually hungry in the morning, it may be a bit more challenging. Try shrinking your eating window one hour at a time.

Once our patients start intermittent fasting or time-restricted eating, many of them find they also eat less. They are less hungry, too. People see their belly fat drop, as well as their blood pressure, blood sugar, insulin, and cholesterol. Many eventually perform time-restricted eating every day, while others do it once or twice a week. You might want to experiment with periodic fasts of up to twenty-four hours. Once you try it, you'll find your groove.

Time-restricted eating makes the "Why are you eating?" question easier, too. Are you eating to nourish yourself, or are you eating because you're bored? Many times, we eat to support our emotions—anger, boredom, depression, or anxiety. If you often find that you are eating for those reasons and not out of true hunger, you are going to need a diversion.

The strategy we often recommend is to do something else. Go for a walk. Get a drink of water. Do some push-ups. Talk to a friend. If you are truly hungry, your body will let you know. But these are the times to fight the urge to eat and let your body burn some of your fat reserves.

How does what I eat make me feel?

Most people eat without paying much attention to how they feel after they've eaten, but it's important. After you eat, notice how you feel. Are you gassy or bloated? Do you feel tired or fatigued? Does your nose run or get stuffy? Do you get a headache or a migraine? Do your ears turn red? Do you develop a rash or itchy skin? Do certain foods increase your bowel movement frequency, cause diarrhea, or leave you constipated?

Many of our patients who have had these kinds of symptoms have been told that they have heartburn or some form of irritable bowel syndrome (IBS). What they are really experiencing, however, is a reaction to the food they've eaten that is caused by low stomach acid, insufficient bile or pancreatic enzymes, microbial imbalances in the GI tract, or a compromised immune system.

Heartburn does not cause gas or bloating. IBS does not cause gas, bloating, or distention. Instead heartburn and IBS are the names of conditions given as a result of having these symptoms. This distinction is a big deal. The diagnosis of heartburn and IBS is based on your symptoms. Heartburn and IBS can't be both the cause *and* the effect. This is the trap in allopathic medicine. Big Pharma drills into our heads that our symptoms *are* the problem, not signs of the problem. Then Big Pharma makes drugs to suppress those symptoms, or the "syndrome," and tells us that their drugs have fixed or managed the problem. This approach creates a few issues:

- It ignores the real causes of symptoms.
- It causes people to become dependent on medications to mask those symptoms.
- People have to deal with the side effects of medications.

Saying that heartburn or IBS is the cause of gas, bloating, diarrhea, or constipation is like saying that "leaky tire disorder" causes nails and screws to become embedded in your tires.

As you follow the dietary fitness steps, you should notice that you have fewer symptoms. You may even see your chronic GI symptoms disappear. Following this cleaner, healthier style of eating will also make you more aware of how some processed foods make you feel when you eat them. When you are eating processed foods on a regular basis, it's hard to determine what is causing symptoms in your GI tract or outside of it. As you scale back on processed foods, eat more whole foods, and eat less frequently, you will be more in tune with the foods that trigger problems.

3. Eat slowly.

Too many people eat in a rush. They eat when they are stressed or gobble down food without really chewing it. To properly produce the acids and enzymes and get your body in digestion mode, you need to activate your parasympathetic nervous system, the rest-and-digest part of your nervous system. As soon as you put food in your mouth, your parasympathetic nervous system goes to work stimulating the digestive system to produce and release acids and enzymes in a systematic sequence throughout your GI tract to properly digest your food.

When you are in a rush and in stress mode, your sympathetic nervous system takes center stage, suppressing the actions of your parasympathetic nervous system. As a result, food doesn't digest properly, which leads to gas, bloating, reflux, changes in GI tract flora, constipation, loose bowels, nutritional deficiencies, and, ultimately, disease. Your body does not efficiently digest food and run around at the same time.

Our advice is to slow down every aspect of eating. First, if you are going to eat, take the time to eat. If you don't have time to sit down, relax, and chew properly, skip the meal. Eating while rushed leads to reduced digestion and absorption of nutrients, and increases GI distress. Putting food into your body without sufficient acids and enzymes is a recipe for problems. (No pun intended.)

Second, take a few minutes before eating to calm your nervous system. Pray, give thanks, or do whatever you need to do to calm your body down. Trying to slam a sandwich between meetings just isn't worth it. You will wind up paying for the meal twice: once when you order it and again when you are dealing with gas, bloating, and indigestion.

Third, once you begin to eat more slowly and chew each bite thoroughly, good digestion can begin. Someone once said that you should chew each mouthful twenty times before swallowing. We're not sure how they arrived at that number, but it's not a bad goal to shoot for.

Chewing each mouthful twenty times breaks down the food into smaller pieces and allows more saliva to be produced and mixed with the contents in your mouth. Saliva serves multiple purposes, from digestion and lubrication to working as an antimicrobial, killing any organisms growing on the food you have consumed. A great indicator that you are eating too fast and not chewing your food thoroughly is thirst when eating. Being thirsty while eating is a sign of insufficient saliva production.

Drinking more fluid with your meals will reduce your thirst, but it works against digestion. This is because it reduces the acidity of your stomach, resulting in reduced bile and pancreatic enzyme secretions. When stomach acid, bile, or pancreatic enzymes diminish, digestion and absorption of nutrients are compromised, and microbial overgrowth becomes more likely.

When you slow down to eat, you will notice that you get the sensation of being satisfied with less food. It takes about twenty minutes from the time you start eating until your brain begins to receive signals of satiety. When you eat quickly, gulping down your food, you get more food into your body before your brain receives those signals. A large volume of food and liquid can cause GI pressure and bloating. So, the simple rule here is to take it slow.

And finally, after you finish eating, take a few minutes to relax. Getting up and rushing around right after a meal pushes you out of rest-and-digest mode, which means incomplete digestion and GI distress.

4. Enjoy your food.

The last principle of dietary fitness is to enjoy your food. Unfortunately, too many people have negative thoughts and feelings about food and their diets. Three things we hear all the time are as follows:

- There's nothing to eat.
- I'm bored with eating the same foods.
- It's too hard to eat healthy.

The purpose of the three-day food log mentioned earlier is to notice what you eat and the variety of foods in your diet. Most people eat the same seven to ten things for breakfast, lunch, and dinner. Your habits may be similar. You may eat the same breakfast every morning—a bowl or two of cereal or oatmeal or a bagel washed down with a cup of coffee or tea. Lunch may typically consist of the same two or three foods. Dinner is usually the meal with the greatest variety, but it's still limited. Most people eat the same five to seven meals for dinner: Monday is taco night. Tuesday is pizza night. Wednesday is spaghetti night. You get the idea.

So the issue isn't boredom with food; it's perception. Most people eat what they've always eaten. They want to stick to their routines. The issue is that routine is the problem. Something in your current diet is causing your symptoms and health problems. Something needs to change, even if that change is temporary.

The idea that there is nothing to eat is, again, all about mindset. Consider searching the internet for Whole30, Paleo, keto, and autoimmune diet recipes. Try a new recipe or two each week until you have a slew of new dishes. As you find ones you like, replace your less-healthy meals with them.

We acknowledge the reality that healthier food, especially organic food, often costs more than processed food. For example, a can of butternut squash soup is probably cheaper than the homemade version. However, there are many ways to make eating organic, nonprocessed food more cost-effective and less time-consuming:

- Join a food co-op.
- Buy food in bulk when possible and freeze what you don't plan to eat soon.
- Cook large batches or multiple servings at one time. This serves two purposes: it is less expensive and saves time. Freeze the extra servings for future meals.

There are nonorganic foods that can be safe to eat, and there are foods you should only buy the organic versions of. Go to the Environmental Working Group's website for their Clean Fifteen (www.ewg.org/

foodnews/clean-fifteen.php) and Dirty Dozen (www.ewg.org/foodnews/dirty-dozen.php) lists.

The challenges most people have with changing their diets are their limiting beliefs. If you believe there is nothing to eat, you will be correct. If you tell yourself you don't like food you've never tried, you'll be right. If you think healthy whole foods are boring and bland, you will be right. But if you believe that changing your diet is easy, enjoyable, and exciting, you'll be right too. If you believe that reducing your intake of processed food and increasing your intake of whole foods is the first step toward improving your symptoms and your health, you'll be right. Changing your diet, lifestyle, habits, and behaviors is as easy or as difficult as you believe it will be. All of the suggestions we make in this chapter are simple changes. They may not be easy for you, but they are simple to perform.

We recommend that you start working on these changes and commit to them for thirty days. You'll be surprised by how much can change in thirty days. If you're doing great after thirty days, fantastic. If after thirty days you are still struggling with chronic symptoms, especially GI symptoms, we suggest that you reach out to a functional medicine practitioner for help. He or she will be able to guide you on tightening up your diet even further and can determine whether functional GI testing is the next logical step. You may learn whether switching to a more restrictive diet—such as the Paleo autoimmune protocol (AIP), a low-histamine diet, or a low-FODMAP diet—is a better option for you. A functional medicine practitioner will evaluate your symptoms and lab test results to determine whether stomach acid, bile acid, or pancreatic support is necessary. A consultation will be money well spent.

We suggest that you set a goal to follow a whole-food diet 80 percent of the time over thirty days. When you do venture into less healthy foods, enjoy the moment. Don't stress about what you're eating, but do be alert to how you feel over the next three days. If your symptoms get worse, you'll know that something in that indulgence did not agree with your system. Decide for yourself whether the indulgence was worth the outcome.

DIETARY FITNESS RECOMMENDATIONS

- Eat more real, whole foods and fewer processed foods.
- Choose a good blend of whole-food proteins, fats, vegetables, and fruits.
- Eat food of the best quality you can afford. Check out the Environmental Working Group's lists of the Clean Fifteen (www.ewg.org/foodnews/clean-fifteen.php) and the Dirty Dozen (www.ewg.org/foodnews/dirty-dozen.php).
- Eat mindfully.
- Eat when you are hungry and need nourishment, not when you are bored or stressed.
- Try practicing time-restricted eating (TRE) for two to five days a week.
- Eat slowly.
- Enjoy your food.
- If you experience no improvement after following a whole-food, time-restricted eating style for thirty days, please consult a functional medicine practitioner.

CHAPTER 15

SLEEP FITNESS

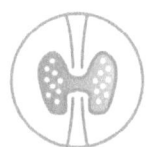

Sleep is one of the most important Fitness Factors that often gets the least amount of attention. Sleep is more than just a time when we close our eyes; it is a critical factor of our overall health.

You may think of sleep as a time of rest, recovery, and recharging, but there is so much more occurring in your body when you have optimal sleep. Sometimes sleep is thought of as a weakness, and time spent sleeping as lost time. You may know of a person, or even be that person, who wears a lack of sleep as a badge of honor, thinking sleep is a total waste of time. Yet these beliefs are the furthest things from the truth. Sleep pays major, sometimes even life-changing, dividends, including decreased risk of cancer and Alzheimer's disease.

There have been many books written on the science of sleep. One of our favorites is *Why We Sleep* by Dr. Matthew Walker, a scientist and professor of neuroscience and psychology at the University of California–Berkeley. In regard to the impact disrupted sleep is having on health Walker states, "We are in the midst of a silent, sleep-loss epidemic that poses the greatest public health challenge we face in the 21st century."

In *Why We Sleep*, Walker masterfully breaks down the most recent scientific findings about sleep and explains them in terms that make sense even if you don't have a PhD. He explains the importance of sleep and why having a high level of sleep fitness is so important. He also details the impact that a low level of sleep fitness can have on every aspect of health and wellness. If you want an extensive understanding of sleep, pick up his book. This chapter will provide a streamlined version of what optimal sleep is, how sleep deprivation can impact thyroid physiology and other aspects of health and function, and what you can do to improve your sleep fitness.

WHAT DOES OPTIMAL SLEEP FITNESS LOOK LIKE?

So what do you need to know about sleep? Let's get into it. Current research suggests that seven to nine hours of quality sleep is optimal for adults; typically longer times are optimal for children, depending on their age. Anything less than six hours is considered a form of sleep deficiency, which encompasses multiple concepts of reduced, inefficient, or poor sleep quality. These concepts include the following:

- **Sleep deprivation, or the elimination of sleep (therefore no sleep) for a period of time:** Sleep deprivation is split into acute sleep deprivation (<7 days of no sleep) and chronic sleep deprivation (>7 days of no sleep).
- **Sleep restriction, or sleeping less than is needed for optimal function:** Research indicates that sufficient sleep time for optimal function is seven to eight hours for the average adult (longer for children). Sleeping less than seven hours may be detrimental to health. Less than six hours of sleep is the line defining sleep restriction.
- **Out-of-sync sleep, or sleeping at a time that doesn't align with the body's natural clock:** Out-of-sync sleep includes sleeping during the day and sleeping at the wrong time of day.

- **Incomplete sleep cycles:** Sleep encompasses multiple ninety-minute cycles during which people experience four phases of sleep (See "Sleep Quality" below.)

Sleep is a natural state of rest occurring at regular intervals. The eyes close, the muscles relax, and responsiveness to external events decreases. Therefore, you may think that the body is in a state of inactivity during sleep. True, muscular activity of the body is mostly still and at rest. Still, the brain and body processes are hard at work, consuming massive amounts of energy to coordinate memory and learning, detoxifying the brain and body, and working on tissue repair and recovery.

There are four key components to optimal sleep: continuity, quality, quantity, and consistency. If any of these are disrupted, your level of sleep fitness declines, and so does your health, function, and memory. Furthermore, disruption of any of these four sleep components increases your risk of developing hypothyroidism, Alzheimer's, and many other chronic diseases.

Sleep Continuity

Sleep continuity is the ability to sleep through the night without disruption.

Sleep is not one long, uninterrupted event, but instead cycles of sleep phases from very light sleep to very deep sleep. Normal sleep may be an almost coma-like state in children, but in adults, short periods of wakefulness are normal with aging. In fact, awakening at night can be normal and even protective in adults. You want to be alerted to signals of danger or concern, such as the sound of a crying child, a window smashing, or needing to go to the bathroom. After that, you should be able to fall back into sleep easily. However, suppose you awaken frequently or have difficulty going back to sleep. In that case, it may be a sign of compromised health caused by inflammation, hormone dysregulation, disrupted breathing, poor glucose regulation, or some other physical problem.

Sleep Quality

Sleep is composed of cycles of two types of sleep: non-REM (non–rapid eye movement) and REM (rapid eye movement) phases lasting approximately 60-120 minutes. If you are sleeping for at least seven hours, you probably experience four to six sleep cycles each night. Each cycle is composed of four stages:

- Non-REM:
    - Stage 1: 1–5 minutes (lighter sleep)
    - Stage 2: 10–60 minutes (lighter sleep)
    - Stage 3: 20–40 minutes (deeper sleep)
- REM
    - Stage 4: 10–60 minutes (deeper sleep)
        - Body paralyzed but brain highly active

How much time is spent in each stage changes from early night to later in the night and early morning. In the first part of the night, you spend more time in the deeper sleep stages. In the second half of the night, sleep is mostly in the lighter stages.

Sleep Quantity

Scientific research indicates that optimal sleep quantity for adults is seven to nine hours, which allows for four to six sleep cycles. Research studies show that health declines when a person gets less than that optimal amount of sleep on a regular basis, especially less than six hours of sleep each night. (Children require more sleep time.)

Maybe this is why we have so many people struggling with chronic health problems. The average American gets less than six and a half hours of sleep each night. Recall that Dr. Walker says sleep loss is a global epidemic.

When you short-change your sleep for just one night—going to bed too late, getting up too early, or awakening for long periods—you severely impact your ability to consolidate what you learned or experienced the previous day. You also disrupt your memory. For example, if you go to bed an hour or two later than normal but awaken at the usual time, you get less deep sleep, which impacts your memory and, more tangibly, affects how alert and energetic you feel during the day. Likewise, when you get up an hour or two earlier than normal, you affect your ability to learn during that day.

Essentially, think of all the things you experience during the day being loaded onto a USB drive in your brain. In the first part of the night, the data is downloaded and organized in your brain. In the second half of the night, the USB drive is erased so that you will have room for new information. If you go to bed too late, the data from the day on your mental USB is not fully downloaded and organized before your mental USB is erased. When you get up too early, your mental USB is not entirely erased, and resource capacity for more data and learning that day is significantly impaired. Even if you could not care less about learning new things, this mechanism is also relevant to brain diseases like dementia and Alzheimer's.

Sleep Consistency

Sleep consistency refers to your sleep schedule. The consistency of going to sleep and waking at about the same times each day is extremely important. Research shows that having a consistent sleep schedule may be the number-one thing to improve sleep fitness. According to these studies, having inconsistent sleep and wake times disturbs the body's circadian rhythms. Circadian rhythms are the physical, mental, chemical, and behavioral changes that naturally occur during a twenty-four-hour cycle. The more consistent your sleep, the better your body functions. If you want to learn more about circadian rhythms, read *The Circadian Code* by Satchin Panda, PhD.

BENEFITS OF SLEEP FITNESS

There isn't a system in the brain or body that is not impacted by sleep. Like other Fitness Factors, sleep fitness is critical to hormone regulation, blood glucose regulation, immune system function, brain function, and detoxification. Every system of the body requires a high level of sleep fitness to work optimally. When you regularly have disrupted sleep, you slowly start the cascade of health deterioration.

THE IMPACT OF DISRUPTED SLEEP

Regardless of the cause of sleep deficiency, its impact is essentially the same. It causes an increase in oxidative stress in the body, especially in the brain. In addition, there are multiple references in the scientific literature to sleep deficiency being a cause of or contributing to all types of chronic illness and disease.

As discussed in several other chapters in *The Thyroid Debacle*, oxidative stress induces or exacerbates a cell danger response. When your cells and tissues are experiencing the cell danger response, normal cell and tissue repair, growth, and development are hindered in favor of an upregulation of immune and inflammatory systems. We also discuss the impact of oxidative stress and the cell danger response on thyroid physiology. Now let us take a deeper dive.

Sleep Deficiency and Thyroid Physiology

When sleep is restricted (<6 hours per night), TSH and fT4 levels drop. That's because the stress of restricted sleep increases T4 and T3 conversion in the hypothalamus of the brain, causing reduced production of TRH. With less TRH stimulating the pituitary gland, it releases less TSH, and so the thyroid gland produces less T4 and T3. One night of restricted sleep may not be that big of a deal, but if you have chronic sleep restriction, you will have lower circulating and tissue thyroid hormone levels, despite a normal or low TSH. You may have symptoms of hypothyroidism, but if you have a blood test for TSH alone and the result is normal, you could be told you do not have a thyroid problem.

Once again, adaptations in thyroid physiology are a protective mechanism to support the physiological changes caused by cell stress. When sleep deficiency occurs, the glial system, the brain's immune system, doesn't work efficiently, impairing the brain's ability to flush away the toxic chemicals produced by normal brain metabolism. (When you have high-quality sleep, the glial system flushes the toxins out of the brain, and your lymphatic and detoxification systems remove them.) Without regular optimal sleep quantity and quality, toxins build up in the brain, increasing oxidative stress and cell-damaging free radicals there and ultimately throughout the body. Eventually this increases T4-to-T3 conversion in the hypothalamus, and that causes the decrease in TRH and TSH described above. Disrupted sleep also increases deiodinase 3, the deactivating thyroid enzyme. (See chapter 8.) As deiodinase 3 increases, more thyroid hormone is deactivated, slowing brain cell metabolism, contributing to symptoms of brain fog and poor memory.

Although the increase in deiodinase 3 activity and decreased thyroid hormone available for the brain may cause unpleasant symptoms, it is actually a protective mechanism. Free radicals are generated as part of normal cell metabolism, and cells produce antioxidants to manage them. But when the toxins can't be flushed out of the brain at night because of sleep deficiency, the amount of free radicals produced overwhelms antioxidant production, leading to oxidative stress and damage to the brain. But deactivating thyroid hormone and slowing brain cell metabolism allows fewer free radicals to form, and less brain damage occurs as a result.

The brain does not rest at night but is extremely metabolically active. It is during optimal sleep that you download and organize information and data from the previous day. You organize what you learn, store the data as memories, and flush the brain to awaken refreshed, with a brain ready to learn new information. The data from the previous day has been neatly organized for future use. Without optimal sleep, learning and memory diminish.

Sleep disruption impacts every system of the body, including thyroid function. In addition, sleep deprivation triggers a stress response on the body, increasing adrenaline and cortisol, which further disrupt sleep and alter homeostatic thyroid regulation.

Reduced sleep suppresses immune system function and your immune system's ability to fight off organisms. Organism overgrowth in the body can activate the cell danger response, leading to cellular hypothyroidism, Hashimoto's thyroiditis, and other immune and autoimmune disorders.

Reduced sleep quality and quantity cause an increased accumulation of reactive oxygen species, or free radicals, in the nervous system, promoting oxidative stress and inflammation, which can activate the cell danger response and cellular hypothyroidism.

In short, when you disrupt your sleep, every system of the body, including thyroid physiology, reacts. Therefore, when you are struggling with sleep deprivation, cellular hypothyroidism is an inevitable consequence.

Optimal Sleep Disruptors

Now that you know how important sleep is, it's time to learn about sleep disruptors so you can make better choices to improve your sleep fitness.

Living in the twenty-first century has many perks: internet, cell phones, time travel (just kidding). But it also has its downsides. For example, many technological advances that people living in a first-world country enjoy are linked to the most significant sleep disruption in human history. According to a study from 2018 on sleep, just one night of sleep deprivation can lead to accumulation in the brain of the beta-amyloid protein, a key component in risk for Alzheimer's disease.[234] That's just one study!

There are piles more that point to the conclusion that getting the best sleep can yield a very high ROI! And there are just as many piles of data pointing toward sleep disruption from extraneous blue light from cell phones, computer screens, and TVs. The blue light emitted from these digital devices suppresses our body's own ability to make the sleep hormone known as melatonin. As the sun sets, the pineal gland in your brain senses the lessening of light, which signals the production of melatonin. Melatonin helps get you to sleep and keeps you asleep. The interference from blue light can be limited by avoiding screens after dusk, which can be difficult, or by wearing blue-light blocking glasses. We both walk-the-walk and use these glasses consistently because we both use sleep-tracking devices, which we cover, that show how blue light can tank our sleep.

When it comes to other things that disrupt sleep, take a peek inside your bedroom. (Your mom told us your bed better be made first, though!)

A thorough evaluation starts with checking your thermostat. Research shows that a bedroom temperature that is too high disrupts sleep. The best range for optimal sleep is between 60°F and 67°F.

Minimize extraneous noise and block out what you can't control with earplugs or mask it with fans, music, and apps or devices (noise machines) that emit soothing sounds, such as those of campfires, waterfalls, rainstorms, and, Dr. Kelly's personal favorite, vacuum cleaners.

Light is not helpful for sleep, so night-lights should be removed or replaced with red lights, as this color has the least negative impact on sleep. If you remove lights that once helped you navigate, be sure to remove potential obstacles in your path so you don't trip when getting up at night. Safety comes first, but it is helpful to know that any light will disrupt your sleep. Therefore, minimize light as best you can.

What do you sleep in and on? Of course, a comfortable, supportive mattress and pillows are musts, but perhaps even more important considerations are their quality and toxicity. Avoid bedding and pillows made with toxic materials, such as formaldehyde. If you don't, you will be absorbing these cancer-causing, endocrine-disrupting toxins all night, every night, which is obviously horrible for your health. Instead choose bedding, mattresses, and pillows made from nontoxic natural materials like wool, natural latex, kapok, buckwheat hulls, and organic cotton. Dr. Kelly owns a wool mattress from Moss Envy, a company that carries organic mattresses and bedding (www.mossenvy.com).

To finish your bedroom evaluation, consider what you do when in bed. Grab a book (using a red bulb instead of white), say a prayer, meditate, or have sex. Some studies suggest that having sex right before bed may disrupt sleep, but the jury is still out on this. (We suggest that you track your sleep to see if sex does or does not help you sleep.) And lastly, do you snore in bed? If so, chapter 16, "Respiratory Fitness" will be of utmost importance to you. And don't forget to leave those blue-light-emitting devices out of the room or turn them off.

Sleep disruptors can start well before you enter the bedroom. What you put into your body during the day and night leading up to sleep can have huge effects—drinking alcohol, for instance. The first thing we put into our bodies—or, better said, expose ourselves to—can be very helpful in getting a good night's rest, and that is bright light. Getting outside in the sunlight or using sunlamps in the morning hours helps prime your body for good sleep and regulates your circadian rhythm by signaling to your pineal gland that now is not the time to produce melatonin, the sleep hormone. Lack of sunlight, especially in the morning, disrupts this natural mechanism.

Lastly, exercising during the day can positively impact sleep, but too much, not enough, or doing it too late in the day can negatively affect sleep.

Alcohol is a significant sleep disruptor. Even a single cocktail, glass of wine, or beer can suppress REM sleep. (During REM sleep, dreaming is used to process unpleasant or traumatic memories and inspire creativity by amalgamating past and present knowledge and experiences.)

Disruptions also occur because sleep pressure, meaning your body's desire to sleep, is lessened. Sleep pressure can be thought of as the brain's need for sleep. It becomes greater the longer you are awake. That's because when you're awake, your body gradually increases the concentration of adenosine in your brain. As adenosine builds, you feel more sleep pressure. The longer you stay awake, the more sleep pressure you experience, which is why you can fall asleep in the middle of the day if you're genuinely exhausted. Caffeine blocks this buildup of adenosine, which can usually be blamed for reduced sleep pressure. Napping has a similar effect. You may want to avoid caffeine (and nicotine) for at least eight hours (or sometimes more!) before bedtime.

Food can also disrupt sleep. Your body wants to detoxify and self-clean at night through a process called autophagy; it does not want to digest food. (Your liver is the organ that works hardest at night doing said functions.) Eating too close to bedtime shifts your body from repair and cleaning mode to digesting food, thereby missing out on important biological functions you need to stay healthy. Stop eating at least two hours before bedtime; four hours is ideal.

Keep your blood sugar steady during the day by avoiding foods that are high in sugar and refined carbohydrates. If you are not metabolically flexible, meaning that your body has a hard time shifting from using glucose (sugar) for fuel to fats and proteins, your sleep can be negatively affected. Intermittent fasting or time-restricted eating can help you become more metabolically flexible so that blood sugar crashes do not occur at night and disrupt your sleep. Using nutrients that help to manage blood sugar may also be worth trying. For example, Dr. Kelly uses Gluco-Beta Stimulator Plus from Professional Health Products.

It is a blend of natural ingredients, such as chromium and cinnamon, that later aid the body in processing and regulating glucose.

Hypothyroidism Can Disrupt Sleep

Cellular hypothyroidism can have a significant impact on your sleep fitness. For instance, people with hypothyroidism are at greater risk of developing sleep apnea.[235] Although multiple factors play a role, obesity is a major risk. People with hypothyroidism have reduced metabolism and tend toward obesity. Edema is another common condition caused by tissue hypothyroidism, and edema is also a primary cause of sleep apnea. Both conditions are associated with higher levels of inflammation.

Hypothyroidism disrupts blood glucose regulation, leading to insulin resistance and diabetes. Each of these conditions can disrupt sleep.

The cell danger response that leads to cellular hypothyroidism often results in an upregulation of the sympathetic nervous system (the fight-or-flight system) and a downregulation of the parasympathetic nervous system (rest and digest system). When you are in a constant state of sympathetic upregulation, sleep disruption is the ultimate consequence.

LIFESTYLE HABITS FOR IMPROVED SLEEP FITNESS

Our habits can make us or break us. Take, for example, the habit of having a glass or two of wine before bed. Although this sounds harmless, alcohol can negatively impact sleep, especially the amount of REM that is achieved each night. On the other hand, the habit of a relaxing bedtime ritual, such as taking a bath, washing your face with cool water, sipping on a warm cup of tea, doing breathing exercises, or reading by red light, can affect sleep in a very positive manner. Other helpful lifestyle interventions include turning off your Wi-Fi router at night so you are not bathing in electric and magnetic fields (EMFs) all night. There are two ways to do so easily. The first is to use a plug-in mechanical outlet timer. The second is to set a timer on your router. Most routers come with the functionality to disable Wi-Fi based on a schedule built into the software. You will need to look up how to use this software in your user manual or on YouTube.

Another excellent lifestyle intervention is to prepare your brain for sleep. Meditation can calm your brain, preparing it for sleep. When you meditate, you are usually working on proper breathing as well. There are a plethora of apps, videos, and books to help you meditate, including

- 10% Happier (www.tenpercent.com),
- Calm (www.calm.com),
- Enso (www.ensomeditationtimer.com),
- Headspace (www.headspace.com),
- Insight (www.insighttimer.com), and
- YogaGlo (www.glo.com).

Proper breathing goes hand in hand with meditation. Most people lose their ability to nose breathe at night, causing them to open their mouths to breathe. The only way to truly improve your nighttime breathing habits is to practice proper breathing during the day, which we discuss in more detail in chapter 16. If you would like to read more about breath training, read *Oxygen Advantage* by Patrick McKeown or *Breathe* by James Nestor. Check out these breathing apps too:

- Breath+
- Breathing Tone
- Heartmath (www.heartmath.com)

HOW TO EVALUATE SLEEP FITNESS

Evaluation of sleep can be tricky unless you use sophisticated technology, which we will present later in this chapter. However, not everyone has the luxury of purchasing such high-tech gear or maybe does not want to. That's where asking the following simple questions can help you figure out whether your sleep fitness is at its highest optimization:

- Do you fall asleep in thirty minutes or less?
- Do you wake up no more than once a night?
- If you wake up during the night, can you fall back asleep easily and in less than twenty minutes?
- Do you wake up refreshed?

If you answered "no" or "not really" or "sometimes" to any of these, it's time to figure out what may be disrupting your sleep and work toward answering "yes" to all. And although these are simple questions, they can also be used on an ongoing basis to gauge your progress.

Another non-techy way of tracking sleep and evaluating sleep fitness is to keep a sleep diary. You can download a free one from the Sleep Foundation at https://www.sleepfoundation.org/nsf-official-sleep-diary. Sleep diaries or journals help you recognize patterns or issues with your sleep or sleeping habits. For instance, one such pattern you may notice is that you may wake up feeling unrested when you've eaten close to your bedtime. This is because digesting food interferes with good-quality sleep, as described above.

Sleep tracking devices are beneficial when trying to measure your sleep objectively. By "objectively" we mean that rather than answering questions (subjective assessment), devices that track sleep and its stages give you measurable data. These numbers document relatively accurately how you sleep. You can then use these data to evaluate the different strategies you are trying to improve those numbers.

The data include amounts in minutes of deep sleep, non-REM sleep, and REM sleep, as well as time spent awake when you should be sleeping. As a rule of thumb, deep sleep should constitute around 25 to 30 percent of your total sleep, REM sleep 20 to 25 percent, and light sleep 45 to 50 percent. Keep in mind that deep sleep seems to play a critical role in fitness, but REM is also important. So aim to hit those percentages, not just to optimize the length of sleep or only one particular stage. Dr. Kelly uses an Oura Ring (www.ouraring.com) to measure all stages of sleep (light, REM, and deep), respiratory rate, body temperature, and heart rate variability (HRV). All this objective data is helpful when trying to gauge whether various sleep interventions are helping her sleep better. There are also other high-tech devices, such as Apple's iWatch, available to track sleep.

NUTRACEUTICALS TO SUPPORT SLEEP

If you have tried everything and are still having trouble getting good sleep, then a trial of nutraceuticals may be warranted. If you do not have a tracking device, such as an Oura Ring, it may be hard to gauge which nutrients work best for you, but sleep journaling is a good alternative. Relying on qualitative data (i.e., how you feel in the morning) versus quantitative data from a device can be difficult. Nonetheless, using natural sleep aids like GABA, L-theanine, jujube (Ziziphus jujube), valerian root, lemon balm, melatonin, magnolia officinalis bark, CBD, magnesium, and 5-HTP is worth a shot. You may need help from a health-care professional to guide your choice of supplements, but most are safe to try to see if they may get you a better night's rest. Also, if you are having frequent waking episodes, a trial of ketone esters, one tablespoon of MCT oil, or collagen before bed works for some people. If nothing you do helps, it may be time to find a functional medicine practitioner to dig deeper into your health. And by the way, please consider the ramifications of sleep medications. Many of the pharmaceutical drugs on the market do not actually improve sleep; they cause sedation. Sedation is not sleep.

SLEEP FITNESS RECOMMENDATIONS

It is our firm opinion that optimizing this Fitness Factor alone is one of the most life- and health-changing things you will ever do for your health. As the great social scientist Brene Brown, PhD, says, "Sleep is the way we love our minds. It is the way we show appreciation to our brains and our lives."

Implementing healthy sleep habits and minimizing those that disrupt sleep do not have to take much time, money, or energy. They simply take you adopting the mindset that good sleep is nonnegotiable.

What we mean by that is that looking at your sleep and recognizing that the things you eat, drink, think, and look at (blue light from phones) determine a good outcome or a bad one. Then choose the good. Choose to balance your blood sugar so you do not have frequent waking. Choose to either put blue-blocking glasses on after dusk or turn your screens off to protect your eyes and melatonin production. Choose not to have that snack before bed, so your body can detox and clean and not spend its sleep time digesting food. Your quality of life is equal to all the small choices you make from day to day. It's just one small, simple choice followed by another.

We also understand there are those of you out there that have less control over your sleep—health-care workers, night shift workers, parents of children with special needs, children of elderly parents, and so on. We urge you, in particular, to implement these techniques as your personal situation allows so you can get the best sleep that is possible for you, especially since you are already a risk for not getting the z's you need.

Sweet dreams!

CHAPTER 16

RESPIRATORY FITNESS

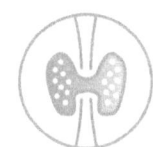

What is respiratory fitness, and why is it important? James Nestor, the author of Breath states, "There is nothing more essential to our health and well-being as breathing: take air in, let air out, repeat 25,000 times a day. Yet, as a species, humans have lost the ability to breathe correctly, with grave consequences." If you search the internet for "respiratory fitness," you will be hard-pressed to find a definition. Instead you will find the term cardiorespiratory fitness (CRF). Cardiorespiratory fitness is the ability of the circulatory and respiratory systems to supply oxygen to the skeletal muscles during physical exercise. It is measured by VO_2 max.

> **VO_2 Max**
>
> VO_2 max is the maximum amount of oxygen the body can utilize during a specified period of usually intense exercise.

Cardiorespiratory fitness is based on two components: the cardiovascular system, which consists of your heart, arteries, and veins, and your respiratory system, which includes nasal passages, larynx, trachea, and lungs. (Notice there is no mention of the mouth. This will be important later.)

From our perspective, cardiorespiratory fitness is your ability to provide a maximal amount of oxygen to your tissues during rest. Basic nonrespiratory fitness is your ability to move air in and out of your body with the least amount of effort and maximal exchange of oxygen and carbon dioxide. These two systems cannot be separated, just as no system in the body can truly be separated from the rest of the body systems. However, we are focusing on the respiratory system and respiratory fitness.

Whether you are at rest or exercising vigorously, your body requires a certain volume of air to support its physiology. Supplying the body with air is critical to survival. You can survive for weeks without food. You can survive days without water. But without air, your life expectancy is measured in minutes. You may think, "What's the big deal? I breathe in and out. It's not that difficult. How could I mess it up?" In reality, more people breathe improperly than get it right.

Does it really matter how we breathe, how frequently we breathe, and how much air we breathe? Does how we breathe make a difference in our health and well-being? I think most people would agree that air quality is important, yet few of us know what the quality of the air we breathe is. In *Particles in the Air: The Deadliest Pollutant Is the One You Breathe Every Day*, Doug Brugge describes how the particles in the air we breathe are responsible for three of the top ten causes of ill health and death worldwide. As we breathe, air carries particulate matter into our lungs and tissues. These potential toxins may trigger chronic low-grade inflammation in our lungs and other tissues that activate the cell danger response, cellular hypothyroidism, glandular hypothyroidism, asthma, allergies, chronic obstructive pulmonary disease (COPD), and a host of other diseases and disorders.

There are four main sources of air pollution:

- mobile sources, such as cars, buses, planes, trucks, and trains
- stationary sources, such as power plants, oil refineries, industrial facilities, and factories

- area sources, such as agricultural areas, cities, and wood-burning fireplaces
- natural sources, such as wind-blown dust, wildfires, and volcanoes

You may have little control over most sources of air pollution. Few of us can pick up and move to the wilderness to avoid air pollution and improve our air consumption. If more of us could do so, those areas would become toxic in time as well. However, having limitations on your ability to control the quality of the air you breathe does not mean you should totally ignore air pollution as a source of cellular stress and a potential factor in your thyroid condition.

WHAT CAN YOU DO?

The best thing you can do to improve your overall health is follow the Strategic Thyroid Solution respiratory fitness recommendations. To the best of your ability, try to control the air quality of the environment in which you spend most of your time. In most cases, this is your home and your car.

Here are our respiratory fitness recommendations:

- Avoid smoke and do not smoke.
- If you use a gas stove, make sure you have a kitchen hood with a fan for ventilation, or replace it with an electric stove.
- Eliminate as much carpet in your home as possible.
- Use dehumidifiers when appropriate.
- Use an air filtration or purifier system in your home and car.
- Eliminate products with artificial fragrances, including cleaning products, dryer sheets, air fresheners, and scented candles, or use them as little as possible.
- Vacuum carpets and floors frequently with a HEPA (high-efficiency particulate air) filter vacuum.

- Reduce or eliminate household products made of petroleum, plastics, and other chemicals that release gas toxins and volatile organic compounds.
- Check the Environmental Working Group's Healthy Living: Home Guide (https://www.ewg.org/consumer-guides/ewgs-top-tips-better-air-quality)
for more information on air pollution and how to control air quality in your home and vehicle.

THE WAY YOU BREATHE MATTERS

Respiratory fitness is the ability to breathe properly for optimal health and function. The higher your respiratory fitness level, the less work it takes for you to breathe in and out. Unfortunately, the reality is that the vast majority of people flat-out breathe incorrectly. How is that possible? Isn't breathing just a natural thing we do? Breathing is natural. It's innate. It should be quiet and effortless, and breath should go in and out through your nose. When you have optimal respiratory fitness, you usually aren't even aware that you are breathing.

How you breathe is an essential aspect of your respiratory fitness. Remember a few paragraphs back where I did not include the mouth as part of the respiratory system? Many people unknowingly breathe through their mouths and not their noses. The nose is the primary passage route for airflow. Yes, there may be times during intense activity that mouth-breathing is important, if not critical, but on a regular basis, airflow should occur through your nasal passages.

Nasal breathing has distinct advantages over mouth-breathing. For one thing, it allows inhaled air to be filtered, warmed, and humidified prior to entering the lungs. These actions don't occur when you breathe through your mouth—at least not to the extent as when you inhale through your nose. Because of these actions in your nasal passage, there is less stress on your physiology and less exposure to toxins and organisms that cause cellular stress, inflammation, stimulate the cell danger response, cellular hypothyroidism, and a host of disorders.

We all start as nasal breathers, but for various reasons—poor posture, inflammation, obesity, stress—we switch to mouth-breathing. Less nasal breathing, especially at night, triggers cell and tissue hypoxia (reduced oxygen), which can stimulate a cell danger response, deactivate thyroid hormone, slow metabolism, and lead to weight gain. In addition, nighttime mouth-breathing is associated with sleep disruption, increased cardiovascular incidents, high blood pressure, and a host of other health conditions.

Here are some additional symptoms and disorders associated with mouth-breathing:

- ADHD
- anxiety
- bad breath (halitosis)
- brain fog
- cellular and glandular hypothyroidism
- chronic fatigue
- dark circles under the eyes
- dental cavities
- dry mouth
- ear and throat infections
- GI disorders
- gum disease
- heart problems
- high blood pressure
- hoarseness
- hypoxia
- sleep apnea and other sleep disorders
- snoring
- TMJ disorders
- waking up tired and irritable
- weight gain

Your mouth is your default alternative respiratory pathway, but when mouth-breathing is chronic, there is less filtration, warming, humidifying, and sterilizing of the air you inhale. Mouth-breathing also causes disordered or dysfunctional breathing, such as hyperventilation, or breathing too fast, and is associated with a number of diseases and disorders.

There are many theories about what causes people to breathe through the mouth at night. At the root of the problem, if we keep it simple, is inflammation. When you have inflammation affecting your nasal mucus membranes, you develop nasal congestion, especially at night. Multiple factors can contribute to increased nighttime congestion, including infections; allergies; reactions to foods; physical narrowing of the nasal passages; systemic inflammation; sleeping on your back, facedown, or with your head lower than your body; and nasal rhythmic cycles, which is an alteration of airflow from one nostril to the other.

The general term for nasal congestion is "rhinitis" or "inflammation and swelling of the nose's mucus membranes." It can be considered allergic or nonallergic. Our thought regarding rhinitis is that whether it is allergic or nonallergic, it is the result of inflammation.

You will read that obesity, hypothyroidism, and chronic diseases can cause or contribute to disordered breathing. But what came first—the obesity, hypothyroidism, or chronic disease, or the disordered breathing? We feel that spending time trying to answer that question is an exercise in futility. It doesn't really matter. You need to restore your nasal breathing *and* address any underlying health conditions, so let's not waste too much time deciding which came first—the chicken or the egg—and simply start working on the fix. You will have to relearn how to become comfortable and efficient at nasal breathing and train your nervous system to make nasal breathing a habit.

There is nothing more essential to our health and well-being than breathing: taking air in and letting air out twenty-five thousand times a day. Yet, as a species, humans have lost the ability to breathe correctly, with grave consequences.

Poor breathing habits aren't all your fault. We're even taught to overbreathe by health, fitness, and medical professionals. How many times have you been told to take some deep breaths to relax or calm down? Unfortunately, taking deep breaths encourages overbreathing. Breathing too much or more than your metabolism requires creates a cascade of events that negatively affect every aspect of your physiology.

Overbreathing is like overeating. If you eat more food than your body needs, given your metabolic state, the extra food and calories become a burden, compromising your health and function. Overbreathing will do the same. Don't believe us? Try this little experiment. Sit up straight and take deep breaths in and out through your mouth for about thirty seconds. Before long, you will start to feel dizzy and lightheaded. Your overbreathing, or hyperventilating, compromises your health and function by negatively affecting the carbon dioxide and oxygen balance.

Once the dizziness has subsided, try to overbreathe again for thirty seconds, but this time, breathe in and out through your nose. Did you get dizzy? Light-headed? You should have noticed that it is difficult to hyperventilate when breathing through your nose but really easy when breathing through your mouth.

Here is what's happening. When you overbreathe through your mouth, you blow off too much carbon dioxide. This loss of carbon dioxide causes your red blood cells to hold on to the oxygen molecules they carry more tightly than they should. This means less oxygen is getting to your tissues, especially your brain. When your brain and nervous system sense a reduction in oxygen, they stimulate a stress response in your body. Your muscles constrict, including the muscles of your airways. Your blood vessels also constrict, increasing your blood pressure, and you start breathing more deeply and frequently to get more oxygen into your body.

Unfortunately, with the increased inhaling, you wind up blowing out even more carbon dioxide through your mouth. This drops the ratio of carbon dioxide to oxygen in your blood, and the cycle continues. So even though you are breathing in more air, you are actually reducing the oxygen in your cells and tissues (cellular hypoxia) and the carbon dioxide in your blood (hypocapnia).

This experiment gives you a sense of what happens in an acute situation. For many people, however, chronic stress and chronic overbreathing at less intense levels are what slowly erode their health.

HYPERVENTILATION, A.K.A. OVERBREATHING

Hyperventilation is breathing beyond the metabolic requirements of your body. If getting air is so vital to our survival, you may wonder how too much air could be a problem. Much like too much food and too much water can be detrimental to our health, so can too much air. The science on this topic can be complex, but too much or too little air can alter your body's chemistry, creating excessive cellular stress.

When you exhale, carbon dioxide from red blood cells in the blood of the lungs releases from the body. When you inhale, you pull oxygen into your lungs. Red blood cells that have released their carbon dioxide now pick up the available oxygen and transport it throughout the body to support cells and tissues. Red blood cells cling tightly to the oxygen they carry. Carbon dioxide (CO_2) is produced as a natural byproduct of cell metabolism. Cells and tissues release the CO_2 into the bloodstream. When the concentration of CO_2 is low in the blood, the red blood cells hold on to the oxygen. As the level of CO_2 rises, it causes the red blood cells to release the oxygen they are carrying in favor of the CO_2. The CO_2 is then transported by the red blood cells to the lungs to be released from the body.

When you breathe through your mouth, you tend to overbreathe. You exhale too much CO_2. Red blood cells will only give up the oxygen to the cells and tissues of the body when there is a high concentration of CO_2. So if you exhale too much CO_2 through your lungs, the CO_2 concentration in your cells, tissues, and body is too low for red blood cells to release oxygen. The end result is that, despite sufficient oxygen circulating in the blood, your cells and tissues are hypoxic.

Overbreathing results in lower levels of CO_2 in the blood, which causes your red blood cells to refuse to release oxygen. As a result, there is a decrease in the level of oxygen available to your tissues and cells—a state called cellular hypoxia.

Occasional mouth-breathing is not the issue. It is chronic mouth-breathing and hyperventilation occurring over weeks, months, and years that ultimately cause distress in the body and alter your physiology. When we discuss respiration and breathing with our patients, most don't believe it is an issue for them. Most of us don't realize that we can overbreathe at two to three times our normal rate without knowing it or that the overbreathing is causing symptoms.

Poor breathing habits aren't all your fault. Health, fitness, and medical professionals may even encourage you to overbreathe by telling you to take deep breaths. However, breathing too much, or more than your metabolism requires, creates a cascade of events that negatively affect every aspect of your physiology.

How Do You Fix Hyperventilation?

When someone is hyperventilating, we ask them to breathe slowly into a paper bag. Why does this technique work? Breathing in and out of the bag causes the person to breathe in CO_2. As CO_2 volume increases in the lungs, their blood vessels and airways dilate. The CO_2-to-oxygen ratio in the blood returns to normal. As a result, more oxygen is released from the red blood cells. An increase in oxygen flow to the tissues, brain, and nervous system reduces the stress response, and breathing returns to normal.

WHAT'S NORMAL, ABNORMAL, AND OPTIMAL BREATHING?

The average adult at rest has a respiratory rate of eight to fourteen breaths per minute. However, what constitutes normal, abnormal, and optimal rates is controversial. An article published by the Cleveland Clinic reported that a respiration rate under twelve and over twenty-five breaths per minute while at rest is abnormal.[236] According to an article in the journal *Breathe*, the average adult respiratory rate is eight to fourteen breaths per minute when at rest.[237] And yet research shows that a respiration rate between six and ten breaths per minute is optimal.[238,239]

Our recommendation is to aim for a respiration rate of ten or fewer breaths per minute, based on a review of studies in *Breathe*.

> *According to the studies reviewed here, "autonomically optimized respiration" would appear to be in the band of 6–10 breaths per min, with an increased tidal volume that is achieved by diaphragmatic activation. Although not reviewed here, nasal breathing is also considered an important component of optimized respiration. This is easily achievable in most individuals with simple practice, and there is yet to appear in the literature any documented adverse effects of respiration in the 6–10 breaths per min range. Controlled, slow breathing appears to be an effective means of maximizing HRV and preserving autonomic function, both of which have been associated with decreased mortality in pathological states and longevity in the general population.*[240]

As you reduce mouth-breathing, increase nasal breathing, and lower your respiration rate to ten breaths per minute or lower, oxygen regulation in your cells and tissues and your thyroid physiology improves, cellular stress lowers, and chronic symptoms, such as fatigue, disrupted sleep, high blood pressure, and anxiety improve. Almost every health condition gets better when breathing improves. And when you breathe better, you actually breathe less.

TESTING YOUR RESPIRATORY FITNESS

How do you know whether you have reduced respiratory fitness? You can use a simple test that we will explain shortly. But sometimes the simplest way is to take notice of your breathing and ask yourself the following questions:

- Are you breathing more than ten to twelve times per minute?
- Are you breathing through your mouth?
- Do your chest and neck move upward when you inhale?
- Do you sigh or yawn frequently throughout the day?
- Do you wake up frequently throughout the night?
- Do you wake up tired in the morning?
- Do you wake up with a dry mouth?
- Have you been diagnosed with sleep apnea?
- Do you snore?
- Do you get out of breath quickly?

Answering yes to several of these questions indicates that you may have impaired respiratory fitness.

Besides these symptoms, you can check your respiratory fitness by determining your controlled breathing hold time (CBHT). Your CBHT is the length of time you can comfortably hold your breath before you have an urge to breathe.

You aren't trying to hold your breath as long as possible. Instead you're paying attention to your first urge to breathe. While holding your breath, you feel a slight panic, a sense of breathlessness, or some movement in your diaphragm or the muscles of your neck. As soon as you get that urge, your CBHT test ends.

The best time to perform this test is when you first wake up in the morning. Because you have no conscious control of your breathing at night, testing first thing in the morning will give you a more accurate measurement of your CBHT. This is because your tissues are more relaxed in the morning and there is less stress and conscious control of breathing than later in the day.

In *The Oxygen Advantage*, Patrick McKeown suggests a method for performing the controlled breath-hold time test:

1. With your mouth closed, take a small, silent breath in through your nose and then give a small, silent breath out through your nose. Make sure you exhale as much air as possible from your lungs.
2. As soon as your exhalation is complete, pinch your nose closed with your fingers to prevent air from reentering your nose and lungs. Make sure that your mouth is closed throughout the process.
3. Start timing from the moment you pinch your nose.
4. Stop timing when you get the first definite desire to breathe, you need to swallow, you feel any panic, or the person watching you sees the vessels in your neck start to pump.
5. Release your nose and breathe normally.
6. If your breathing volume after the test is the same as it was before you did the test, you probably performed the test correctly. However, if you need to recover with rapid breaths, as you might do after exercise, you likely held your breath too long. Try the test again.
7. We recommend performing the test three times and taking the average of the three attempts. Of course, you won't have to do this every time, but just until you get the hang of determining your CBHT.

How did you do? Here are some ranges to gauge your level of respiratory fitness:

- CBHT greater than 40 seconds = optimized breathing
- CBHT between 20 and 40 seconds = mildly reduced respiratory fitness

- CBHT between 10 and 20 seconds = moderately reduced respiratory fitness
- CBHT less than 10 seconds = severely reduced respiratory fitness

Research shows that a CBHT of greater than forty seconds is optimal. Less than forty seconds is associated with hyperventilation, low blood CO_2, a host of metabolic and neurologic disorders, and generally reduced health. Hyperventilation is associated with cellular hypoxia, elevated hypoxia-inducible factor 1 alpha, and increased deiodinase 3. (Elevations in deiodinase 3 are associated with increased deactivation of cellular thyroid hormone and cellular hypothyroidism. [See Chapter 6.])

HOW TO BREAK THE HABIT OF MOUTH-BREATHING AND INCREASE YOUR CBHT

If you are going to come back to the world of nasal breathers, it isn't going to happen without some time and effort. The first thing you need to do is accept the reality that you are more of a mouth-breather than a nasal breather. So many of our patients fight the notion that they breathe through their mouths at night. Until you embrace this fact, your behavior will be difficult to change.

If you answered yes to many of the questions in the respiratory fitness test, you are a mouth-breather at night. If your CBHT was less than forty, you are likely a mouth-breather at night. If you are still not convinced, here is another easy test. Take a piece of hypoallergenic medical tape (or use the fancy SomniFix tape described below) and place it across your mouth before going to bed. We know what you're thinking: your spouse is going to think you are nuts. Perhaps if you explain that this little experiment might lead to a reduction in your snoring, your spouse will be thrilled instead.

If you wake up in the morning and your lips are still taped shut, you are likely not a mouth-breather. If you wake up and the piece of tape is somewhere other than your lips, however, you probably pulled it off during the night to breathe, confirming that you are a mouth-breather.

Now that we've got you convinced, let us introduce our two-pronged approach to improving your breathing.

Encourage Unconscious Nasal Breathing

The first step in encouraging unconscious nasal breathing is to use mouth tape, nasal strips, or both. There are many other options for keeping your mouth closed and your nasal airways open at night, but these two are the easiest to use. You can opt for Velcro straps that keep your mouth shut at night and intranasal devices that keep your nasal passages open, but our patients have found those devices a bit uncomfortable.

You can purchase tape designed for mouth-taping called SomniFix Strips. These hypoallergenic strips cover your lips. While they help keep your mouth closed and reinforce nasal breathing, they have a slit that allows for some mouth-breathing. The other option is simple medical tape. Try using nasal strips as well to keep your nasal passages open, which discourages mouth-breathing. If you think having tape over your mouth will be uncomfortable or cause you to feel anxious, try mouth-taping in the evening while watching TV or reading to get used to the sensation.

Breathing Exercises

The second step to improving your breathing is to perform basic breathing exercises during the day to make the transition to nasal breathing at night easier. For a more in-depth discussion of breathing, the CBHT test, and simple breathing exercises, see *The Oxygen Advantage* by Patrick McKeown.

The goal of doing breathing exercises is to train your body, brain, and nervous system to work harder at lower oxygen levels to maximize metabolic function. The less you breathe, the less damage you do to your body! (If your CBHT is less than ten seconds or you have asthma, wheezing, COPD, or heavy coughing, consult your medical doctor before performing these exercises.)

If your CBHT is greater than ten seconds, start utilizing the exercises below. Test your CBHT at the same time every morning to gauge your progress. The goal is to increase CBHT by a couple of seconds every week.

- **Exercise 1:** Spend between one and five days getting used to the concept of breathing in and out only through your nose. During the day, make a conscious effort to keep your mouth shut and breathe only through your nose.
- **Exercise 2:** Walk with your mouth closed, breathing only through your nose. Start with short durations and build up to twenty minutes of nose-only breathing. Then pick up your pace to the point where you feel you almost have to open your mouth for air.
- If you are a runner or jogger, we urge you to slow your pace so that you can breathe in and out through your nose during runs longer than twenty minutes. We will talk more about this in chapter 19, "Physical Fitness," but for now, if you are going to run, you should run at a pace where you can keep your mouth shut unless you are performing short, intense bursts or sprint workouts.
- **Exercise 3:** Once you can perform exercise 2 for twenty minutes, start walking with one nostril plugged. A cotton ball works well to block one nostril. Go only as fast as you can to maintain breathing through your nose. After ten minutes, block the other nostril and walk for twenty minutes.
- **Exercise 4:** This exercise helps you work on creating a greater CBHT capacity. With your mouth closed, take a shallow breath in through your nose, followed by a shallow breath out. Next, pinch your nose closed and walk as many steps as you can

while holding your breath until you feel a strong need for air. Release the pinch on your nose and breathe in and out through your nose, trying to decrease the depth of your breath and your breath rate while continuing to walk. After thirty seconds to a minute, or once your breathing has returned to a calm state, repeat this exercise five more times.

These exercises are relatively simple to perform. As you become more proficient at nasal breathing, you should see improvements in your CBHT, your ability to sleep through the night without interruption, your energy level upon waking and throughout the day, your weight, and your hypothyroid symptoms.

RESPIRATORY FITNESS RECOMMENDATIONS

- Perform an initial, controlled breath-hold time test.
- Focus on nasal breathing during the day.
- Start nasal breathing exercises, progressing from exercise 1 to exercise 4.
- Use mouth and nose tape at night to prevent mouth-breathing while sleeping.
- Retest your CBHT test weekly to ensure you are improving.

CHAPTER 17

EMOTIONAL FITNESS

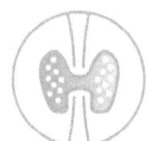

Your thoughts and emotions can have a tremendous effect on your overall health. Scientific evidence suggests that how you think and feel daily can trigger either a positive or negative inflammatory stress response in your body.[241] Mark Hyman, MD the founder of The UltraWellness Center has stated, "I truly believe that if your spirit is broken, and if your connection to yourself and your values has been shaken, you can become ill even if you're eating the right foods, taking the right supplements, and moving."

Emotional stress can take the form of worry, fear, nervousness, anxiety, sadness, or depression. Sometimes it is brought on by a traumatic event, such as an injury, the loss of a loved one, a divorce, or financial turmoil. However, it is often your *perception* of the emotional stressors you face that determines their impact on your overall health.

For instance, if two people are fired from their jobs, one may feel inspired and hopeful about seeking a new position that will better accommodate his or her skills. The other may feel worthless, sad, or afraid that he or she may never find another suitable job. Same scenario, different perception of the stressor. For both individuals, losing a job may be a dramatic and life-changing event. Still, based on how each person interprets the situation, the stress from that event may result in increased determination and a positive outcome or increased negativity and a poor outcome.

Emotional stress, including consistently negative or fearful thoughts, can increase the activation of the sympathetic nervous system and upregulate the HPA axis.[242] The upregulation of these two systems for sustained periods triggers chronic inflammation, excessive cortisol production (the body's stress hormone), and activation of the cell danger response. As explained in part 2, the cell danger response is a protective mechanism against a perceived threat. The threat can come from a stimulus within the cell or a stimulus external to the cell.

The problem with emotional stress is that there is no toxin or organism for the body to fight and destroy. Instead, because the threat is in the form of thoughts and perceptions, which tend to hang around longer than, say, a virus, the inflammatory response, oxidative stress, and cell danger response become chronic—unless we change those thoughts and perceptions.

The result of psychological stress is the same as for other types of stressors: the sufferer starts to develop signs and symptoms of cellular hypothyroidism, such as fatigue, constipation, dry skin, thinning hair, weight gain, low libido, aches, and pains. These signs and symptoms are not the problem but are the result of excessive cellular stress and the innate intelligence of our cells to alter thyroid hormone for only the most critical need in times of excessive stress, which is cell defense. The goal is to minimize cell metabolism to keep cells alive, with the rest of the thyroid hormone used to support cell defense—similar to how food and other resources are rationed during wartime.

Your body responds to the way you think, feel, and act. The word "responds" is key. When you feel stressed, your body reacts by producing cortisol and other stress hormones, triggering inflammation and increasing physiological stress on your body. The first step in managing your emotional health is to become aware of your thoughts and feelings. Red flags that your emotional health is being negatively impacted include poor sleep, frequent infections, irritability, lack of energy, and depression or anxiety. Remember: stress left unmanaged or unaddressed can lead to actual physiological disease. That's why it's crucial to implement strategies and practices to manage stress, especially if you have a chronic health condition, such as hypothyroidism.

People who have sound emotional health try their best to be aware of their thoughts, feelings, and behaviors and have learned healthy ways to cope with the stress that is a normal part of life. They consistently try to employ practices that increase their bandwidth for stress and lessen their reactivity to situations that are considered to be negative. They build resilience. These practices include meditating, yoga, breathing exercises, listening to music, and engaging in tai chi to bring themselves into the present. It may also include the use of technology to help better manage emotional stress.

HIGH-TECH SOLUTIONS FOR EMOTIONAL STRESS

Not too long ago, even the most advanced doctors and neuroscientists believed that the brain could not be changed. For example, the thought was that if someone had a brain injury or a stroke, the damage was permanent. However, neuroplasticity offers real hope to everyone, including stroke victims, those with dyslexia, and those with emotional trauma and anxiety. Many of the trainings and therapies we will discuss in this chapter have to do with taking advantage of this amazing process and using it to improve your emotional fitness.

We have personally used many of the tools and techniques in this chapter, putting them into action. We believe personal experience is helpful and essential when making recommendations. We also want you to be able to have options when it comes to improving your emotional health.

Like almost all other Fitness Factors, one size (technique or diet) does not fit all. We are not into protocols, but principles, and the principle that serves as the foundation for this chapter is that your emotional health is not separate from your physical health. Not addressing your mental state and psychological stress can and will prevent you from living your best, fullest, and healthiest life. So either find something in this chapter that resonates with you and try it or keep looking for a practice that keeps your emotional fitness a priority.

We also include the caveat in this chapter that we are not opposed to medications or any other allopathic treatment that may be needed to help with depression and anxiety. However, we urge you to work with a licensed health care practitioner to help guide your choices and decisions when dealing with any serious illness, including those under the mental health umbrella.

Heart Rate Variability (HRV)

Managing stress, resolving trauma, and addressing issues like anxiety and depression may include using a plethora of technology, such as apps that help you meditate (Ten Percent Happier, Calm); technology, such as neurofeedback; therapy; or techniques that are free and easy, such as tapping. Whichever you choose, using HRV is a great way to measure and track your progress. HRV is one of the best objective markers of emotional health and the state of the autonomic nervous system. It can be assessed using devices such as an Oura Ring, Biostrap, Whoop, or Apple Watch. Obtaining objective data is different from obtaining subjective data in that objective data typically involve factors that can be assigned numbers and values. This is helpful, as using data helps you see whether something is or is not working to improve your emotional fitness, akin to having a scale to measure weight loss.

What Is HRV?

A healthy heartbeat contains healthy irregularities. Even if your heart rate is sixty beats per minute, it doesn't mean that your heart beats at 1-second intervals like a metronome or a clock. The intervals between your heartbeats vary. For example, there may be 0.8 seconds between two beats and 1.5 seconds between another two beats. Even though the difference is measured in parts of seconds, you can feel the difference by gently placing a finger on your wrist and finding your pulse. You should feel the shortest intervals when you inhale and the longest intervals when you exhale.

HRV can be traced to the autonomic nervous system, which regulates such things as heart rate, respiration rate, and digestion. The autonomic nervous system has two branches: parasympathetic (rest) and sympathetic (activation). HRV is an indicator that both branches are functioning properly and that one is not more dominant than the other. You want to be especially aware of a predominating sympathetic nervous system. That is because the sympathetic regulation elevates your heart rate, leaving less room for variability between beats.

The lower your HRV score, the more likely it is that your sympathetic nervous system is more active than your parasympathetic nervous system. Your fight-or-flight response is engaged, which affects your sense of well-being as well as your physiological state. Sympathetic dominance can lead to such symptoms as anxiety, obsessive thoughts or behaviors, insomnia, digestive issues, and inflammation. (Parasympathetic activation lowers your heart rate, thus allowing more room for variability between heartbeats.)

HRV is a marker of physiological resilience and behavioral flexibility, and it reflects your ability to adapt effectively to stress and environmental demands. HRV scores can be obtained from the devices mentioned or from more sophisticated ones your health-care practitioner has in the office, such as HeartQuest. They all give reliable results.

When you measure your HRV, the first thing to pay attention to is your HRV baseline—that is, your HRV score when you're feeling average. Your baseline is the starting point for your HRV explorations. If your HRV baseline is low (less than thirty), consider implementing lifestyle changes that will increase it, which will be discussed further in this chapter. Although having an HRV score that is less than thirty can be concerning, there are no published reference ranges for what is normal versus what is abnormal.

It is also important not to get hung up on whether your score is lower than, say, that of your significant other. Anyone reading this book, no matter his or her HRV score, will benefit from improving it by using all the Fitness Factors in part 3. However, it is best to learn your baseline first and then learn what makes it go up and down. The things that make ours personally go down are stress, alcohol, overexercising or underexercising, poor sleep, and unhealthy food. The things that make them go up are meditation, breathing exercises, exercise, proper supplementation, and a healthy diet.

Do keep in mind that HRV is just one indicator of the state of your emotional fitness and overall health. Many factors contribute to your HRV score, so also pay attention to how you feel as a whole—that is, your subjective data. Keeping a journal can help with this effort. Most HRV training apps have places to record how you feel on a particular day so that you can keep all of your data in one place.

You can also do HRV training. The most well-known platform for HRV training is HeartMath. Studies conducted on more than 11,500 people have shown improvements in mental and emotional well-being in just six to nine weeks of using HeartMath technology.[243] This training involves purchasing a heart rate sensor (that costs about $100) that clips onto your earlobe. The sensor plugs into a cell phone and uses a free app called Inner Balance. The app directs you to breathe in and out at the same pace as an image on the screen, which encourages your brain to get into proper coherence.

Practicing being in coherence, where your nervous system—and thereby your body—is operating most efficiently is extremely relevant to good health. The company recommends doing a session each day for at least five minutes and adding a fifteen-minute session once a week to build higher coherence. You can find more information at www.heartmath.com.

BrainTap: Meditation on Steroids

BrainTap is a revolutionary and powerfully effective tool designed to help you achieve balanced brainwave states. It is a headset that comfortably delivers light and sound to affect the brain in positive ways. Healthy brainwaves enhance the production of neurotransmitters that are needed for optimal function of the body and mind. After decades of research, Patrick Porter, PhD, developed this exclusive technology that has been extensively tested to create the perfect symmetry of sound, music, and spoken word for the ultimate in brainwave training and relaxation, providing your mind and body with all of the benefits of meditation without the disciplined effort.

Unlike meditation apps, BrainTap uses a neuro-algorithm to produce brainwave entrainment—the synchronization of brainwaves to specialized sounds—with no effort from the user required. The result is full-spectrum brainwave activity, which leads to a more flexible and resilient brain.

BrainTap relies on four key elements to induce brainwave entrainment:

- Binaural beats: When two different tones, separated in frequency by only a few hertz, are introduced—one in each ear—the brain perceives a third, unique tone. Binaural beats work by creating this phantom frequency, which the brain then mimics. As a result, you experience deep relaxation.
- Guided imagery: Visualization has been studied for decades; it has been shown to positively affect mental states, improve physical and athletic performance, and even heal the body.[244]

When combined with the other elements of BrainTap, these effects are increased and optimized.
- Ten-cycle holographic music: BrainTap technology produces a 360-degree sonic environment. In this environment, visualizations become more real to the mind, helping you take full advantage of the power of visualizations by creating a more receptive learning state.
- Isochronic tones: These are regular beats of a single tone used alongside monaural beats and binaural beats in brainwave entrainment. The discrete nature of isochronic tones makes them particularly easy for the brain to follow. This is one of the reasons why the proprietary algorithms incorporate both types of tones.

More information about BrainTap can be found at www.braintap.com.

Limbic System Retraining

Becoming aware of the status of your nervous system is essential, as the seat of your emotions lives deep inside your brain. This seat of emotions is called the limbic system, and it is a complex set of structures that includes the hypothalamus, hippocampus, amygdala, and cingulate cortex. It is responsible for the formation of memories and is continually determining your level of perceived safety. The limbic system assigns emotional significance to everything you hear, see, smell, feel, and taste. Interestingly, the limbic system is closely tied to the immune, endocrine, and autonomic nervous systems. (The autonomic nervous system is responsible for regulating automatic body processes, such as heart rate, breathing, and digestion.)

Many things can impair limbic system function, including psychological and emotional trauma, ongoing stress, chemical or heavy metal exposure, mold toxicity, microbial infection, inflammation, and physical or head trauma. When it's not functioning correctly due to assaults, the limbic system becomes oversensitive and begins to label things that would usually be considered safe, such as foods or scents, as threats. This results in inappropriate activation of the immune, endocrine, and autonomic nervous systems, leading to many widespread downstream effects that can confuse patients and their doctors. Why would walking down a laundry detergent aisle cause someone to have a panic attack? Limbic system overactivation, that's why.

If the limbic system remains in this state of oversensitivity, it can weaken the immune system, detoxification, digestion, and overall brain function. So the first step is to determine whether an overactive limbic system is playing a role in your current state of health. In her groundbreaking book *Wired for Healing*, Annie Hopper has a questionnaire that can help you determine whether you may need limbic system retraining. You can access that questionnaire at https://retrainingthebrain.com/wp-content/uploads/2017/08/DNRS-Self-Assessment-Questionaire.pdf. The book also discusses in depth Hopper's limbic system retraining program, which she calls the "Dynamic Neural Retraining System." Dramatic results have been produced from using this system for people across the globe for over a decade.

Eye Movement Desensitization and Reprocessing (EMDR)

Eye movement desensitization and reprocessing (EMDR) is a form of psychotherapy that enables people to heal from the symptoms and emotional wounds of disturbing life experiences or trauma. Multiple studies show that EMDR therapy can quickly heal emotional pain that in the past would have required vast amounts of time and numerous therapy sessions. EMDR therapy effectively helps people recover from psychological or emotional trauma because it removes blocks that impede healing. It does so by using a set of eye movements or physical stimulation administered by a trained professional to naturally uncover and process the traumatic event, thereby setting in motion an innate therapeutic process.

More than thirty positive, controlled-outcome studies have been done of EMDR therapy. One study showed that 84 to 90 percent of single-trauma victims no longer had post-traumatic stress disorder (PTSD) after only three ninety-minute sessions of EMDR. Another study, funded by Kaiser Permanente, found that 100 percent of single-trauma victims and 77 percent of multiple-trauma victims no longer were diagnosed with PTSD after only six fifty-minute sessions of EMDR. A study done on combat veterans found that 77 percent were free of PTSD after twelve EMDR sessions. EMDR is recognized as an effective treatment for trauma and other disturbing experiences by organizations such as the American Psychiatric Association, the World Health Organization, and the US Department of Defense. More than one hundred thousand clinicians worldwide use this therapy, and millions of people have been successfully treated over the past twenty-five years.[245]

EMDR therapy is done in different phases of treatment. For example, eye movements (or other bilateral stimulation, such as from handheld vibration devices) are used during one part of the session. At the start of a session, the therapist determines which memory to target first. He or she then asks the client to hold different aspects of that event or thought in mind and use his or her eyes to track the therapist's hand as it moves back and forth across the client's field of vision. As the client does so, he or she begins to process the memory and the disturbing feelings associated with it.

In a successful EMDR session, the meaning of a painful event is transformed on an emotional level. For example, a child abuse victim will shift from feeling at fault and shameful to a new belief, such as, "I survived the event, and I am strong and not at fault." Unlike traditional cognitive-based therapy (CBT), clients can shape their own interpretations (not clinicians') and process experiences in a new framework. In a sense, the clients' wounds are opened, exposed, processed, and healed.

Emotional Freedom Technique (EFT)

Emotional Freedom Technique (EFT) is a technique for healing that draws on various theories of alternative medicine, including acupuncture, neurolinguistic programming, energy medicine, and

Thought Field Therapy (TFT). It is best known through Gary Craig, a Stanford engineering graduate specializing in healing and self-improvement who wrote the *EFT Handbook*. EFT has also been popularized by other related books and workshops conducted by various teachers and authors. EFT and similar techniques are often discussed under the umbrella term "energy psychology." Energy psychology uses a form of psychological acupressure, based on the same energy meridians used in traditional acupuncture to treat physical and emotional ailments for over five thousand years. The energy is stimulated via tapping energy meridians, which replaces the invasiveness of needles.

Recent research has found that, compared to a control group who did not perform the EFT tapping sequence, EFT significantly increased positive emotions and decreased negative emotional states.[246] The method involves tapping specific points on your head and chest with your fingertips while thinking about your specific problem and voicing positive affirmations. The problem can be anything from a traumatic event to back pain. This can be done alone or under the supervision of a qualified therapist. The combination of tapping on the energy meridians and voicing positive affirmation is said to work by clearing the emotional block from your body's bioenergy field and thereby restoring your mind–body balance.

While energy psychology is still not completely accepted and sometimes criticized by mainstream medicine, EFT has actually met the criteria for evidence-based treatments set by the American Psychological Association for a number of conditions, including PTSD.

Demonstrations of how to perform EFT can be found on www.youtube.com. However, we strongly recommend you watch videos done only by professional EFT practitioners, such as Julie Schiffman. A general demonstration of EFT can be tailored to many problems. Keep in mind that while easy to do, EFT is not a treatment for serious medical conditions. We strongly encourage you to seek out a licensed therapist or doctor for more severe or complex issues. That being said, EFT can be used for deep-seated issues, though this typically requires assistance from a skilled practitioner. If you try to self-treat, you may end up concluding that EFT doesn't work, though research suggests otherwise.

There are also many different EFT apps available for both Apple and Android phones in their respective app stores. Again, please be sure to download and use only those created by professionals. The apps range from EFT basics to a virtual coaching app from professionals.

The Manifesting All Possibilities (MAP) Method

The MAP Method is an advanced neural retraining method to help resolve both emotional and physical symptoms of all kinds. Unwanted memories, traumas, beliefs, and negative emotions can be neutralized in minutes with this therapy. This is done by working with your subconscious, leveraging the latest discovery in neuroscience—that the brain can be rewired, which is also called neuroplasticity. The process of MAP is fast, gentle, and permanent.

Why haven't you heard of this, you may ask? Because it is a relatively new form of therapy built on techniques like EMDR and tapping (TFT, EFT). MAP can systematically explore the entire mental, emotional, and even energetic blueprint of the client. Most MAP practitioners use the method to rewire subconscious programming for better mental health. This treatment method can also be used to address chronic health issues, such as allergies and sensitivities, irritable bowel syndrome, chronic fatigue, chronic pain, and sleep issues.

The sessions are systemized to be client-centered, enabling the client's innate wisdom to guide the session itself and allow the MAP coach to act as a facilitator for the process. The system is taught to coaches and therapists around the world as a powerful adjunct to their practice.

> "We believe, and we have seen, that our brain can actually heal itself on instruction in minutes."
>
> —Colette Streicher, founder of the MAP Method

Once your brain is initiated to the process, it is instructed to heal specific negative memories, emotions, and patterns, and it can do so quickly, easily, and gently. With the MAP Method, you can rewire the mind to release unconscious negative, sabotaging beliefs, emotions, and patterns impacting your health. It is not necessary to discuss or relive painful memories. There is also no need to know what the underlying issues may be for the process to work. Instead, the MAP Method enables the client's superconscious mind to identify the relevant issues. Sometimes the client will experience an insight during the process, but at other times the emotional trauma is released without conscious awareness.

The MAP Method is not psychotherapy, cognitive behavioral therapy, hypnosis, NLP, EMDR, or tapping. You will be awake and aware throughout the session. No equipment is needed, and the process can be facilitated at a distance via videoconference. Sessions typically last ninety minutes and, on average, are done initially every one to two weeks, depending on the need and response. Personally, Dr. Kelly used the MAP Method, and after one session, her lingering issues with fatigue resolved. While this is not usually the norm, it is not unheard of to have such incredible improvements with such a small amount of therapy. She continues to use this type of therapy for other symptoms and has had great personal success.

To learn more about The MAP Method, go to www.mapcoachinginstitute.com.

EMOTIONAL FITNESS RECOMMENDATIONS

You may not be used to talking to your doctor (or yourself!) about problems with your emotional health or what's stressing you out. But remember, emotional stress is a huge component of what might be causing your cellular hypothyroidism, autoimmunity, and a host of related problems we call multisystem adaptive disorder. (See chapter 10.)

Most doctors are ill-equipped to help patients address emotional stress other than by making referrals to psychiatrists or psychologists, which may be entirely appropriate. Therefore, creating a plan of action to manage emotional stress and heal from emotional trauma, if needed, is imperative. We suggest choosing from this list of action steps:

- Keep a gratitude journal. Gratitude journaling is the simple process of writing down everything you are grateful for in your life. It is a helpful tool for becoming more focused on and present with what is good in your life and keeping positive emotions flowing. Journaling is an excellent habit at the start and end of every day.
- Make a "Be, Do, Have" list. This is a simple habit of defining what you want to have in your life and then making a list of what you need to do to achieve those things. The last step involves asking yourself who you need to be to do the things you need to do in order to have the things you want to have. You then need to behave like that person.
- Write out your long-term and short-term goals. This strategy goes along with the "Be, Do, Have" list. To get where you want to go in life, you need a direction. You need a goal. If you don't know what you want, how will you ever get it?
- Use affirmations. Affirmations are positive statements that you write and repeatedly say to help fight off the self-sabotaging thoughts and emotions that can cloud your mind.
- Apply the 30/30/30 rule. It has been said that we are the average of the five people with whom we spend the most time. You will hear people say that you should try to associate with people

who are happier, healthier, and more successful than you. That might sound good on paper, but it doesn't really work in real life. Why not? Because the people doing better than you would be breaking the rule. Instead we suggest you spend 30 percent of your time with people above you, 30 percent of your time with people like you, and 30 percent with people below you. We find that some of the most rewarding times in life involve helping those worse off than we are. Sometimes the feeling associated with helping others is the best way to improve your own thoughts and feelings about yourself and your circumstances. So what happens to the final 10 percent? That's the time you spend alone, learning about yourself and improving yourself.

Do not skip these action steps to boost your emotional fitness. You can do it without spending a lot of money or committing massive amounts of time.

Remember: you can't medicate or supplement yourself into health, especially if you don't address your emotional health. It also goes without saying that all of the practices and technologies discussed in this chapter are best used in conjunction with other healthy lifestyle routines, such as eating healthy meals, getting enough sleep, maintaining healthy connections to others, and having an attitude of gratitude and stewardship. As the great Neil Nathan, MD, author of *On Hope and Healing*, says, "Be kind. Be grateful. Be of service."

CHAPTER 18

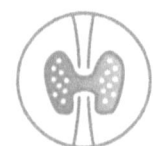

PHYSICAL FITNESS

There is almost as much confusion about what physical fitness means as there is about a healthy diet. The common definitions of physical fitness include the following:

- "the ability to carry out tasks without undue fatigue"
- "good health and strength achieved through exercise"
- "the heart, blood vessels, lungs, and muscles having the capacity to function at optimal efficiency"
- "the capacity to meet physical demands in an emergency situation"
- "the ability to function efficiently and effectively in work and leisure activities regardless of age"

We don't know about you, but these descriptions don't really tell us what physical fitness is. So we came up with our own definition: Physical fitness is the ability to perform daily physical activities and be moderately adaptable to unfamiliar physical activities without fatigue, pain, or restriction of movement.

You must possess physical strength, flexibility, mobility, cardiorespiratory and muscle endurance, and good posture to meet this definition. We think most people could agree with this simple definition of physical fitness; however, each person's level of fitness will be defined by his or her unique reality.

Depending on your current health, physical demands, perspective, and goals, you can define your physical fitness for yourself. People who run a 5K in under twenty minutes may consider themselves physically fit, for example. Still, they may not be physically fit enough to compete in a hundred-mile endurance race or a CrossFit competition.

A FEW DISTINCTIONS

When it comes to strengthening your Fitness Factors, we suggest you focus initially on general daily physical fitness. Anything above that is a massive bonus. To begin, here are a few distinctions between the different types of fitness.

Health versus Fitness

Health is a composite of all your Fitness Factors, and physical fitness is but one component. The higher your level of fitness in each factor of the Strategic Thyroid Solution, the greater your level of health. You might assume that your friend who trains for marathons is healthy. You're probably correct, but your friend could be significantly unhealthy. Many athletes and weekend warriors focus aggressively on just one Fitness Factor or even a single aspect of physical fitness. She may be a great distance runner but have limited physical strength. He may be extremely strong but have limited flexibility and poor balance. Both may put a ton of time into their physical appearances, endurance, and strength but put little time into their emotional fitness and suffer from depression and anxiety. Because of their narrow focus, they may be very physically fit but in poor overall health.

Let's use the example of a bodybuilder. The bodybuilder's strength training creates muscle mass and definition, but a bodybuilder may still struggle with high blood pressure, high cholesterol, and other disorders. Similarly, many endurance athletes can run, bike, and swim like nobody's business, yet they suffer from chronic GI, adrenal, hormone, and thyroid disorders. So being physically fit does not guarantee health. However, if done frequently and correctly, exercise and training can significantly boost the other Fitness Factors and your health in general.

Activity versus Exercise

Physical activity is movement your skeletal muscles perform, and it requires energy. For example, standing up, walking to the fridge, and sitting down on the couch are physical activities. Exercise is planned, structured, repetitive, and intentional movement you do to improve or maintain some aspect of physical fitness. Running, lifting weights, and yoga are examples of exercise.

Exercise versus Training

Exercise is physical activity done for its own sake or general wellness. Training is performing exercise with the purpose of achieving a specific fitness or performance goal. For example, if you go for a five-mile run every day with no specific goal or expected outcome, that is exercise. On the other hand, if you are running every day with the goal of running a marathon in three months, that is training. If you are playing pickup basketball with friends in the neighborhood, that's exercise. If you are going to organized basketball practices in preparation to compete in a tournament, that's training.

Flexibility versus Mobility

These two terms are often used interchangeably, but they differ quite a bit. Flexibility is a muscle or muscle group's ability to lengthen or stretch *passively* through a range of motion. For example, your ability to bend and touch your toes or reach behind your back are indications of your level of flexibility.

Mobility is the ability of a joint to *actively* move through a range of motion. Mobility requires muscle and joint movement, strength, and flexibility.

You can increase the flexibility of your hamstring by stretching it, but your ability to perform a squat may be hampered by a lack of hip and knee mobility. A squat is a movement that requires both lengthening of muscles and connective tissue but also the strength to move through the motion.

Put simply, flexibility is the ability of a muscle to stretch, and mobility is the ability of a joint to move. Therefore, you could have good flexibility without good mobility. So if you work on your mobility with activities like yoga, Pilates, tai chi, and dynamic stretching, you are often improving your flexibility at the same time.

Are all of these definitions important? Yes and no. We really don't care if one term is used in place of another, but we often have to differentiate these things for our patients to help them better understand what we are asking them to do. For example, we have patients who assume that they are exercising because they go up and down the steps a few times, do three loads of wash or walk 150 feet from their car to the office every day. We don't consider that exercise; we consider it activity. You should be active every day. The goal in most fitness apps is ten thousand steps per day, but ten thousand steps is a minimum. Simply taking ten thousand steps without putting much stress or strain on your system via exercise may not significantly improve your physical fitness.

Our goal is not to judge you, not to tell you that you need to achieve a specific level of physical fitness. Instead we want to help you understand that there are a few key components of physical fitness to incorporate into your physical fitness regimen as often as possible. Focusing on one component may make you really good at that skill, but ignoring the others ultimately reduces your level of physical fitness and overall health.

COMPONENTS OF FITNESS

The essential elements of foundational, functional physical fitness are the following:

- muscle strength
- muscle endurance
- mobility
- flexibility
- cardiorespiratory endurance
- posture

We recommend that you incorporate exercises and activities into your daily life that encompass all six components. Attending to them all regularly will improve your overall physical fitness, lower your risk of injury, and enable you to physically adapt to most situations. Of course, how you perform each component and what types of exercises and activities you choose depends on your current health and fitness goals.

Muscle Strength

Strength exercise, or strength training, is working your muscles against some form of resistance. The resistance could be your body weight, bands, or physical weights. Strength training should be a vital component of any physical fitness program. Building lean muscle mass is critical to your overall health. Numerous studies are showing that strength or resistance training has a beneficial effect on health and longevity.[247,248,249,250]

Because there are so many options, many people who are new to strength exercise may be confused about what to do. They ask what exercises to do, how many reps and sets to perform, whether to use light weights or heavy weights, whether to opt for bodyweight exercises or free weights, and whether to do CrossFit or powerlifting. Unfortunately, you, too, may have asked these questions and not received clear answers, which prevented you from getting started.

There isn't a canned answer to each of these questions for every person. The type of strength training that is best for you will be based on your current level of strength, state of health, and goals. Regardless of your health or level of physical fitness, there is a strength-building option for you.

We recommend working with a personal trainer to help you get started. A trainer tailors a program to your individual goals and time commitments. he or she will evaluate your current state of health and develop a strength program that emphasizes proper movement, form, and rate of movement. The weights you use should provide a challenge, but even if you're lifting light weights, moving them slowly and with control gives you a great workout.

If you are struggling with chronic injuries or joint or muscle pain, it is best to be evaluated by a chiropractor, physical therapist, or orthopedist before starting any strength-training program.

We love a style called slow or super-slow strength training for people new to strength training or with preexisting injuries. This type of strength training uses a technique in which you lift and lower weight very slowly. The benefit of super-slow strength training is that you use weights that are often much lighter than traditional strength training uses. As a result, slow or super-slow strength training limits the risk of injury while developing strength through a full range of motion. It also shortens the time needed for an effective workout.

For example, you may take about ten seconds to lift the weight and another ten seconds to lower the weight. Most super-slow routines work five large muscle groups once a week. There is one set of four to nine repetitions for each muscle group. An effective weekly workout can be performed in less than thirty minutes. Check out *Body by Science* by Doug McGuff, MD, for more information. You can also find lots of great content online and on YouTube.

If you are doing super-slow strength training for the whole body, perform the exercises once a week. Other types of strength training can be done daily, depending on the muscles you are exercising.

Muscle Endurance

Muscle endurance is the ability of your muscles to do work overtime. It's important to be strong, but you should also have some level of endurance. It's about balance with these concepts. If you can lift a car but can't walk a mile without fatiguing, you are strong but have poor endurance.

Just as with strength training, there are multiple ways to improve your muscle endurance. Building both muscle strength and muscle endurance should be part of your regular exercise routine. We recommend looking into high-intensity interval training (HIIT) or a form of it called Tabata Training. Both of these styles of endurance training are effective, require less time than other types of endurance workouts, and create little impact on joints.

Mobility and Flexibility

We're lumping mobility and flexibility together because it's difficult to separate one from the other. One of the best ways to increase mobility and flexibility is yoga. Yoga also improves strength, balance, coordination, endurance, and posture.

If strength training, running, biking, or even walking is difficult for you, there is a foundational level of yoga that you can start with. Then, as you get stronger and develop better endurance, balance, mobility, and flexibility, you can progress into more challenging yoga disciplines and poses.

Cardiorespiratory Endurance

Cardiorespiratory endurance is typically defined as the ability of the circulatory and respiratory systems to supply oxygen to the skeletal muscles during sustained physical activity. The more familiar term is "cardio."

To keep things relatively simple, your cells and tissues can generate energy either with the use of oxygen (aerobic system) or without oxygen (anaerobic system). Therefore, when building up your cardiorespiratory endurance, you need to improve both your aerobic and anaerobic systems.

Both systems are constantly working. Your aerobic system is more efficient at making energy and burning fat but is a slower-working system. It works well in situations of low stress and lower energy demand. Your anaerobic system can generate energy quickly, and without oxygen, so it predominates during periods of stress. Its primary energy source is glucose, or blood sugar.

Ultimately, you want your aerobic system to predominate. Why? Because its primary fuel is fat, which many people have too much of in storage. Optimal fat metabolism requires a high level of oxygen. When you improve your aerobic capacity, you become more efficient at burning fat as a fuel source. This can reduce your body fat as well as curb your cravings for sweets. Which system predominates for you? If you are constantly craving sugar and carbohydrates, you are likely favoring your anaerobic system. You are putting on fat around your midsection and struggling with chronic hypothyroid symptoms.

Consider a fireplace in a house. What is the better source of fuel, paper or logs? It depends on what you are trying to do. If you want to start a fire quickly, paper is preferable. On the other hand, if you are trying to maintain a fire with little work, wood is the better choice once the fire is started.

Paper ignites quickly, but it also burns quickly. If you tried to maintain your fire with paper only, you would need a ton of paper. You would have to be putting paper on the fire constantly to keep the fire going. You would also need to ask your friends to bring you more paper so as not to run out. Think of glucose as being like paper. If you have a constant craving for it, you want as much as you can get. You use some of the paper to support the fire and keep it going, and you store the rest in a closet. Your body does something similar with excess glucose from food. If it can't use the glucose immediately, it is stored as fat.

The body tends to use the glucose coming in before using the stored fat. Similarly, you would likely use the newspaper someone just dropped off at your door over the newspaper you stored in a closet. Burning glucose provides quick energy, but it takes a lot of work to maintain a constant supply of glucose.

Now consider wood logs. Getting them to burn takes a bit more work, but once they start burning, you can place a couple of logs on your fire and it will burn for hours with little attention. You don't need the same volume of wood as you would paper to keep your fire burning because wood burns slower. Think of fat as being like the wood logs. It is more efficient for your muscles and tissues to burn fat as their primary fuel source. If you are leaner in your midsection and don't crave carbs and sugar, you are probably efficient at burning fat.

Now, when it comes to improving your cardiorespiratory endurance, you need to train both systems by performing both aerobic and anaerobic exercises. Traditional cardio exercise, such as running, can train both systems, but the way you conduct your cardio exercise can make all the difference.

If your primary goal is to improve your overall health and physical fitness, you should consider two principles:

- If you are going to perform less than twenty minutes of cardio exercise, high-intensity interval training (HIIT) is excellent for your anaerobic system. The training period is short, and there is less potential for stress and strain on your joints. However, the activity phase must be at your maximum capacity to make this exercise effective.
- If you are going to perform over thirty minutes of cardio exercise, you want to make the exercise more aerobic in nature. To do so, you need to monitor your heart rate so that you stay within your optimal aerobic fat-burning range. Long cardio sessions that are too intense will push your body out of its aerobic fat-burning capacity and drive it into its glucose-dominant anaerobic capacity.

After decades of working with elite athletes, Phil Maffatone, PhD, developed a relatively simple formula for determining a person's optimal fat-burning aerobic range, called the "180 Formula." We recommend that you visit his website, philmaffetone.com, for an in-depth discussion, but following is our short version.

When you perform cardio exercise for thirty minutes or more, you want to keep your heart rate below 180 minus your age and no lower than 170 minus your age. So, for example, if you are forty years old, the upper limit of your optimal aerobic fat-burning range is 140, and the lower end is 130. Now, this isn't exactly true to Dr. Maffatone's calculations, so we encourage you to check out his website, but it is close enough for our purposes.

You might be wondering how to measure your heart rate. There are many devices for measuring heart rate, from inexpensive chest straps to high-end watches. A quick search on the web of heart rate measuring devices will provide the best options and their prices.

When your heart rate remains within your optimal aerobic range during extended cardio training, you are in an efficient fat-burning state. Efficient fat-burning, which is the goal for most people, is best performed in an oxygen-rich aerobic state, in which the mitochondria of the cells initiate a process called "oxidative phosphorylation" to generate massive amounts of ATP, or energy, from fat. However, if your heart rate rises above your optimal aerobic threshold during long bouts of cardio training, your cells will favor anaerobic respiration. That means they will prefer using glucose over fat. You can still improve your cardiorespiratory endurance in an anaerobic state, but there is a price to pay long-term.

Our concern is not one or two days of improper cardio training, but weeks, months, and years of long-duration anaerobic cardio. People who chronically train in an anaerobic range typically become insulin resistant, put on belly fat, and show signs of HPA axis dysregulation. (Some people refer to signs and symptoms of HPA axis dysregulation as adrenal fatigue.) Research indicates that distance runners tend to develop type 2 diabetes. Whether it is caused by the training or the high-carbohydrate diet that most endurance athletes follow is debatable. In our opinion, both are contributors. Years of this type of training caused Dr. Eric to become insulin resistant and contributed to his developing Hashimoto's thyroiditis. Thankfully, following the concepts presented in this part, part 3, has led to the resolution of his health challenges.

Adrenal Dysregulation

Adrenal Dysregulation is an adaptive response of the adrenal glands to chronic or excessive levels of cellular stress. People struggling with adrenal dysregulation have symptoms including exhaustion and fatigue, difficulty falling asleep, fatigue upon waking, substance dependency (caffeine, alcohol, nicotine, and so forth), brain fog, dizziness, nausea, low appetite, low blood pressure, increased sugar or salt cravings, unexplained weight loss or gain, unexplained hair loss, and hormone imbalances.

Prolonged training in an anaerobic range will cause your body to become more efficient at using glucose. You essentially train your cells and tissues away from being efficient at using fat as a fuel source. Because you become inefficient at burning fat and your cells want glucose, you constantly crave and consume carbohydrates. When you aren't exercising, any excess carbohydrate is converted to fat.

Because you are inefficient at burning fat even in an aerobic state, your body will crave sugar, which you will consume instead of using your stored fat. In addition, training anaerobically for extended periods increases cellular hypoxia, which impairs cellular thyroid physiology and cell metabolism. The shame is that you start exercising in an effort to improve your health, but because you are exercising inefficiently, it only contributes to your cellular stress, inflammation, cellular hypothyroidism, and reduced health.

If you aren't planning to participate in endurance events, then one of the best ways to increase your cardiorespiratory endurance is to strength train, following the principles of slow fitness discussed earlier in this chapter.

Posture

Everything you do from a fitness perspective—activity, exercise, or training—should take into account your body posture. If you exercise with bad posture or bad form, you are bound to sustain injuries.

You want to ensure that the exercise or activity you are doing is helping to improve your posture, not making it worse. For example, many people who sit all day focus on enhancing their abs by doing lots of crunches. They hook their feet onto something and curl up. This makes their hip flexors, or the muscles toward the front of the hip, which are already short and tight from sitting all day, even tighter. Tight hip flexors cause the lumbar or lower back muscles to become chronically tight, pulling the back into hyperextension. Hyperextension is excessive curvature in the lower back, sometimes referred to as "swayback."

When your hip flexors and lumbar muscles are chronically tight, your abdominal and gluteal muscles become weak. The long-term consequences are chronic back pain and weak posture. So in this situation, your attempt to strengthen your abs actually causes more postural distortion and sets the stage for chronic back problems. Therefore, we recommend seeking out a reputable chiropractor, physical therapist, or both to evaluate your posture and provide some guidance as you begin working on your physical fitness.

MAKING TIME FOR REST AND RECOVERY

You must allow yourself time for rest and recovery. If you don't, all of your hard work to improve your physical fitness may be for naught. You might look fit, lean, and strong but still struggle with chronic health conditions. Many athletes who appear healthy only look that way. Chronic stress in the form of too much strenuous exercise without proper recovery breaks their bodies down on the inside. To achieve true health, you must follow *all* of the Fitness Factors, not just one.

But how do you determine how much rest is appropriate? One great tool to use is HRV, which is the variation in time between each heartbeat. Basically, the higher your HRV, the more variability in the time between heartbeats. The higher your HRV, the better your recovery from the previous day's stress and the more capable your body should be to cope with added stress. The lower your HRV, the less capable your body is of adapting to more stress, and generally, the lower your state of health. When your HRV is back to baseline, you have recovered sufficiently. If you do not have a device to track your HRV, there are other ways to determine whether you haven't recovered from your last workout.

Here are some examples of indications that you need more recovery time.

- You can test your waking pulse daily. No tool is needed other than your fingers and a watch. Test your resting pulse every morning to get a good baseline. If your waking pulse rate is more than ten points over your normal or baseline pulse rate, you may not be fully recovered.
- Your muscles are still painful or sore.
- Your muscles feel tired or weak.
- You wake up tired and fatigued.
- You try to work out, but you feel unusually winded or weaker than you did after your last similar workout.

GAUGING YOUR EXERCISE NEEDS

By nature, humans are lazy. It's not our fault. We are evolutionarily geared toward conserving energy. Physical fitness is important, but our lazy nature can make doing what it takes to achieve it challenging.

Exercise is great. It improves your anatomy and physiology as well as your mood, leading to the release of feel-good hormones called endorphins. In order to maintain health, you need to move your body. The million-dollar question is: How much should you move your body, especially if you suffer from hypothyroidism or other chronic health conditions?

> **Yes, You Can Overdo It**
>
> An effort to boost her physical fitness backfired on Dr. Kelly. In 2012, she was trying to get in shape for an upcoming beach trip with her husband. She was getting better than she had been during the worst of her health issues, but she was not in what we would consider good health. So she decided to start getting up extra early to do high-intensity interval training (HIIT) on an elliptical trainer—a piece of equipment that she had been using mostly as a clothes rack. She was excited to get back into exercising, and she committed to doing HIIT four times a week and using free weights on the other days. Suffice it to say that her body revolted. She became more tired, had more brain fog, and ended up gaining weight. (No, it was not muscle mass; it was fat. She used a bioelectrical impedance analysis [BIA] to measure changes in her body composition. BIA is a method used to measure body composition by sending a low-strength [safe] electrical current through the body. The current passes freely through the fluids in muscle tissue but encounters resistance when it passes through fatty tissue. The level of resistance to the current is termed "bioelectrical impedance," and when set against a person's height, gender, and weight, it can be used to compute body fat percentage.)

> The key to physical fitness is finding the sweet spot where your body is under just enough positive stress to improve your respiratory, cardiovascular, and musculoskeletal systems. Overdoing exercise can put more stress on an already overtaxed system and make cellular hypothyroidism worse.

HRV can be a great tool to gauge how well your body is tolerating your workouts. In addition, tracking devices such as the Oura ring or Biostrap can help you decide whether your body is ready for a workout by giving you a "readiness" or "recovery" score. This score, created first thing in the morning, is based on your overnight sleep quality, respiration rate, heart rate, body temperature, and HRV score. Exercising when you're not ready can lead to exacerbations in cellular stress, which can end up making you feel worse, as Dr. Kelly did.

PHYSICAL FITNESS RECOMMENDATIONS

- Create a daily habit of engaging in daily exercise of twenty to sixty minutes based on the type and intensity of exercise and your level of fitness.
- Vary the types of exercises you engage in each week to include strength, cardio, mobility, and flexibility training.
- Use a tool like your HRV to monitor your recovery.

CHAPTER 19

HABITUAL FITNESS

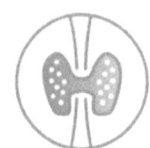

Your habits define you. The things you say and do on a daily basis shape the outcome. People who come to our offices looking for a way to improve their thyroid physiology are often surprised to learn that the most important thing we do is work with them to change their habits.

Your habits—the things you say, think, do, and believe—play such a massive part in why you are healthy or unhealthy, obese or fit, happy or sad, or in a good marriage or a bad one. Yes, it's easier to blame the environment, people, parents, and microbes for our ills, but often, if we are honest, we must look in the mirror first.

One of the things we love to have our patients do is keep a three-day log. We ask them to write down everything they do, eat, and drink each day. Very few people like to do this. And very few people write down everything they do. No one ever notes time spent in front of the TV or on Facebook, Instagram, email, and Twitter. Yet these are the time sucks of life. If you don't monitor and measure that time, you can't manage it. Most people fail to write down the snacks, the M&M's, the Skittles, and the handfuls of nuts, pretzels, and chips they eat throughout the day. They think it's only a little snack and ask, "How important could it be?"

However, when people take the time to track everything—what time they get up, the time they spend on their devices and social networks, their time at work, their time being active, what they eat and drink, and what time they go to bed—they are often shocked by what their habits are and the time they consume. They are surprised to learn they have daily habits and rituals that are probably part of the reason they have problems with health, wealth, happiness, work, and relationships. They realize they have few habits that improve their overall health and fitness. For example, people say they want to lose weight, but their habit is eating lots of toxic, highly processed, high-carbohydrate foods. They say they want to lose weight or tone up, but they don't do any physical activity.

People say that they don't have time to exercise, but somehow they can spend an hour and a half on social media. People say, "I don't have time to cook," but they have time to drive to a fast-food restaurant, stand in line, sit and eat, and then drive home.

We all have time for the things that are most important in our lives. We use the excuse that we don't have time. Time is a limited commodity, but we do get to choose how we spend the time. I don't have time to _____. Fill in the blank. But if I said I would pay for you to go to France, I bet you could find the time. If I said your favorite band was in town and I would pay for the ticket, you would find the time to go.

You make time for what is most important in your mind right now. If you want to know what is most important to you right now and is taking up all your precious time, write out everything you do for the next three days. Write down what you eat and drink. Write down what times you get up and go to bed. Get an app that logs how much time you spend on social platforms. When you write it all down, when you track all that you do, you will see what's important to you. You will see where your priorities lie. You will quickly see why you don't achieve what you say you want.

Our actions often are not congruent with our goals. We see in our patients and ourselves a disconnect between what we want—our goals—and our daily actions. We don't have habits, behaviors, or actions that are congruent with our professed goals. We spend a lot of time with emotional diversions from the truth.

Where do you stand? Do you have a diet and a lifestyle that is health-promoting? Do you have a diet and lifestyle that is helping you reach your stated goals? Or is the real problem that you don't know what you want? Is the problem that what you say you want is something you truly are not passionate about?

Most of us are passengers in life. Becoming the driver of your future, the driver of your destiny, the driver of where you are headed with your life, is possible but can be challenging. We say this from humble experience, not from a lofty perch. It's easy to be a passenger. You always have someone else to blame when you don't wind up where you wanted to go. But the reality is that you are often where you are in life because of the things you do or don't do every day, the things you focus on and think about regularly, and the people you surround yourself with. You are the sum total of your habits.

I know you might be thinking you had bad parents or that an accident or illness led you to be where you are. Absolutely, those things are real. They suck. But is your habit to focus on the negatives of those things or to use them as motivation to grow and become stronger?

Do you pay more attention to your illness and poor health than on what you do to get better? Do you try to figure out how to eat healthier or complain about what junk food you can't eat? Do you tell yourself you don't have time or figure out how to make time? Do you contemplate what you don't have or think about how to get what you want? Do you complain about your spouse, or do you consider how lucky you are to have him or her in your life every day? It's all about choices and habits.

Here are some strategies for improving your habitual fitness.

3-DAY SELF-ASSESSMENT

For the next three days, write down everything you do, eat, and drink. Next, write down what time you get up and what time you go to bed. Finally, track how much time you spend checking and answering email, interacting on social media, watching TV, working out, associating with family, working, and engaging in downtime. There are plenty of free apps you can download on your phone to see how much time you spend on social platforms.

Next, evaluate how much time you devote to things to improve your health and quality of life and how much time you're spending doing things that have no real value in improving your time on this planet, improving your health, family relationships, and quality of life. It's not until you start measuring what you do every day that you can see what your habits are and what needs to change.

EMOTIONAL SCORECARD

Whom do you talk to the most on any given day? It's you. We often complain about how other people treat us or that they say nasty or inappropriate things. We take offense to negative or demeaning comments, yet the person who often treats you the worst and says the worst things about you is you. Most people have no idea that the thoughts and feelings reverberating in their own minds are either the things that bring them out of despair or drown them in it.

One of my favorite strategies is to have people keep emotional scorecards. Keep track of all your positive and negative thoughts, feelings, emotions, actions, and what you say for one day. Every time you have a positive thought, feeling, emotion, or action, score it on the positive side. Every time you laugh or make a positive comment to yourself or someone else, score it on the positive side too. Every time you do something nice for yourself, your family, a coworker, or a perfect stranger, score it on the positive side. Do the same for every negative thought, feeling, emotion, action, and comment you have or make to yourself or someone else.

At the end of the day, total your scorecard. Which side wins, the positive or the negative side? If you find the negative side is winning in your life, it's no wonder your life, your health, and your relationships are not where you would like them to be. It is easy to wind up with the negative side winning. Watch the news, check out Facebook, get on Twitter. You will find it's the negative things that get the most attention. It's easy to be attracted to the negative. But when it dominates your life, it has serious consequences on your health.

Many patients tell us that after performing this exercise, they realized that some of what is causing their cell stress, what is responsible for their hypothyroidism, is the negative emotional stress in their lives. Let's face it; bad things happen. That is a reality. But those bad things don't have to destroy your health and your life if you don't let them.

For years I, Dr. Eric, carried a foam clown nose in my pocket. When I was stressed or angry, I would put my hand in my pocket and squeeze the clown nose. It would make me smile and remember a story I heard from someone regarding the nose. The story went something like this.

A woman was scheduled to leave town for a business meeting. She knew the best option was to leave the day before a meeting in Philadelphia so she would not have to deal with flight delays and traffic on the day of her meeting. She had previously planned to take her daughter to the circus on the day she planned on leaving. When she told her daughter they would have to cancel the trip to the circus because of her trip, her young daughter was devastated.

The woman decided to change her plans and travel early in the morning the day of her meeting so she could take her daughter to the circus. At the circus, they were all given foam clown noses. She placed hers in her purse and forgot about it. The next morning, she was up early and at the airport. Unfortunately, her flight was delayed. She was starting to stress. The meeting in Philadelphia was really important to her company's future, and being late could have profound implications.

When she finally arrived in Philadelphia, she knew that she would have little time to spare to get to her appointment. Unfortunately, the traffic leaving the airport was a disaster. It was backed up for miles because of an accident. She grew more stressed. She started second-guessing her decision to take her daughter to the circus. She said all kinds of not-so-nice things to herself as she sat in traffic that wasn't moving an inch.

At some point, she realized she would never make it to the meeting in time. She was distraught, as she knew that missing the meeting would significantly impact her company and probably cost her her job. As she reached a boiling point of frustration, she reached into her purse for her phone. Instead of finding her phone, she found the clown nose.

For some crazy reason, she put on the nose and looked in the rearview mirror. It made her laugh. It made her think of the joy of going to the circus and getting the clown nose brought to her daughter. At that moment, she realized that she had made the better decision. The time with her daughter was precious, and she would never get that time back. She calmed down.

Out of the corner of her eye, she caught the woman in the car next to her staring at her as if she were crazy. She looked at her and made a silly face. The woman had her husband turn to look at the crazy lady wearing the clown nose. Before he could see her, she took off the clown nose and acted as she had never worn it. When the husband turned away, she put the clown nose back on and made more silly faces at the woman. Again the woman had her husband look her way, and again she took the nose off before he could see her wearing it.

She continued to have fun with this game for the hour she was stuck in traffic. By the time she reached her destination, she was beside herself with joy and emotion. Unfortunately, she missed the meeting and lost her job, but the lesson was learned. The lesson was that life is precious. It's too short to be upset about things we cannot change.

When I heard that story, it changed me. I took its lesson to heart. I bought myself a foam nose and kept it in my pocket. Whenever I was stressed or got upset, I would squeeze the foam nose, which reminded me of the story. I gave foam noses to some of my patients. One patient was a principal at a local junior high school. I was asked to come and speak about health to the student body.

I chose to tell the story of the clown nose. I gave every student a clown nose with instructions on how to use it. The school staff may not have been as happy with the story and the noses, as the kids wore them the rest of the day. There was a bit of disruption, but the kids were happy. However, you never know how something you say or do will affect the lives of those around you.

One day a new patient, a police officer, came to my office, and sometime during the appointment, he realized that I was the guy that had passed out clown noses at his son's school. The man said that the nose changed his life.

He came home one day from work feeling angry and agitated. His son and wife were arguing, and his son was being disrespectful. The man became angry, lost control of his emotions, and got ready to hit his son. His son cowered and tipped his head down. As his son's head popped back up, the man saw his son had put on the clown nose. At that moment, he was taken aback. He didn't hit his son, and instead, they all started to laugh.

This silly foam clown nose defused what could have been a violent altercation. As the patient told me the story, tears rolled down his face. They ran down my face too. We often take our thoughts and feelings out on the wrong people. We take life too seriously. Sometimes we just need to pause and realize that what we are thinking and what we are fixated on are things that aren't helpful. Indeed, they may even contribute to our demise.

We urge you to check your emotional scorecard. See where you are putting your emotional energy. If you need a clown nose, get one.

DEFINE YOUR DAILY ROUTINE

The most successful people tend to be those with structured daily routines. Their habit is structure and organization. They plan their days. They make sure that the things that are most important in their lives take priority. You might be thinking that organizing your day doesn't leave time for play, fun, and free time. But the opposite is true. When you structure your day, when you have a routine, it's easier to get things done. You can even schedule in TV and social media time if you choose. Just organize your day. If you do, you'll realize you get more things accomplished.

You already have a daily routine. The problem is that your daily routine may be full of activities that are not beneficial or don't help you achieve your goals and desires. In addition, your routine may be filled with habits that waste time and divert your attention from the things you desire, including improved health and well-being.

When people plan their days, they wind up being more efficient with their time. More of their priorities get accomplished. Think about it. If we told you we were leaving for a trip tomorrow, you would probably make a list of everything that needed to be done in order to be ready to go. You would likely get a massive number of things accomplished because you organized and scheduled your time. If it works when you are under a deadline, why not do it daily? You are on a deadline, by the way. You have a limited time on earth—a limited time with your spouse, kids, and friends. Don't you want to squeeze every moment available out of it?

So plan out your day from the time you get up to the time you go to bed. Make sure to schedule time for your Fitness Factors, including downtime to rest, recover, and have fun.

REVIEW, PRUNE, REPLACE

Regularly perform RPR, which stands for "review, prune, and replace." Periodically, about every sixty days, you should take a step back and review your daily habits and routines. This review is similar to the three-day log we discussed previously. Why?

Because stuff happens. Life gets in the way. We lose focus. It's natural to find that some less-healthy habits replace your well-intentioned good ones in time, or that habits you have and regularly perform no longer match up with your current goals and desires.

Every sixty days, review your goals in conjunction with your daily routine and habits. Track your day. Are your daily habits congruent with your current goals? Does something need to change? Do you need to change your habits? Do you need to change your goals? What needs to be pruned? Do you have some less-productive habits that have crept into your routine? As you prune habits that are not congruent with your goals, replace them with new, more congruent habits. It's hard to quit a habit unless you replace it with something else.

AFTER-ACTION REPORT

This sounds like a military saying, right? It is. For us, an after-action report is one of the best ways to end your day. Review your daily routine. Did you get all your priorities handled? If not, it's time to break down why this is so. This is not meant to be done to beat yourself up. It's intended to keep you focused and to allow you to see what's taking you off your task. It can also be used to encourage yourself and to show yourself that you can achieve anything you set your mind to.

This is different from your RPR. With your RPR, you are reevaluating your goals and habits. Your after-action report is just a way to make yourself more accountable for your day and prevent you from getting too far off track. Think about this in the same way you might use "catch and release." That is a fishing term, but it works well here. You want to catch the less-productive habits early and then release them from your routine.

HABITUAL FITNESS RECOMMENDATIONS

- Perform a three-day assessment of your life. Identify what you do on a daily basis. What are your habits and behaviors? Are the majority of them helping you achieve your goals?
- Define your routine. Determine and plan out your daily activities so they align with your goals. By planning out your day, you cause your actions to become habits that don't require motivation to perform.
- Review, prune, and replace. Regularly (we like a period of every sixty days to take a broader look at your life) review your goals, habits, and behaviors. Remove those that are no longer relevant or have sneaked their way inappropriately into your life. Then replace what is being removed with new goals, actions, and behaviors.
- Make an after-action report. Take time at the end of each day to assess your day's successes so you can end the day on a positive note.

CHAPTER 20

ENVIRONMENTAL FITNESS

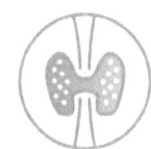

There is a growing concern in both public and scientific communities about the increasing number of chemicals and toxins we are exposed to daily throughout our lives. Moreover, the concern is growing regarding the potential and probability of many of these chemicals contributing to, if not causing, excessive cellular stress, dysfunction, disease, and death. According to a 2019 Environmental Protection Agency (EPA) report, consumer products in the United States contain more than forty thousand chemicals.[251] And only a small fraction of the chemicals we are exposed to have been rigorously tested for human safety.[252]

Chemical exposures are just part of the issue. Our exposure to electromagnetic radiation from various sources, including cell phones and Wi-Fi, has risen dramatically in the past decade. Research is showing that such exposure is contributing to cell stress, damage, and poor health.[253] For example, multiple scientific papers indicate a direct impact of cell phone radiation on thyroid function.[254,255,256]

Many of the chemicals we encounter daily are harmless, but many are carcinogenic, neurotoxic, and endocrine disrupting. Unfortunately, the reality is that you can't avoid all the toxic or potentially toxic chemicals you come across in your water, your food, the air, and personal and household products. There are just too many.

Instead of increasing your anxiety by worrying about all the potential threats and trying to become toxin-free, it's best to put your energy into reducing your burden by leading a "low-tox" life. Our friend Alexx Stuart has done a great job of presenting strategies to reduce your toxic burden in *Low Tox Life: A Handbook for a Healthy You and a Healthy Planet*. If you desire more information than what is provided in this chapter, Stuart's book is an easy read and is loaded with great tips, strategies, and resources.

This chapter gives you a simple strategy for reducing your toxic exposure and improving your environmental fitness in six aspects of your life: air, water, food, personal and household products, and work. Before describing the Strategic Thyroid Solution for reducing your environmental stress and improving your environmental fitness, we need to define these two terms: "environment" and "environmental fitness."

Your environment is the complex physical, chemical, and biotic (climate, soil, and living things) factors you encounter that may impact you physically, chemically, and emotionally. Your environmental fitness is your ability to adapt and stay healthy within your environment. For example, if you are sensitive to smells, have allergies, or react to foods, light, or Wi-Fi, your level of environmental fitness is lower than that of a person without these sensitivities or allergies.

Your environmental fitness is determined by your fitness level in the other components of health and the level of exposure to environmental stressors. Have you ever noticed that pollen does not seem to affect all people the same? Have you ever noticed that some people are extremely sensitive to electromagnetic radiation and others aren't? The lower your environmental fitness, the more sensitive you are likely to be to your environment. Can you improve your environmental fitness? Absolutely.

Over the last three decades, we have worked with hundreds of patients and have seen their allergies and immune responses to environmental stressors diminish or disappear. The environmental stressors didn't go entirely away. Sure, the people limited some of their toxic environmental exposures, but to think that you will eliminate all toxic exposure is wishful thinking and unrealistic. Instead the goal is to reduce the accumulated exposure or load. The goal should be a "low-tox" life, not an unrealistic "no-tox" life.

We think Alexx expresses her concept of living a low-tox life beautifully.

> *If we strive for 'no tox' or 'toxin free' we run the risk of believing "I'm not good enough" because you're inevitably going to walk past a car's tailpipe or need to use the restroom and one of those horrible air fresheners is going to go off while you try desperately to hold your breath, and despite all the excellent things you did to be low tox that day, you'll be angry about the exposures you came across. This is not a time for a small select group of people to achieve a completely non-toxic life because that isn't possible. We have to let that go. What we need right now for the health of people, animals, and the planet to improve pronto is everyone feeling that they can hit their next plastic reduction goal, find the perfect non-toxic deodorant for their pits (at last!) or finally make that important investment in a natural-fiber, fair trade mattress and pillow ... or whatever it is their next goal to kick might be. Every positive step we take to improve our health and choose better products for our planet is something to be celebrated, not something to keep beating yourself up about because you're not 'there' yet; you still haven't swapped the kettle or your mascara. You've got this, and the more people that believe doing something is better than nothing, the sooner we'll look around and think, "Wow, can you believe so many people used to suffer from chronic illnesses?" I want that day to come soon, and I know you do too.*[257]

When our patients lower their overall stress loads and improve their levels of fitness in a few or all of their fitness factors, their bodies adapt to their environments better. Therefore, we suggest that how well you adapt and perform in your environment directly reflects your overall health and success in improving all the Fitness Factors.

THE FREE STRATEGY

Since most of us won't be moving into a nontoxic snow globe any time soon, we recommend putting the FREE strategy into action now. "FREE" is an acronym for "filter, reduce, exchange, or eliminate." This is the approach to coping with environmental toxins that we teach our clients and is an integral part of the Strategic Thyroid Solution. We recommend using FREE to evaluate and reduce toxic exposure in those six critical areas mentioned earlier. You can use the FREE strategy in every fitness factor category, but we have found it especially helpful when helping our clients work on their environmental fitness.

Figure 1: The FREE strategy.

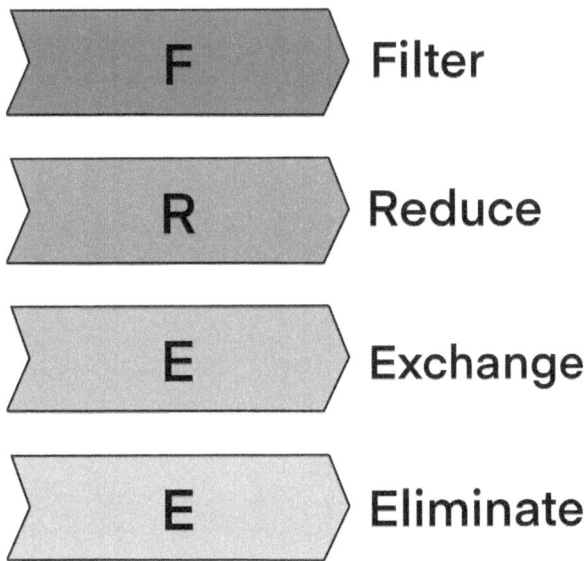

Filter

The first component of the FREE strategy is to determine whether you can filter out the unwanted environmental stressors and reduce your environmental stress load. For example, filtering the air in your home, car, and work is a simple strategy for eliminating some of the particulate materials, chemicals, organisms, and toxins in your environment. Filtering your water is another simple strategy.

Reduce

There are many things that we can't or don't want to remove from our environment and our lives. For example, you can't eliminate all unhealthy food all of the time. Likewise, in today's world and in the future, you will not be able to entirely give up Wi-Fi, social media, or TV. Similarly, you may not want to remove alcohol from your life altogether. But you can limit all these things, reducing the degree and frequency of your exposure. In helping many people improve their environmental fitness over the years, we have learned that eliminating the things that create stress can be challenging initially. However, most people can make positive changes if they begin by minimizing their exposure before eliminating it entirely. So start today, and look for ways to lower your exposure to environmental stressors.

Exchange

Exchange is one of the most helpful strategies. It means replacing one thing with another. For example, if you drink a lot of soda, exchange it for carbonated water and remove some of the sugar and chemicals in your diet. You then still get the soda feel without the negatives. Exchange "dirty" foods (those with high levels of pesticides, herbicides, and other toxic chemicals) for "clean" versions of the same foods. As mentioned in chapter 15, the Environmental Working Group has two lists that are updated every year: the Dirty Dozen and the Clean

Fifteen. When buying foods on the Dirty Dozen list, opt for organic versions of the foods.

Eliminate

Your goal might be to eliminate toxic mold, margarine, the herbicide glyphosate, cigarettes, and the nasty chemicals in your personal and household products. That's difficult with some toxic things (yes, relationships fit in this category at times). If you are sensitive to gluten, dairy, scented candles, a cleaning product, or your pillow, it is best to eliminate the item. Curtailing your exposure to it is a start, but flat-out removing some things is necessary.

PUTTING THE FREE STRATEGY INTO ACTION

There are six critical areas of your life where you want to reduce your environmental stress: the air, your water, your food, your personal use products, household products, and your work. Remember: you can use the FREE strategy for every Fitness Factor, but definitely use it to lower your environmental stress and improve your environmental fitness.

Both the quantity and quality of our air, food, and water are critical to survival. We can live for weeks without food, and for days without water, but for only minutes without air. Because of the importance of air, this is where we start.

Figure 2: Implementing the FREE strategy in your environment.

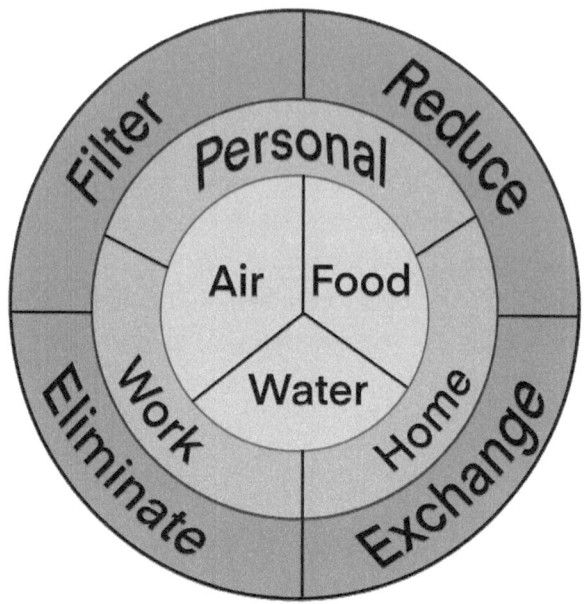

Air

It's thought that the average human cannot live longer than three minutes without air. But we often don't give much thought to the quality of the air we breathe. In chapter 16, "Respiratory Fitness," we suggested how to improve your air quality because research shows that poor air quality has a massive impact on your health and quality of life.

Poor air quality has been directly related to the thyroid gland and thyroid physiology dysfunction, thyroid autoimmunity, thyroid nodules, and thyroid cancer.[258,259,260,261] Filtering the air in your home, car, and work environment can go a long way in reducing your cellular stress and your risk of developing hypothyroidism.

Air filtration can be inexpensive or extremely expensive, depending on the challenges your environment presents and your needs. There are filtration systems that can filter your entire home or individual rooms.

Any filtration is better than no filtration in most cases, so consider your needs and work within your budget to improve your personal air quality. According to the EPA, the air quality inside homes can be two to five times more polluted than the outdoors. This becomes a huge issue when you consider we spend 90 percent of our lives indoors. The combination of energy-efficient building construction, synthetic building materials, furnishings, personal care products, pesticides, and household cleaners contributes to our homes' declining air quality.[262]

If you spend a significant amount of time in your car, your exposure to auto exhaust rises dramatically the longer you are in the car. We don't always realize the impact auto exhaust has on our health or how quality air cabin filters improve the environments of our vehicles. At our places of work, many of us have little control. We see reports of people developing "sick building syndrome" because of the poor air quality in their workplaces. Even though your control at work is limited, there are still things you can do to improve the air quality there, such as using a Molekule air purifier.

Symptoms of Poor Air Quality

You may not think your indoor air quality is a contributing factor to your chronic health challenges, but think about whether or not you experience any of the following symptoms of poor air quality:

- asthma, allergies, or respiratory disorders (especially if they worsen when you're indoors)
- headaches and nausea
- shortness of breath
- sinus congestion, coughing, or sneezing
- eye, nose, throat, or skin irritation
- memory loss
- fatigue
- dizziness
- depression

Symptoms may be mild or severe. You might be surprised how much these symptoms improve when you breathe cleaner air.

Evaluating Air Quality

The difficulty with evaluating air quality is that you can't see the particulate matter. So it is best to have your air quality measured by a professional. They can identify particulate matter, chemical pollutants, carbon monoxide, carbon dioxide, formaldehyde, radon, and mold. A professional can also assess humidity and temperature.

There are devices to help you check your air quality regularly. Their cost varies from under a hundred dollars to a few hundred dollars. The more expensive the device, the more it can typically measure. There are always new products coming onto the market, so do some homework and research, and get the best tool for your budget.

Food

We discuss foods to avoid in chapter 15, "Dietary Fitness," but the FREE strategy works well when evaluating all foods. Depending on how you shop, food may be a significant source of chemical and toxic exposure in your life. So look at what you are purchasing. Can you eat fewer processed foods? Can you consume fewer foods that are known to have high levels of contaminants, pesticides, and herbicides?

Consider how you can exchange some of your favorite foods for less toxic, healthier versions. If you can't go completely organic, take a copy of the Clean Fifteen and Dirty Dozen lists with you when you go shopping to help you make the healthiest choices. Use them to help you determine which foods you should purchase organic versions of to reduce your exposure to toxins. For example, consider exchanging farm-raised salmon and shrimp for healthier wild-caught versions. And of course, look at those foods that are just flat-out not needed and eliminate them from your home. Highly processed foods, oils, and artificial sweeteners are a few to banish.

Water

Water is one of the most essential life requirements, yet it is one of the most contaminated things we consume. A 2019 EWG report identifies 517 contaminants or contaminant groups in the US water supply.[263] Pesticides, herbicides, fertilizers, disinfectants, medications, organisms, and a host of other substances are hidden in the water we consume.

While there are existing legal limits for many water contaminants, some have no restrictions at all, including the highly toxic fluorinated compounds known as perfluoroalkyl and polyfluoroalkyl substances, or PFAs. PFAs have been shown to disrupt thyroid physiology[264] and overall health.[265]

Apply the FREE strategy to your water supply. Filter your water. There are simple systems like filtered pitchers and filters that can be placed on your kitchen faucet or refrigerator, as well as more expensive systems for your entire home. Again, what is best for you will be based on your budget and needs. We like the ECHO H2 Water Machine from Synergy Science (go to www.drkellyhalderman.com for more information) and the Berkey Water Filters system.

The EWG has an excellent resource for helping you learn what might be in your local water supply and the best filter to support your needs. Head over to www.ewg.org/consumer-guides and click on the National Tap Water Database. Plug in your zip code and find your water supplier, and you can see what contaminants are in your local water supply. At the bottom of the page are the types of water filters that reduce your particular contaminants. In addition, the guide indicates both the health impacts and legal limits of chemicals. The EWG also has a water filter guide to inform you of the types of filters available and help you choose one most appropriate for your needs and budget.

You should also limit your use of plastic water bottles. Research has shown that bisphenol A (BPA) and other phenol compounds are known to be endocrine disruptors. As a refresher, your endocrine system is composed of glands (such as your thyroid gland) that produce hormones. Endocrine-disrupting chemicals mimic or disrupt the actions of your hormones, contributing to numerous disorders and diseases. For example, BPA and similar compounds can disrupt thyroid physiology at every level of thyroid physiology.[266] So while we feel it is best to eliminate drinking from plastic water bottles both for your health and the health of our planet, that may not be practical in some situations. So at least exchange plastic water bottles for stainless steel or glass ones whenever possible. Bring your water with you instead of purchasing bottled water. Not only are you likely to get cleaner water, but you will also save a small fortune. The markup on bottled water is thought to be approximately 4,000 percent.[267] The average two-dollar bottle of water costs the manufacturer five cents to produce.[268] In most areas, the cost of bottled water is more expensive than gasoline.

Personal Care Products

Personal care products are another source of toxic and potentially toxic chemicals. The average male uses about seven or more personal care products a day, and the average female uses twelve or more. Some of the most common include toothpaste, mouthwash, soap, shampoo, conditioner, deodorant and antiperspirant, shaving creams, lotions, creams, cologne and perfume, and cosmetics. By the end of a day, you can easily expose yourself to hundreds of chemicals, depending on the products you use.

Are they all problematic? No. But don't assume that all the chemicals in these products are safe. There is research showing that many of the chemicals below, alone or in combination with other products, could potentially be toxic and disrupt endocrine pathways and are therefore considered the "Dirty Dozen" of personal care products by the David Suzuki Foundation[269]:

1. butylated hydroxyanisole (BHA) and butylated hydroxytoluene (BHT)[270]

2. P-phenylenediamine[271]
3. diethanolamine (DEA) and DEA-related ingredients[272,273]
4. dibutyl phthalate[274]
5. formaldehyde and formaldehyde-releasing preservatives[275]
6. parabens[276]
7. parfum (a.k.a. fragrance)[277]
8. polyethylene glycols (PEGs)[278]
9. petrolatum
10. siloxanes
11. sodium laureth sulfate
12. triclosan[279]

Clinical research indicates that all of these ingredients are potentially toxic to your cells and tissues. For more information on these and other potentially harmful chemicals in your personal care products, again go to www.ewg.org. In addition, the EWG has a great resource called "Skin Deep," where you can check the potential toxicity of the products you currently use or would like to use.

Once again, apply the FREE strategy when you start evaluating your personal care products. There are many great ones now on the market that are "cleaner" and less toxic. For almost every personal care product you can think of, there is a healthier alternative to one containing harmful ingredients.

Don't panic. Don't think you have to change everything tomorrow. Just start making changes as your current products run out. There will definitely be some duds. For example, we went through half a dozen natural deodorants before finding one that did the trick. Some companies not only make their products from natural, nontoxic substances but also use eco-friendly packaging.

Household Products

They say home is where the heart is. Unfortunately, what no one says is that home is also where the toxins are. Today homes are being built more energy-efficient than ever before, which is excellent from a heating and cooling standpoint. But energy efficiency also creates a new health issue—that is, a condition called sick building syndrome (SBS). SBS is caused by a combination of factors, including airtight construction; the off-gassing of particulates and chemicals from construction materials, carpet, paint, furniture, and appliances; poor ventilation; and mold growth. Unfortunately, most of us don't have the luxury of rebuilding our homes with toxin-free materials. Instead we must do the best we can to reduce the chemical load and exposure in our current home.

Home furnishings are a potential source of chemical exposure. You may not be able to replace all the furniture and carpeting in your home with less-toxic versions in one fell swoop, so we recommend starting with a few things and making steady changes over time.

One of the best places to start is where you spend about a third of your life—your bed. After all, you spend a lot of your time with your face buried in your bedding. We think of our beds as sanctuaries—places where we can cuddle up and feel safe. But what if your bed is one of the most toxic things in your home? Many conventional mattresses are made with unhealthy or potentially harmful chemicals, including polyurethane foam, synthetic latex, flame retardants, and vinyl.

There are many "clean" mattresses, pillows, and bedding products available today. The nice thing is that many of the manufacturers allow thirty-to-ninety-day trials with free returns. In addition, the cost of many of the "cleaner" bedding products has come down, bringing them closer in price to conventional mattresses, which makes the purchase a bit easier to swallow. If you are on a tight budget, try switching out your pillow with a cleaner version. You might be surprised how your sleep improves and how much better you feel having changed just your pillow.

Once you've addressed your bedding, start working on some of the other furnishings in your home that may be contributing to your chemical burden. Work on things that you can manage. Switch out your Teflon pans for aluminum, cast iron, ceramic, or carbon steel versions. Switch out your cleaning products for less-toxic versions as they run out. You can order wool dryer balls to replace the dryer sheets that damage you and your dryer. Exchange your conventional dishwasher detergent for one that is not toxic to you and your gut flora.

None of these changes are terribly difficult, and the overall expense of making some of them may be less than you might think. The EWG has a section titled "Healthy Home" that contains a guide for almost every product in your home. Check it out at https://www.ewg.org/healthyhomeguide.

We almost feel lazy for repeatedly encouraging you to go to www.ewg.org, but this group has done a great job putting together resources for cleaner living. It would be a shame for you not to take advantage of what EWG has to offer.

CHECK YOUR WORK ENVIRONMENT

Work is the environment where you may have the least control, but there are still things you can do to lower your environmental stress. Use the FREE strategy at work. What can you filter, reduce, exchange, or eliminate? Here are some suggestions:

- If you drive to work, exchange your current cabin filter with a HEPA cabin filter. Change the filter frequently based on your driving and the manufacturer's recommendations.
- Use a portable air filtration system to improve air quality in your office if you work in one. You can't control the air filtration in the whole building, but there are devices that can measure and filter your office air.
- Plug in your devices versus using Bluetooth whenever possible to reduce exposure to electromagnetic radiation (EMFs).

- Put a screen filter on your work computer to reduce blue light exposure.
- Open your windows. If possible, open the windows at your office to increase the flow of fresh air.
- Get up and out of the building. Use your breaks to get outside. When possible, take your lunch and eat outside of the office.

We can't give this topic nearly the attention it deserves, and space doesn't permit a complete guide to low-tox living. So our goal is to provide you with a rough framework of what to consider and resources to investigate.

ENVIRONMENTAL FITNESS RECOMMENDATIONS

- Incorporate the FREE strategy into your life to reduce your environmental burden.
- Look for ways to reduce the toxins in your air, food, and water.
    - Use the www.ewg.org resources.
    - Have your home air quality measured by a professional and consider buying a home device.
- Look for ways to reduce the toxins in your personal products, home, and work environments.
    - Use the health guides at www.ewg.org.
- Limit the use of plastic containers, wraps, and bottles.
- Grab a copy of *Low Tox Life* by Alexx Stuart to help make your transition to cleaner living easier.
- Make gradual, steady changes.
- Get to work making your internal environment as healthy as possible by improving all of your fitness factors so that environmental toxins impact you less.

CHAPTER 21

METABOLIC FITNESS

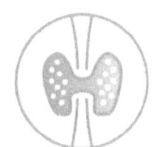

Most people think about metabolism in the context of eating. They are under the impression that metabolism has to do with the speed at which they burn calories, as in fast or slow metabolism, and its impact on body weight. That's true, but metabolism is much more than that. It encompasses all the chemical processes that occur within the body that sustain life.

We define metabolic fitness in terms of how well your body chemistry functions in relation to your diet, lifestyle, and environment. The higher your level of metabolic fitness, the more adaptable and resilient you are and the less need there is for outside interventions, such as medications. While all the body's systems are important for determining your metabolic fitness, some of the most essential include the following:

- digestive system
- detoxification system (liver and gallbladder)
- blood glucose (sugar) regulation
- adrenal system
- immune system
- iron regulation
- hormone physiology
- neurotransmitter physiology

How well each of these systems works determines your level of metabolic fitness.

Figure 1: Factors influencing your metabolic fitness.

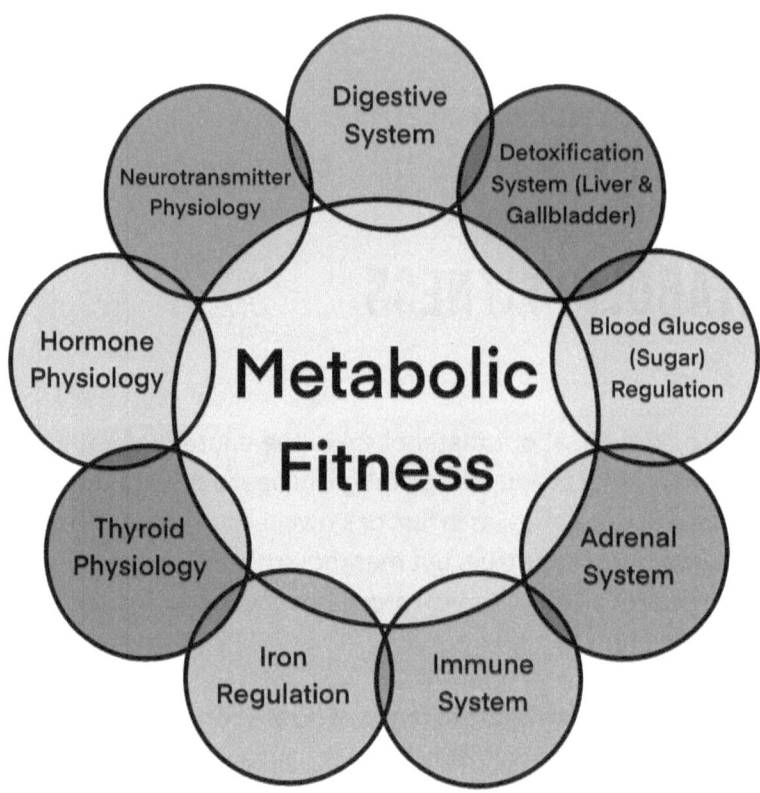

METABOLIC FITNESS CONTINUUM

Like all Fitness Factors, metabolic fitness ranges along a continuum. People with average metabolic fitness typically do not need daily medication. They have no chronic diseases or disorders and can function well in their environments. People with below-average metabolic fitness have at least one disease, condition, or disorder that requires some level of ongoing treatment or medication. Someone with above-average metabolic fitness not only has good metabolic function in his or her everyday daily life, but he or she can adapt to a temporary increase in physical, emotional, or environmental demand without excessive cell stress or injury.

Figure 2: The Metabolic Fitness Continuum

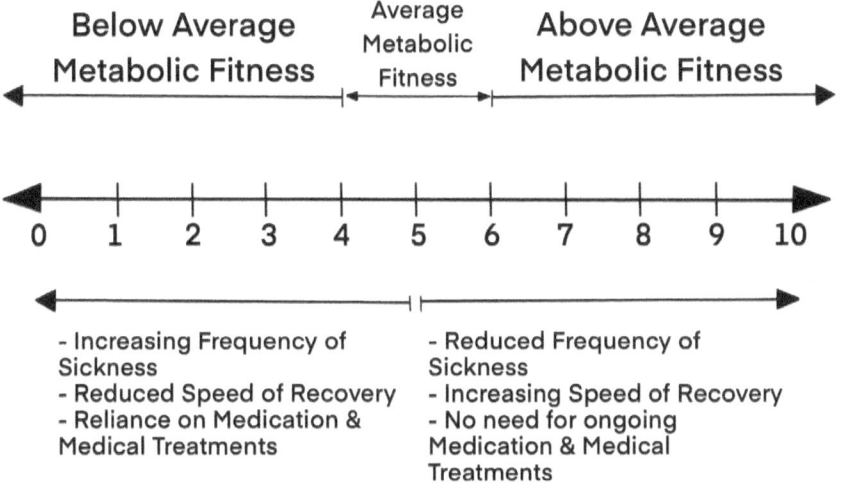

In chapter 7, "A New Perspective," we discussed how excessive cell stress can initiate a cell danger response. The questions you might ask are, What does excessive mean? Is the same amount of stress excessive for everyone? Excessive cell stress is defined as more stress than your cells and your metabolism can adapt to in order to maintain homeostasis. The more fit your metabolism, the more stress your cells can adapt to before initiating a cell danger response. For example, if three people hike the same trail for two days without sleep or food, the person with the highest level of metabolic fitness will probably manage the best, since he or she has the most efficient metabolism to drive energy production.

All the Fitness Factors impact your metabolism. While allopathic medicine compartmentalizes human physiology into distinct separate systems, the functional medicine concept is that we are a physiological web. All our cells and tissues communicate in an integrated way when we're in good health. You cannot impact one area of the body without a ripple effect on all the body's cells and tissues. Dysfunction and disease begin when that interconnected communication becomes compromised. You are either a web of physiological function or a web of physiological dysfunction. The state of your physiology is often determined by the levels of your fitness factors.

Eliminating stress from your life will never happen, so our goals are to enable you to make small strides to lower your excessive stress and allow your body to recover quickly when the stress is unavoidable. Being able to adapt to the challenges of various forms of stress has a hormetic effect. In other words, some stress can make you stronger. As your resilience increases, you can use cellular stress and recovery as tools to make you healthier and more adaptable and resilient than you have ever been.

EVALUATING YOUR METABOLIC FITNESS

A metabolic assessment questionnaire (MAQ) is a survey of your signs and symptoms organized by body systems. It helps identify the tissues, organs, and systems struggling with excessive cellular stress. The questionnaire is broken down into organs and systems in the body, such as the digestive, immune, and adrenal systems and the others in the list above. There are numerous versions of these forms available.

In addition to the MAQ, we prefer to use a combination of other tools, such as lab test results, data from wearable technology, and an evaluation of signs and symptoms, to determine metabolic fitness. Go to www.thyroiddebacle.com and download our metabolic assessment form to assess your multisystem adaptive disorder today. You can also sign up for a complimentary class to understand the metabolic assessment form in detail.

A metabolic assessment questionnaire is a great tool to evaluate which of your body systems may have become compromised and help you or your functional medicine practitioner understand your multisystem adaptive disorder (MSAD). (See chapter 10, "Hypothyroidism Is a

Spectrum Disorder.") Chronic cell danger response causes adaptive shifts in the body's physiology. The allostatic shift leads to dysfunction or breakdown (allostatic overload) in various tissues, organs, and systems, creating the signs and symptoms you experience. Both allopathic and functional medicine practitioners diagnose symptoms as separate conditions, but they are really part of your adaptive response.

On most MAQs, the higher your total score, the lower your metabolic fitness. The higher your score in a particular category on the MAQ, the more likely that system is struggling and will require support. Understanding your unique MSAD helps you and your doctor determine what tissues and systems need support. Together you can develop a strategy for recovery.

We ask our patients to complete a MAQ every few months and each time we order a comprehensive metabolic panel of blood tests. The MAQ is an invaluable tool for developing a strategic plan to address a patient's health challenges for a functional medicine practitioner. The MAQ also helps determine what functional or pathology-based testing to order.

While the MAQ is an excellent tool for those with signs and symptoms, what if you don't have any consistent symptoms? If you don't have obvious signs and symptoms, the MAQ is of less value for evaluating your metabolic fitness. For example, if you have no diagnoses, no disorders, no need for daily medication, and no chronic, persistent symptoms, it's likely your metabolic fitness is average or higher. However, the absence of apparent signs and symptoms does not always indicate above-average metabolic fitness. You can still complete a MAQ on a regular basis, but you need to use additional tools to evaluate your metabolic fitness.

Pathology-based tests and lab reference ranges are often inappropriate for evaluating optimal function or dysfunctional states that may eventually lead to disease. This creates a problem for many people. Here are a couple of examples.

First, as earlier chapters explain, TSH is often the only test used to evaluate thyroid physiology. Yet it usually does not rise above the reference range until 90 percent of the thyroid gland has been damaged. Therefore, it is an indicator of late-stage thyroid disease, not early dysfunction.

Second, gluten intolerance is a growing problem. When many allopathic doctors are looking for gluten intolerance, they perform the standard celiac panel of blood tests available at most conventional labs. For a long time, it was taught that a person could not be gluten intolerant unless he or she had celiac disease. Celiac disease is caused by immune damage to the intestinal villi as a consequence of gluten exposure and reactivity. (Intestinal villi are tiny hairlike projections lining the small intestine that contain blood vessels and help absorb nutrients.) People develop celiac disease because of an intolerance to gluten. So the celiac panel of blood tests run in allopathic medicine doesn't show reactivity or gluten intolerance (dysfunction) until after one has the disease. It detects not the beginning of a gluten intolerance problem but the late stage.

Also, the conventional celiac panel often does not include tests for gluten reactivity, such as an antigliadin antibody test. Your doctor has to order that test separately. The standard allopathic tests that include gluten testing typically assess only one of ten components of wheat that sensitive people react to. This often results in a physician telling someone who is clearly symptomatic when eating wheat or gluten-based foods that he or she is not reactive or intolerant to gluten.

One of my patients was told that she was not gluten intolerant for years because all the measures on her celiac panel were negative. Her doctor said she could and should continue to eat gluten-containing foods. She struggled with severe health problems for eight more years. Finally, after taking more tests for celiac disease, her results were positive. She was told to stop eating gluten, and almost overnight, her symptoms started to improve.

Third, many people who suffer from chronic GI symptoms like gas, bloating, pain, constipation, and diarrhea are evaluated with conventional allopathic, GI pathology–based testing. However, when scopes, imaging tests, and biopsies don't turn up any overt pathology, doctors often tell them they have a "functional" GI disorder like irritable bowel syndrome. This means that the doctors understand the GI tract is not functioning appropriately; they just cannot determine what is causing the signs and symptoms. The reason for this is that they are looking for diseased tissue that has not developed yet. Thus, they are using tests that measure disease, not function and dysfunction.

The good news is that there are some fantastic labs that provide functional lab testing. Some of our favorites include the following:

- Precision Analytical: https://dutchtest.com/
- Genova Diagnostics: https://www.gdx.net/
- Diagnostic Solutions: https://www.diagnosticsolutionslab.com/
- Great Plains Labs: https://www.greatplainslaboratory.com/
- HDRI Labs: http://www.hdri-usa.com/
- Cyrex Labs: https://www.cyrexlabs.com/
- Vibrant America: https://www.vibrant-america.com/

These labs provide cutting-edge tests that help practitioners find early dysfunction and dysregulation often long before disease develops. However, it is best, in our opinion, to work with an experienced clinician. If you are not a health-care provider, you may be able to purchase some of your own laboratory assessments online at companies such as www.requestatest.com and www.everylwell.com

ADDITIONAL TOOLS TO MONITOR METABOLIC FITNESS

Today it is easier than ever to monitor your metabolism. We've entered the world of wearable devices that can provide data on how our metabolism is functioning on a daily and up-to-the-minute basis.

Wearable devices like the Oura Ring, Biostrap, some smart watches, and Whoop provide information on your respiration, sleep, heartbeat, oxygen saturation, and HRV. In addition, these devices provide information that allows you to monitor where you are compared to population data or even to your own history.

HRV is one of our favorite tools. (See chapter 17, "Emotional Fitness.") What's great about HRV is that it is a measurement of your body's restoration and recovery from day to day. The higher your HRV, the greater the balance between your sympathetic and parasympathetic nervous systems. In other words, the higher your HRV, the better. As a result, HRV is widely considered one of the best objective measurements of physical fitness. But HRV provides more information than that; it really is a measurement of metabolic fitness and recovery.

We often see those with less-than-average metabolic fitness having low HRV levels. What's neat is that if a patient has a wearable device that was tracking HRV before and during the time they developed health challenges, we can look at the patient's data and see his or her HRV declining before metabolic problems were apparent to the patient.

One of my patients came to see me, Dr. Eric, after struggling with a hyperthyroid episode caused by a Hashimoto's thyroiditis storm. Such a flare-up of inflammation causes a large amount of thyroid hormone to be released, causing hyperthyroidism. I asked her when the problem started. As she was telling me her story, I noticed she was wearing a smart watch. I asked her whether it tracked her HRV. She did not know what HRV was or whether her watch could track it. We looked at her data, and, sure enough, unbeknownst to her, it was tracking her HRV. Her HRV data showed that forty-five days before she sought medical help, her HRV started to plummet. That was an indicator that her metabolic fitness was being challenged long before she realized it. We discussed what was happening around that time that may have caused excessive cell stress. We were able to piece together the triggering factors—work and family stresses and lack of sleep—that ultimately led to her thyroid condition. Addressing the triggering factors led to improving her thyroid condition, HRV, metabolic fitness, and health.

Many people mistakenly believe that metabolic fitness declines or health problems develop when signs and symptoms develop. Unfortunately, this is often not the case. Almost all disorders and diseases are developing long before your body lets you know that something is amiss.

If you are currently struggling with metabolic challenges, please consider adding a functional medicine practitioner to your healthcare team. Your functional medicine practitioner will likely have a totally different evaluation and treatment strategy than your allopathic providers. This does not make either approach wrong, but it provides you with options. Your allopathic physician's job is to manage your diseases, disorders, and lab reference ranges. Your functional medicine practitioner identifies issues that create health challenges. Your functional medicine practitioner will be working to take you from disease and illness management to above-average metabolic fitness, health, and wellness.

METABOLIC FITNESS RECOMMENDATIONS

- Add a functional medicine practitioner to your health team.
- Have a functional medicine practitioner interpret your lab test results utilizing functional ranges.
- When trying to identify underlying causes of thyroid and other disorders, consult a functional medicine provider to perform functional diagnostic tests.
- Complete the metabolic assessment questionnaire or symptom surveys your practitioner provides. Your practitioner will interpret it, and along with your lab results, the medications, and supplements you are taking, and your history, the practitioner will map your multisystem adaptive disorder.

- Work with a functional medicine practitioner to modify your diet, lifestyle, habits, and environment to improve metabolic fitness.
- Work with a functional medicine provider to utilize supplements and nutraceuticals to strategically support functional lab test results and metabolic assessment form findings.
- Use a wearable device to track metrics like HRV, heart rate, oxygen saturation, respiration, sleep, and recovery.

CHAPTER 22

GENETIC FITNESS

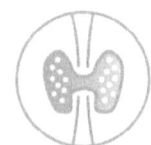

You might be wondering how, if you can't change your genes, you will improve your genetic fitness. And while you are right that you can't change your genes, you sure can influence how they are expressed and function. Improving your genetic fitness is the premise of the book *Dirty Genes* by our friend and colleague Dr. Ben Lynch.

GENETICS 101

Genetics is a branch of biology concerned with the study of genes, genetic variation, and heredity. Genetics and its application to health has become a popular subject in functional and integrative medicine. Owing to the work of functional medicine pioneers such as Ben Lynch, ND; Gordon Crozier, DO; and many others, we are beginning to apply cutting-edge research to genes and, more importantly, their expression in our everyday lives to make personalized, health-promoting changes.

Figure 1: Chromosomes to nucleotides.

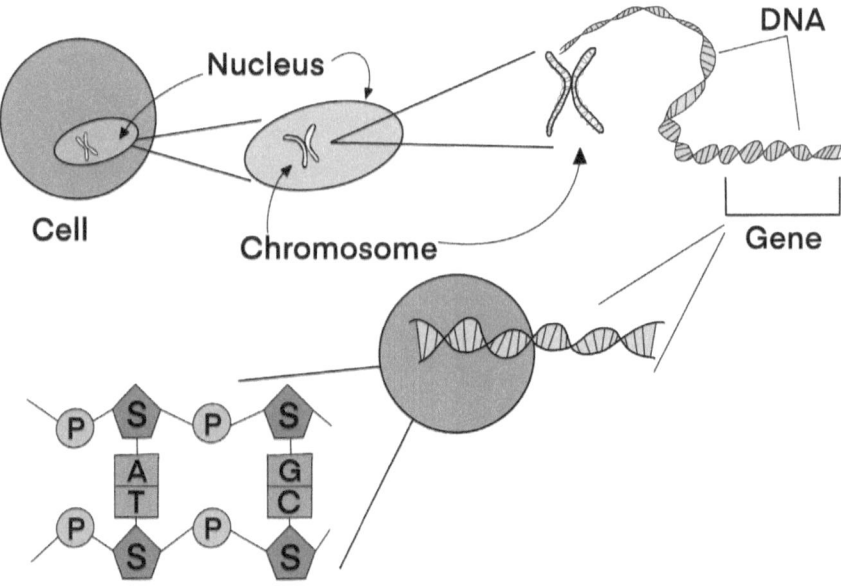

Nearly everyone has heard the terms "chromosomes," "DNA," "gene," and "gene expression" at some time or another. But let's give all these words some context. We are made of trillions of cells. Within most of the cells of your body is a structure called the "nucleus." The nucleus houses twenty-three pairs of chromosomes. Chromosomes are composed of tightly wound genetic material called "deoxynucleic acid" (DNA). DNA is the hereditary material that contains the blueprint for making you. It includes the code for making everything your body needs.

DNA is a double-stranded string of nucleotides. A nucleotide consists of a base of one of four chemicals: adenine (A), thymine (T), guanine (G), and cytosine(C), plus a molecule of sugar and phosphoric acid. Genes are specific sequences of DNA. In the double strands, A pairs with T, and C pairs with G.

Sections of the DNA string are called "genes." Each gene is composed of nucleotides in a specific sequence. DNA carries genetic information, and genes provide instructions for making proteins—a process called "gene expression." Those protein products can be enzymes, protein channels in cell membranes, or structures, such as collagen. We inherit two copies of each gene, one from each biological parent.

The most prevalent nucleotide sequence seen is called the "wild-type gene." However, occasionally one of the nucleotide bases—A, T, C, or G—within a gene is replaced by one of the other three nucleotide bases. This is referred to as a "single-nucleotide polymorphism," or SNP (pronounced "snip"). The gene, now called a "genetic variant," will produce a variation of the protein from the most prevalent or wild-type gene.

You inherit a gene from each parent. If the gene from one parent contains the wild-type sequence and the gene from the other parent has a polymorphism (SNP) in the same gene, you are said to be heterozygous (–/+) for that genetic variant. If the same genes from both parents have a polymorphism, you are said to be homozygous (+/+). The variation of the gene can potentially impact the end product. Homozygosity is thought to have a more significant impact on the end product than heterogenicity.

We like to use the analogy of Legos because we both have children and have built many Lego sets. The car kits always come with building instructions (think of this as the DNA). Following them produces a Lego car (the protein).

Imagine that you and your child are going to build two identical cars. You buy two of what you think are identical Lego car kits off the internet. Each kit comes with a set of instructions. The instructions are a bit different because the kits were manufactured in two different facilities. You follow each set of instructions, and one car ends up looking great, but the other is a bit clunky and doesn't work as well. This same sort of thing happens in real life because you receive one set of DNA from Mom and another from Dad. Like the instructions for the Lego car kits, the DNA instructions you receive from your parents are similar but have some differences.

There are literally millions of instances in which the directions to build products in the human body vary from what is considered normal. Of the millions of SNPs in an individual's genetic code, most have zero ramifications, meaning that the protein produced is normal. But other SNPs can alter the way the end product works, as in our Lego car example. For example, a SNP in the gene containing instructions for making the MTHFR enzyme (the methylenetetrahydrofolate reductase gene) may occur at the 677th nucleotide. As a result, thymine (T) is replaced for the normal cytosine (C).

Figure 2: An example of a polymorphism of the MTHFR gene.

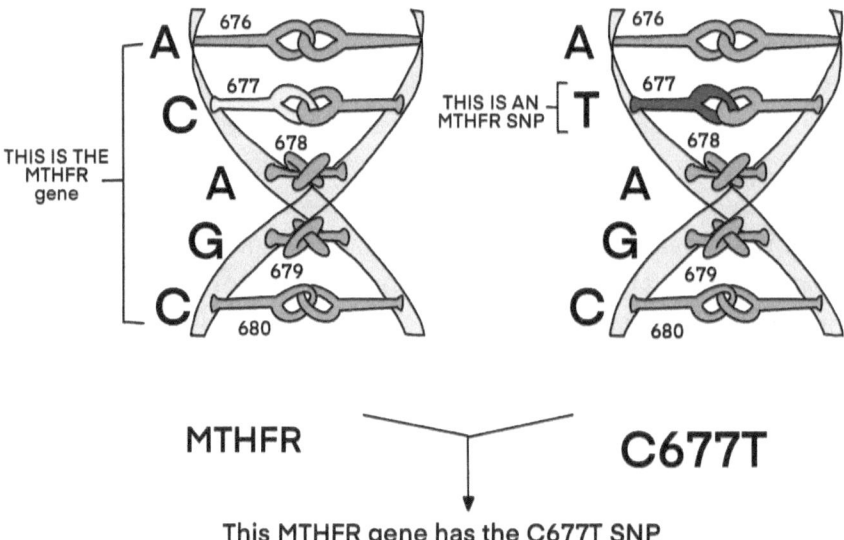

This single change can decrease the ability of the MTHFR enzyme to do its job. This can translate into significant health issues, such as problems repairing your DNA, difficulty with detoxification, or hormone regulation. Other SNPs alter the formation of transporters, which are the doors that let substances into your cells so that key nutrients, such as magnesium, can't enter. That alteration may lead to many health problems. Science is uncovering SNPs associated with thyroid physiology, and we are still learning of its impact.

Genetic information is a valuable piece of the clinical puzzle but is not the golden ticket to health. A polymorphism in a gene does not necessarily alter its function. Often, the gene sequence alterations occur in an area of the gene that never expresses.

THE SNP ADVANTAGE

If you are born with SNPs in genes like MTHFR, you can find information on supporting those genes that may need help to function better. Notice we used "may." Seeing a SNP on a genetic report does not necessarily mean that you should do something to support its function. Unfortunately we see many people in our practices who have experienced the negative consequences of these efforts. For example, excessive amounts of vitamin B6 may cause clumsiness, burning pains, loss of muscle coordination, paralysis, dyspnea, pain and numbness in the arms and legs, and rapid breathing.

Some SNPs may parlay an evolutionary advantage. For example, having a SNP in the gene that makes the instructions to produce the catechol-O-methyltransferase (COMT) enzyme, which slows the deactivation of dopamine and epinephrine, may help you focus better and be more productive.

Understanding which SNPs may negatively impact your health and need support and which may not is not a simple, straightforward science. It usually takes a seasoned professional who understands how to interpret your genetic reports in conjunction with your health history, health assessment forms, and functional medicine test results to guide you in making correct choices for your body. There are several books on this topic. One of the best is *Dirty Genes* by our friend and colleague Dr. Ben Lynch.

Think about your genetic SNPs or polymorphisms like road construction. Construction has the potential to slow traffic significantly, but it doesn't always do it. For example, consider construction on a four-lane highway, with two lanes moving southbound and two moving northbound. The construction is on one of the southbound lanes. If you are traveling to work in the southbound lane at rush hour, there is a high probability that the roadwork will slow you down. During an off-peak time when there is little traffic, however, the construction may cause little, if any, disruption in the traffic.

Genetic polymorphisms have a similar effect. During times of high demand for a particular enzyme, a polymorphism in the gene that contains instructions for that enzyme may slow enzyme production. It's possible you may experience the impact of the reduced enzyme production as overt symptoms. However, during times of expected demand for the enzyme, you may not notice that production is slower.

Some polymorphisms cause pathways to move faster, and others cause pathways to move slower. Therefore, when looking at their genetic reports, many people focus on which supplements make a polymorphism work faster, which they assume is better.

There are a few problems with this thinking. The first is the assumption that putting more of an enzyme cofactor into your body will support the particular gene polymorphism that concerns you. For example, let's say you have a polymorphism of the COMT gene, which slows its action. Since the cofactor is S-adenosylmethionine (SAMe), you might assume that putting more SAMe into your body makes the enzyme work better.

Some of the early work on polymorphisms revolved around the idea that providing more of a particular cofactor enables a polymorphism to work more efficiently. This works well on paper and in a research lab where one pathway can be isolated, but it doesn't often work well in practice. Why?

To continue with the same example, SAMe is the primary methyl donor in the body, and hundreds of reactions in the body require it. Your cells and tissues determine how to use the available SAMe. However, when you take a SAMe supplement, you can't choose which of the myriad reactions in the body the SAMe will affect. It's like throwing food to a crowd of starving people and thinking that the person with whom you make eye contact will get it. It's unrealistic.

The body uses nutrients to support what it sees as the most critical processes occurring at any given moment. Therefore, it is naive to assume that taking a supplement of SAMe (or B6, B12, or magnesium), will have the effect you want.

THE IMPORTANCE OF EPIGENETICS

Genes are commonly referred to as units of heredity because their transmission to offspring is the basis for the inheritance of traits ranging from hair and eye color to the production of antioxidants. Most traits are under the influence of many genes, as well as the interaction between genes and the environment. This interaction between genes and the environment is called "epigenetics."

Epigenetics is the science of how genes are influenced by lifestyle choices, diet, supplements, and environmental factors. Epigenetics was introduced in 1942 by embryologist Conrad Waddington. Since then, "epigenetics" has become a more well-known term, implying that laypeople are starting to understand how their daily choices influence their genes and contribute to how their bodies function. For example, it doesn't take a rocket scientist to figure out that when we eat or sleep poorly or are stressed over the hassles in our lives, we feel terrible. Epigenetic factors, such as diet, sleep, and stress, directly affect how our genes express themselves and influence our overall health.

People who obtain their genetic data from places like 23andMe.com and Ancestry.com should understand that even if one is born with "normal" genes, poor lifestyle choices compromise how the genes express. Having normal or wild-type genes does not absolve you of the responsibility of taking care of your body and environment to stay healthy.

In *Dirty Genes*, Dr. Lynch discusses many common polymorphisms that may contribute to health problems. The important word here is "may." Dr. Lynch does not suggest taking supplements for gene polymorphisms; rather, he suggests improving your diet and lifestyle so gene polymorphisms can work better.

A problem with thinking that supplements fix your polymorphisms is that external factors influence functions of many genes, polymorphisms or no polymorphisms. Inflammatory cytokines, microbial toxins, and toxic substances often have a more significant influence on how a gene functions than whether or not there is a polymorphism in that gene. Unless you reduce the inflammation, microbial toxins, or toxic substances, the gene may not work efficiently regardless of the supplements with which you flood your system.

Let's return to our traffic analogy. Road construction can slow traffic, but an accident could slow traffic as well. When the traffic on your drive to work is backed up for miles, you might assume that the backup is due to construction. You might think the answer is to have more construction workers come to the area of congestion. But if the cause is an accident, bringing in more construction workers (the cofactors, such as SAMe, B12, and folate) would be useless and may only worsen the situation.

For many of our patients, polymorphisms are not the cause of their health issues or illnesses. They may be likely areas where biologic congestion occurs, but the real problems are the things causing the congestion in the first place.

We agree with Dr. Lynch that for most people, getting a genetic profile and "treating" gene SNPs with supplements is not the place to start improving health and function. Instead, gene reports should be used as tools only by health-care providers with the training to understand what polymorphisms mean in relation to a specific person.

In *Dirty Genes*, Dr. Lynch does a great job of explaining how genes function and express. He explains that some of us are born with "dirty genes" and some create them with their diets, lifestyles, and environments. If you are born with dirty genes, it means you have a polymorphism that is impacting function. When he says you develop dirty genes, he is referring to the epigenetic influences that negatively impact gene function. However, regardless of your situation, Dr. Lynch asserts there is something you can do. Many of the suggestions and recommendations we outline in part 3 are Dr. Lynch's strategies for cleaning up your genes.

BEWARE THE QUICK FIX

Today, people who know nothing about how some genes work are making recommendations based on genetic reports. They are providing generic information about how to fix genes, which is close to utter nonsense. The motive is profit. Many so-called experts are from the same companies that sell bottles of supplements for every polymorphism you have. Not only is this strategy ineffective, but it's also often harmful.

We've seen reports stating that a person needs to take B6 because he or she has a polymorphism of "x" gene and then, in another area, telling the person to avoid B6 because he or she has a polymorphism of "y" gene. There are companies touting that they can formulate a multivitamin that is custom-tailored to a person's genetic profile. Please don't buy into this nonsense regardless of the retired superstar who endorses it.

Each person's gene polymorphisms are unique to that person. Two people can have the same MTHFR gene SNP, but the SNP doesn't affect each one to the same degree. People often come to our offices who are following the advice of some online expert. They are taking five to fifteen supplements for their polymorphisms and still feel awful. To make matters worse, they are living in a state of fear that they must take the supplements to support their polymorphisms. The so-called expert's advice is causing more stress, which negatively impacts all of their genes, with and without SNPs. How could experts who know little or nothing about your life, diet, and stressors possibly provide you with customized advice? They may be helping you, but not with your health. They are helping you empty your wallet.

Supplements cannot overcome a compromised diet and lifestyle. There aren't enough supplements to target specific genes to fix you. So don't waste your money. Instead, start by addressing your diet and lifestyle. If you want to get genetic testing and obtain a genetic report, that is fine. We use these reports all the time as a tool, but not as *the* tool. We strongly advise that you leave it up to a person trained in genomics to determine the significance of your gene polymorphisms and guide you on how to support them best. You can go to Dr. Lynch's website, http://go.strategene.org/genetic-analysis, for a list of professionals who have undergone his training.

GENETIC TESTING

Using genetic testing to reveal biological weaknesses to which you may be predisposed can be helpful when optimizing your diet and lifestyle. In some instances, this can mean the difference between suffering from depression, anxiety, ADHD, insomnia, heart disease, obesity, food cravings, addictions, and a hundred other disorders and living a healthy and energetic symptom-free life.

However, trying to learn more about your genes, how they work, and what you should or should not do to support them can be confusing, even for doctors. There is a mass of conflicting information and contradictory recommendations out there. Health-care providers can use StrateGene from Seeking Health (www.go.strategene.org) or MaxGen Labs (www.maxgenlabs.com) to obtain raw data (from saliva), process it, and produce a personalized report. Laypeople can take genetic data obtained from companies like 23andMe and pay another fee for a report about their genes from a reputable company such as StrateGene, MaxGen Labs, Livewello (www.livewello.com), or Promethease (www.promethease.com).

The latest and most reliable science backs the reports these aforementioned companies produce from individuals' genetic data. That's why we use them.

The gene SNPs that impact thyroid hormone production, thyroid hormone transport, and thyroid hormone conversion by the deiodinases aren't available on most reporting systems. We debated whether to detail what those gene polymorphisms are, but after consideration, we decided not to include them in *The Thyroid Debacle*. We made this decision not because they aren't important, but because the best way to support gene polymorphisms is to address your lifestyle and fitness factors—not take more supplements.

The most significant gene polymorphisms typically result in congenital defects like congenital hypothyroidism and Down's syndrome. Living your best life is possibly the most impactful way to affect your SNPs. If you've done the work on your fitness factors and want to look into the role that a gene polymorphism might play in, say, your deiodinase activity and the conversion of T4 to T3, work with a professional who understands both cellular thyroid physiology and genetics.

WHAT SHOULD YOU DO?

The field of genetics is growing and evolving every day. Surrounding this growth is a lot of excitement regarding our ability to assess genetic information. However, the extent to which this information can guide diagnosis and treatment is still unclear. In other words, how can what you learn about your unique genetic fingerprint help you lose weight, have more energy, and recover from hypothyroidism?

That is the genetics world's million-dollar question. And people are literally making millions by cashing in on the public's excitement to tailor their diet and exercise regimens to their genetic profiles. You need to be careful about relying on recommendations based solely on your genes.

Genes don't work in isolation; they work in tandem with other genes. When one gene turns off, another might turn on. Case in point: just because a person has an MTHFR polymorphism or variant does not mean that he or she will have an issue. It means that the person has a variant in his or her MTHFR gene or that his or her variation is different from that of the general population. Other people without an MTHFR variant may still have the symptoms of an MTHFR SNP. That is why it is essential to look at genes and how they communicate with each other and, even more importantly, understand how lifestyle affects our genes.

All of the "lifestyle influences" that affect your genetics are addressed in part 3—that is, how you feed your body, how you sleep, how you breathe, your mindset, and your environment. Don't make the mistake of inundating your body with supplements based on genetic reports without evaluating your Fitness Factors. Instead, do the best you can with them every day. Then fill in any gaps with superior nutrition from companies like Professional Health Products, US Enzymes, Seeking Health, and Sophia Nutrition, to name a few.

GENETIC FITNESS RECOMMENDATIONS

- If you are curious about your genetic profile, check out one of the companies that provide an analysis for a fee, such as 23andme or MaxGen Labs or StrateGene.
- Don't rely on genetic reports alone to determine what supplements you need.
- Improve your fitness in each of the Fitness Factors in part 3.
- Have the genetic information interpreted by a provider trained in doing genetic assessments.
- Grab a copy of *Dirty Genes* for an easy-to-follow explanation of some of the most significant genes that influence your everyday life and function.

CHAPTER 23

EPILOGUE

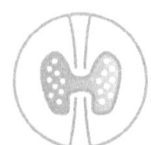

You did it! You made it through the book. We urge you not to put this book too far out of reach. Do not make it another book that you read and find interesting but doesn't change your actions. Change is the only thing that will fix your chronic thyroid symptoms, your health and quality of life.

We fully realize that restoring your thyroid physiology would be much easier if we could provide you with a step-by-step strategy. It would be so much easier if you could change just one thing, or you could take one supplement that would reverse months, years, or decades of chronic cellular stress and altered thyroid physiology. We would do it if we could. But regardless of what you might have heard or read elsewhere, the magic pill doesn't exist. If it did, you wouldn't have picked up this book. If it did, the supplement protocols for fixing thyroid physiology that you read about on blogs or in other books would have worked. If a drug or supplement could fix the physiology of the body, we wouldn't have a thyroid debacle, an obesity crisis, a diabetes crisis, a cardiovascular disease crisis, a dementia crisis, or a chronic disease crisis in general in this country.

New drugs are constantly being put on the market and pumped into our bodies. We are toxic with drugs and other chemicals. The United

States population consumes the vast majority of prescription drugs,[280] yet our health continues to decline.

Studies report that about 10 percent of the adult population struggles with hypothyroidism. However, the estimates are skewed by the way hypothyroidism is determined. The statistics are based on the faith in TSH as a valid marker of thyroid disease, and now you know that it most certainly is not a reliable marker. How can we put one test on such a high pedestal when its value can be manipulated and suppressed by many of the medications we take and by the number-one problem adults struggle from, which is chronic inflammation?

We believe that the numbers of people struggling with thyroid physiology problems are grossly underreported. Why? Because the tools used to assess thyroid physiology are lacking. Are there better tools? Yes. We have reviewed better ways to evaluate thyroid physiology in this book. And we hope that in the not-so-distant future, even better, more accurate tools will be developed.

Why are the allopathic hypothyroid treatments you have been receiving not making you well? Don't blame your doctors; they are working within a system that dictates how to evaluate and treat patients. The problem is the paradigm. The problem is a system that:

- Never determines the cause of hypothyroidism
- Fails to identify tissue and cellular dysfunction until tissues and cells become diseased
- Fails to consider that normal TSH and T4 may not equate to optimal cellular thyroid physiology
- Fails to consider that what is causing hypothyroid symptoms may not be mistakes of physiology but a protective mechanism
- Has become complacent with managing symptoms, disorders, and diseases rather than identifying and correcting the causes of those symptoms, disorders, and diseases

- Has become biased and blinded by the profitability of treating symptoms and managing disease
- Deceptively promotes to the public that the acute-care crisis model of medical care is the same thing as healthcare

We've been educated by Big Food, Big Pharma, Big Media, and Big Medicine. We've been brainwashed to believe that processed food is the same as or better than real food. We've been brainwashed to believe that symptoms are the disease or disorder instead of being signposts that our cells are under stress. We've been led to believe that chronic illness is a normal part of aging versus a sign of chronic cellular stress and dysfunction that can be reversed.

We've been led to believe that the solution is a pill or potion and that suppression of symptoms is the equivalent of health. We are being told by advertising that pills and medications are the key to greater longevity and a healthier life. We have companies and media manipulating data and research to further their agendas at our expense.

You will not find the solution you seek outside you; it is within you. There are no shortcuts in life. You must constantly work on yourself, your habits, your behaviors, your emotions, and your fitness if you want to be healthier than you are right now.

We've both experienced health challenges, including Hashimoto's, and overcome them. At 54 years of age my thyroid panel is normal, my thyroid antibodies are non-existent, my insulin resistance is gone, and my episodes of Raynaud's a thing of the past. But the work is not over. We are constantly seeking to improve every aspect of our health and fitness. If we do not stay on top of our game and our cellular stress, signs and symptoms will return. We overcame our own illnesses and thyroid challenges by working on the things we've outlined in this book. But we know that this is a journey, and we have to individually decide where our weaknesses are and address them as best we can every day. Optimal health is not a destination. If you do not work at it constantly, your health is sure to decline.

Yes, there are great tools available for purchase to improve every aspect of your health and fitness. There is a supplement to replace nearly every food if you choose. But none of those things will be as effective or as beneficial if you don't work on the free things first. Your diet, you sleep, respiration, habits, mindset, and physical fitness. There are things you can and should do that cost nothing but can radically reduce your cellular stress and improve your health and quality of life. Do those things first.

If you are already doing those things and you're still struggling with chronic signs and symptoms, seek the appropriate advice. Maybe your metabolism has been too far compromised and the diet and lifestyle modifications you've done on your own just aren't enough, and you need crisis medical care. Maybe. Or maybe you need guidance from a functional medicine doctor who can help you fine-tune your fitness factors.

If you want to take a natural approach, seek out a functional medicine practitioner who understands the concepts we've laid out in this book. And when you do, get engaged. Ask the question "why" often. You need to ask why because getting the answer to the "why" is where your strategic thyroid solution lies.

We urge you not to take any of the fitness factors lightly. For example, many people are doubtful at first about how their breath could impact their thyroid physiology and their overall health. Some of those same people are later diagnosed with sleep apnea and are amazed by how much better they feel when their cells, tissues, and brain begin receiving more oxygen. Many of our patients swear that they are not mouth-breathers until they are tested and find out that they are.

Some of our most difficult patients are the ones who have the worst mindset. They are often the ones who do not believe that there is a connection between emotions, mindset, and cellular stress. They are stuck in a cycle of negative thoughts and emotions. They are paralyzed by a fear of change. Dr. Eric had a patient tell him that her negative attitude does not impact her health, and then later in the same visit told him that when she is stressed, she becomes incontinent and has difficulty sleeping. Sleep quality and duration are critical to reducing cellular stress and restoring cellular health. Cheating yourself out of sleep will have a detrimental impact on your thyroid physiology. We can both personally attest to that.

Many people want to take probiotics to improve their GI discomfort, failing to realize that probiotics are not very effective at restoring bacterial balance in the GI tract. What works better: a quality diet, exercise, emotional fitness, proper sleep, and proper respiration. Improving any or all your fitness factors works better and is cheaper than a single bottle of probiotics.

The diet craze du jour or a meal replacement shake or bar is not a substitute for good food. Almost anything of value in one of those things can be found in real food in its natural state.

You are the most valuable resource to yourself, your family, your kids, your spouse, your friends, your coworkers, and thousands of strangers as well. You may not realize it, but you have influence. You leave an impression in this world. You have more value than you allow yourself to take credit for. Realize that. Also understand that everyone in your circle of influence gets a vibe from you. You either emit positive energy, happiness, and joy or you are a black hole that robs those things from others. So you matter.

Why is this important to say? Because people are often so busy, so focused on others that they don't take time to care for themselves. They think they are not important enough to commit time to their diet, fitness, and health. They are too devoted to tending to the needs and desires of their family and friends that their own health and quality of life slowly but steadily diminish.

Don't be that person. If you want to be the best for everyone else, start by working on being your best you. Don't the flight attendants tell us to put our own oxygen masks on first? That's a lesson for your life. You are not ignoring those around you; you are just putting yourself first. It sounds pompous, but it's not. You can't give what you don't have.

You are the best thing to happen in your life and the lives of those around you. Make time for yourself. Commit to improving your fitness factors. Encourage the people around you to do the same. Small, incremental changes in a positive direction are what make good things happen in life and health. Sometimes those changes seem insignificant, yet those small, incremental changes create the ripple that becomes a tidal wave!

We hope that you have gotten value from this book. We hope that this book will help you make the changes you need to start improving your chronic hypothyroid symptoms and cellular stress so that you can turn your health and your quality of life around. We will continue to stay in touch and keep you updated on all our new research, educational opportunities, personal consultations and more at www.thyroiddebacle.com as well as on our social media. We look forward to hearing about your individual success stories, just like you've heard about our own using The New Model of thyroid care.

We sincerely appreciate you and hope you will share our message.

ENDNOTES

INTRODUCTION

1. R. K. Naviaux, "Metabolic Features of the Cell Danger Response," *Mitochondrion* 16 (May 2014): 7–17, doi:10.1016/j.mito.2013.08.006.
2. R. K. Naviaux, "Metabolic Features of the Cell Danger Response," *Mitochondrion* 16 (May 2014): 7–17, doi:10.1016/j.mito.2013.08.006.

CHAPTER 3

3. Winnifred Frolik and M. Kresimira, "What Is Hashimoto's Thyroiditis?" Endocrineweb, November 8, 2021. https://www.endocrineweb.com/conditions/hashimotos-thyroiditis/hashimotos-thyroiditis-overview
4. J. G. Hollowell, N. W. Staehling, W. D. Flanders, et al., "Serum TSH, T(4), and Thyroid Antibodies in the United States Population (1988 to 1994): National Health and Nutrition Examination Survey (NHANES III)," *Jof Clin Endocrinol Metab.* 87, no. 2 (2002): 489–99.
5. Y Aoki, R. M. Belin, R. Clickner, et al., "Serum TSH and Total T4 in the United States Population and Their Association with Participant Characteristics: National Health and Nutrition Examination Survey (NHANES 1999–2002)." *Thyroid* 17, no. 2 (2007): 1211–23.
6. V. Kumar, A. Abbas, and J. Aster, *Robbins Basic Pathology*, 10th ed. (Philadelphia, Pennsylvania: Elesvier, 2018), 749–96.
7. C. T. Sawin, W. P. Castelli, J. M.Hershman, et al., "The Aging Thyroid: Thyroid Deficiency in the Framingham Study," *Arch Inter Med* 145, no. 8 (1985), 1386–8.
8. Robert S Porter, *Merck Manual of Diagnosis and Therapy*, 19th ed. (West Point, Pennsylvania: Merck, Sharp & Dohme Corp; 2011), 755–901.
9. Ibid.

CHAPTER 4

[10] Bickley, L. *Bates' Guide to Physical Examination*, 12th edition (Philadelphia, Pennsylvania: Wolters Kulwer, 2017), 215–66.

[11] Gesunhdheit, N, "Thyroid Exam," *Stanford Medicine* 25, accessed [date], https://stanfordmedicine25.stanford.edu/the25/thyroid.html.

[12] Garber, J. R.; Cobin, R. H.; Gharib, H.; et al., "Clinical Practice Guidelines for Hypothyroidism in Adults: Cosponsored by the American Association of Clinical Endocrinologists and the American Thyroid Association," *Thyroid* 22, no. 12 (2012), 1200–35.

[13] Ibid.

[14] Ibid.

[15] Fatourechi V., "Subclinical Hypothyroidism: An Update for Primary Care Physicians," *Mayo Clin Proc.* 84 (2009), 65–71.

[16] Garber, J. R.; Cobin, R. H.; Gharib, H.; et al., "Clinical Practice Guidelines for Hypothyroidism in Adults: Cosponsored by the American Association of Clinical Endocrinologists and the American Thyroid Association," *Thyroid* 22, no. 12 (2012), 1200–35.

[17] Ibid.

[18] Ibid.

[19] Ibid.

[20] Ibid.

[21] C. Marcocci and M. Marino, "Thyroid-Directed Antibodies," in L. E. Braverman and R. Utiger, editors, *Part II Laboratory Assessment of Thyroid Function* (Philadelphia, Pennsylvania: Lippincott Williams and Wilkins, 2005), 360–72.

[22] V. Fatourechi, "Subclinical Hypothyroidism: An Update for Primary Care Physicians," *Mayo Clin Proc.* 84 (2009), 65–71.

[23] Wartofsky L, Dickey RA. The evidence for a narrower thyrotropin reference range is compelling. J Clin Endocrinol Metab. 2005;90:5483-5488.

[24] Garber, J. R.; Cobin, R. H.; Gharib, H.; et al., "Clinical Practice Guidelines for Hypothyroidism in Adults: Cosponsored by the American Association of Clinical Endocrinologists and the American Thyroid Association," *Thyroid* 22, no. 12 (2012), 1200–35.

[25] S. M. Abdalla, A. C. Bianco. "Defending Plasma T3 Is a Biological Priority," *Clin Endocrinol (Oxf)* 81, no. 5(2014), 633–41, doi:10.1111/cen.12538.

[26] Garber, J. R.; Cobin, R. H.; Gharib, H.; et al., "Clinical Practice Guidelines for Hypothyroidism in Adults: Cosponsored by the American Association of Clinical Endocrinologists and the American Thyroid Association," *Thyroid* 22, no. 12 (2012), 1200–35.

[27] Ibid.

[28] S. M. Abdalla, A. C. Bianco. "Defending Plasma T3 Is a Biological Priority," *Clin Endocrinol (Oxf)* 81, no. 5(2014), 633–41, doi:10.1111/cen.12538.

CHAPTER 5

[29] Sarah J. Peterson, Elizabeth A. McAninch, Antonio C. Bianco, Is a Normal TSH Synonymous With "Euthyroidism" in Levothyroxine Monotherapy?, The Journal of Clinical Endocrinology & Metabolism, Volume 101, Issue 12, 1 December 2016, Pages 4964–4973, https://doi.org/10.1210/jc.2016-2660

[30] Saravanan P, Chau WF, Roberts N, Vedhara K, Greenwood R, Dayan CM. Psychological well-being in patients on 'adequate' doses of l-thyroxine: results of a large, controlled community-based questionnaire study. Clin Endocrinol. 2002;57:577–585.

[31] Samuels MH, Kolobova I, Smeraglio A, Peters D, Purnell JQ, Schuff KG. Effects of levothyroxine replacement or suppressive therapy on energy expenditure and body composition. Thyroid. 2016;26:347–355.

[32] Wiersinga, W. (2017). THERAPY OF ENDOCRINE DISEASE: T4 + T3 combination therapy: is there a true effect?, European Journal of Endocrinology, 177(6), R287-R296. Retrieved Jan 11, 2020, from https://eje.bioscientifica.com/view/journals/eje/177/6/EJE-17-0645.xml

[33] Saravanan P, Chau W-F, Roberts N, Vedhara K, Greenwood R, Dayan CM. Psychological well-being in patients on 'adequate' doses of L-thyroxine: results of a large, controlled community-based questionnaire study. Clin. Endocrinol. 2002;57:577–585. doi: 10.1046/j.1365-2265.2002.01654.x

[34] Wekking EM, Appelhof BC, Fliers E, Schene AH, Huyser T, Tijssen JGP, Wiersinga WM. Cognitive functioning and well-being in euthyroid patients on thyroxine replacement therapy for primary hypothyroidism. Eur. J. Endocrinol. 2005;153:747–753. doi: 10.1530/eje.1.02025.

[35] Panicker V, Evans J, Bjoro T, Asvold BO, Dayan CM, Bjerkeset O. A paradoxical difference in relationship between anxiety, depression and thyroid function in subjects on and not on T4: findings from the HUNT study. Clin. Endocrinol. 2009;71:574–580. doi: 10.1111/j.1365-2265.2008.03521.x.

[36] Sanjay Kalra and Sachin Kumar Khandelwal, "Why Are Our Hypothyroid Patients Unhappy? Is Tissue Hypothyroidism the Answer?" Indian Journal of Endocrinology and Metabolism 15, Suppl 2 (2011): S95–8, doi:10.4103/2230-8210.83333

[37] Hannoush ZC, Weiss RE. Thyroid Hormone Replacement in Patients Following Thyroidectomy for Thyroid Cancer. Rambam Maimonides Med J. 2016;7(1):e0002. Published 2016 Jan 28. doi:10.5041/RMMJ.10229

[38] Wiersinga WM. T4 + T3 combination therapy: any progress?. Endocrine. 2019;66(1):70–78. doi:10.1007/s12020-019-02052-2

[39] Mullur R, Liu YY, Brent GA. Thyroid hormone regulation of metabolism. Physiol Rev. 2014;94(2):355–382. doi:10.1152/physrev.00030.2013

[40] Chatzitomaris A, Hoermann R, Midgley JE, et al. Thyroid Allostasis-Adaptive Responses of Thyrotropic Feedback Control to Conditions of Strain, Stress, and Developmental Programming. Front Endocrinol (Lausanne). 2017;8:163. Published 2017 Jul 20. doi:10.3389/fendo.2017.00163

[41] Hoermann R, Midgley JEM, Larisch R, Dietrich JW. Recent Advances in Thyroid Hormone Regulation: Toward a New Paradigm for Optimal Diagnosis and Treatment. Front Endocrinol (Lausanne). 2017;8:364. Published 2017 Dec 22. doi:10.3389/fendo.2017.00364

42. Kalra S, Khandelwal SK. Why are our hypothyroid patients unhappy? Is tissue hypothyroidism the answer?. Indian J Endocrinol Metab. 2011;15(Suppl 2):S95–S98. doi:10.4103/2230-8210.83333
43. Johannes W. Dietrich, Gabi Landgrafe, and Elisavet H. Fotiadou, "TSH and Thyrotropic Agonists: Key Actors in Thyroid Homeostasis," Journal of Thyroid Research, vol. 2012, Article ID 351864, 29 pages, 2012. https://doi.org/10.1155/2012/351864
44. Sheehan MT. Biochemical Testing of the Thyroid: TSH is the Best and, Oftentimes, Only Test Needed - A Review for Primary Care. Clin Med Res. 2016;14(2):83–92. doi:10.3121/cmr.2016.1309
45. Toft AD, Beckett GJ. Thyroid function tests and hypothyroidism. BMJ. 2003;326(7384):295–296. doi:10.1136/bmj.326.7384.295
46. Salman Razvi, Sindeep Bhana, and Sanaa Mrabeti, "Challenges in Interpreting Thyroid Stimulating Hormone Results in the Diagnosis of Thyroid Dysfunction," Journal of Thyroid Research, vol. 2019, Article ID 4106816, 8 pages, 2019. https://doi.org/10.1155/2019/4106816
47. Pahwa R, Singh A, Jialal I. Chronic Inflammation. [Updated 2019 Dec 13]. In: StatPearls [Internet]. Treasure Island (FL): StatPearls Publishing; 2019 Jan-. Available from: https://www.ncbi.nlm.nih.gov/books/NBK493173/
48. Straub RH. Interaction of the endocrine system with inflammation: a function of energy and volume regulation. Arthritis Res Ther. 2014;16(1):203. Published 2014 Feb 13. doi:10.1186/ar4484
49. E. M. de Vries, S. Nagel, R. Haenold, S. M. Sundaram, F. W. Pfrieger, E. Fliers, H. Heuer, A. Boelen, The Role of Hypothalamic NF-κB Signaling in the Response of the HPT-Axis to Acute Inflammation in Female Mice, Endocrinology, Volume 157, Issue 7, 1 July 2016, Pages 2947–2956, https://doi.org/10.1210/en.2016-1027
50. Leung AM. Thyroid Emergencies. J Infus Nurs. 2016;39(5):281–286. doi:10.1097/NAN.0000000000000186
51. Marcocci C, Marino M. Thyroid-directed antibodies. In: Braverman LE, Utiger R, editors., editors. Part II Laboratory Assessment of Thyroid Function. Philadelphia, PA: Lippincott Williams and Wilkins; (2005). p. 360–72.
52. Fröhlich E, Wahl R. Thyroid Autoimmunity: Role of Anti-thyroid Antibodies in Thyroid and Extra-Thyroidal Diseases. Front Immunol. 2017;8:521. Published 2017 May 9. doi:10.3389/fimmu.2017.00521
53. Gomes-Lima C, Burman KD. Reverse T3 or perverse T3? Still puzzling after 40 years. Cleveland Clinic Journal of Medicine. 2018 Jun;85(6):450-455. DOI: 10.3949/ccjm.85a.17079.
54. Robert Udelsman and Yawei Zhang.Thyroid.Mar 2014.ahead of printhttp://doi.org/10.1089/thy.2013.0257
55. https://columbiasurgery.org/thyroid/thyroid-cancer-diagnosis
56. Bianco AC, Kim BW. Deiodinases: implications of the local control of thyroid hormone action. J Clin Invest. 2006;116(10):2571–2579. doi:10.1172/JCI29812
57. Hoermann R, Midgley JEM, Larisch R, Dietrich JW. Recent Advances in Thyroid Hormone Regulation: Toward a New Paradigm for Optimal Diagnosis and Treatment. Front Endocrinol (Lausanne). 2017;8:364. Published 2017 Dec 22. doi:10.3389/fendo.2017.00364

58 Bianco AC, Kim BW. Deiodinases: implications of the local control of thyroid hormone action. J Clin Invest. 2006;116(10):2571–2579. doi:10.1172/JCI29812
59 Chatzitomaris A, Hoermann R, Midgley JE, et al. Thyroid Allostasis-Adaptive Responses of Thyrotropic Feedback Control to Conditions of Strain, Stress, and Developmental Programming. Front Endocrinol (Lausanne). 2017;8:163. Published 2017 Jul 20. doi:10.3389/fendo.2017.00163
60 Peterson SJ, McAninch EA, Bianco AC. Is a Normal TSH Synonymous With "Euthyroidism" in Levothyroxine Monotherapy? J Clin Endocrinol Metab. 2016 Dec;101(12):4964-4973. doi: 10.1210/jc.2016-2660. Epub 2016 Oct 4. Erratum in: J Clin Endocrinol Metab. 2017 Apr 1;102(4):1406. PMID: 27700539; PMCID: PMC6287526.
61 Hoermann R, Midgley JE, Larisch R, Dietrich JW. Relational Stability in the Expression of Normality, Variation, and Control of Thyroid Function. Front Endocrinol (Lausanne). 2016;7:142. Published 2016 Nov 7. doi:10.3389/fendo.2016.00142
62 Ibid.
63 Franco JS, Amaya-Amaya J, Anaya JM. Thyroid disease and autoimmune diseases. In: Anaya JM, Shoenfeld Y, Rojas-Villarraga A, et al., editors. Autoimmunity: From Bench to Bedside [Internet]. Bogota (Colombia): El Rosario University Press; 2013 Jul 18. Chapter 30. Available from: https://www.ncbi.nlm.nih.gov/books/NBK459466/
64 Hoermann R, Midgley JEM, Larisch R, Dietrich JW. Individualised requirements for optimum treatment of hypothyroidism: complex needs, limited options. Drugs Context. 2019;8:212597. Published 2019 Aug 13. doi:10.7573/dic.212597
65 Razvi S, Bhana S, Mrabeti S. Challenges in Interpreting Thyroid Stimulating Hormone Results in the Diagnosis of Thyroid Dysfunction. J Thyroid Res. 2019;2019:4106816. Published 2019 Sep 22. doi:10.1155/2019/4106816
66 Ibid.
67 Hoermann R, Midgley JEM, Larisch R, Dietrich JW. Individualised requirements for optimum treatment of hypothyroidism: complex needs, limited options. Drugs Context. 2019;8:212597. Published 2019 Aug 13. doi:10.7573/dic.212597

CHAPTER 6

68 National Institute of Diabetes and Digestive and Kidney Diseases (NIDDK). U.S. Department of Health and Human Services. August 2016. https://www.niddk.nih.gov/health-information/endocrine-diseases/hypothyroidism
69 Moncayo R, Moncayo H. Applying a systems approach to thyroid physiology: Looking at the whole with a mitochondrial perspective instead of judging single TSH values or why we should know more about mitochondria to understand metabolism. BBA Clin. 2017;7:127–140. Published 2017 Apr 4. doi:10.1016/j.bbacli.2017.03.004
70 Brown BT, Bonello R, Pollard H. The biopsychosocial model and hypothyroidism. Chiropr Osteopat. 2005;13(1):5. Published 2005 Apr 12. doi:10.1186/1746-1340-13-5
71 https://thyroidpatients.ca/2019/06/01/question-pilos-study-thyroid-hormone-reductionism/

72 Sheehan MT. Biochemical Testing of the Thyroid: TSH is the Best and, Oftentimes, Only Test Needed - A Review for Primary Care. Clin Med Res. 2016;14(2):83-92. doi:10.3121/cmr.2016.1309

73 Sheikh SI, Parikh TP, Kushchayeva Y, Stolze B, Masika LS, Ozarda Y, et al. TSH Should not be used as a Single Marker of Thyroid Function. Annals Thyroid Res. 2018; 4(2): 151-154.

74 Ling C, Sun Q, Khang J, et al. Does TSH Reliably Detect Hypothyroid Patients?. Ann Thyroid Res. 2018;4(1):122–125.

75 Hoermann R, Midgley JE, Larisch R, Dietrich JW. Homeostatic Control of the Thyroid-Pituitary Axis: Perspectives for Diagnosis and Treatment. Front Endocrinol (Lausanne). 2015;6:177. Published 2015 Nov 20. doi:10.3389/fendo.2015.00177

76 R. Hoermann, J. E. M Midgley, R. Larisch, and J. W. Dietrich, "Individualized Requirements for Optimum Treatment of Hypothyroidism: Complex Needs, Limited Options," *Drugs Context.* 8, no. 212597 (2019), doi:10.7573/dic.212597.

77 Razvi S, Bhana S, Mrabeti S. Challenges in Interpreting Thyroid Stimulating Hormone Results in the Diagnosis of Thyroid Dysfunction. J Thyroid Res. 2019;2019:4106816. Published 2019 Sep 22. doi:10.1155/2019/4106816

78 Lewandowski K. Reference ranges for TSH and thyroid hormones. Thyroid Res. 2015;8(Suppl 1):A17. Published 2015 Jun 22. doi:10.1186/1756-6614-8-S1-A17

79 Midgley, J.E.M., Toft, A.D., Larisch, R. et al. Time for a reassessment of the treatment of hypothyroidism. BMC Endocr Disord 19, 37 (2019). https://doi.org/10.1186/s12902-019-0365-4

80 Kalra S, Khandelwal SK. Why are our hypothyroid patients unhappy? Is tissue hypothyroidism the answer?. Indian J Endocrinol Metab. 2011;15(Suppl 2):S95–S98. doi:10.4103/2230-8210.83333

81 Hoermann R, Midgley JEM, Larisch R, Dietrich JW. Individualized requirements for optimum treatment of hypothyroidism: complex needs, limited options. Drugs Context. 2019;8:212597. Published 2019 Aug 13. doi:10.7573/dic.212597

82 Hennemann G, Krenning EP. The kinetics of thyroid hormone transporters and their role in non-thyroidal illness and starvation. Best Pract Res Clin Endocrinol Metab. 2007;21(2):323–338. doi:10.1016/j.beem.2007.03.007

83 Fu J, Dumitrescu AM. Inherited defects in thyroid hormone cell-membrane transport and metabolism. Best Pract Res Clin Endocrinol Metab. 2014;28(2):189–201. doi:10.1016/j.beem.2013.05.014

84 Rosalia Lavado-Autric, Rosa Maria Calvo, Raquel Martinez de Mena, Gabriella Morreale de Escobar, Maria-Jesus Obregon, Deiodinase Activities in Thyroids and Tissues of Iodine-Deficient Female Rats, Endocrinology, Volume 154, Issue 1, 1 January 2013, Pages 529–536, https://doi.org/10.1210/en.2012-1727

85 Larsen PR, Zavacki AM. The role of the iodothyronine deiodinases in the physiology and pathophysiology of thyroid hormone action. Eur Thyroid J. 2012;1(4):232–242. doi:10.1159/000343922

86 Hoermann R, Midgley JE, Larisch R, Dietrich JW. Homeostatic Control of the Thyroid-Pituitary Axis: Perspectives for Diagnosis and Treatment. Front Endocrinol (Lausanne). 2015;6:177. Published 2015 Nov 20. doi:10.3389/fendo.2015.00177

CHAPTER 7

[87] Luongo, C., Dentice, M. & Salvatore, D. Deiodinases and their intricate role in thyroid hormone homeostasis. Nat Rev Endocrinol 15, 479–488 (2019). https://doi.org/10.1038/s41574-019-0218-2

[88] Abdalla SM, Bianco AC. Defending plasma T3 is a biological priority. Clin Endocrinol (Oxf). 2014 Nov;81(5):633-41. doi: 10.1111/cen.12538. Epub 2014 Aug 7. PMID: 25040645; PMCID: PMC4699302.

[89] Larsen PR, Zavacki AM. The role of the iodothyronine deiodinases in the physiology and pathophysiology of thyroid hormone action. Eur Thyroid J. 2012;1(4):232–242. doi:10.1159/000343922

[90] Kalra S, Khandelwal SK. Why are our hypothyroid patients unhappy? Is tissue hypothyroidism the answer?. Indian J Endocrinol Metab. 2011;15(Suppl 2):S95–S98. doi:10.4103/2230-8210.83333

[91] Ferrandino G, Kaspari RR, Spadaro O, et al. Pathogenesis of hypothyroidism-induced NAFLD is driven by intra- and extrahepatic mechanisms. Proc Natl Acad Sci U S A. 2017;114(43):E9172–E9180. doi:10.1073/pnas.1707797114

[92] Midgley, J.E.M., Toft, A.D., Larisch, R. et al. Time for a reassessment of the treatment of hypothyroidism. BMC Endocr Disord 19, 37 (2019). https://doi.org/10.1186/s12902-019-0365-4

[93] O'Reilly DS. Thyroid function tests-time for a reassessment. BMJ. 2000;320(7245):1332–1334. doi:10.1136/bmj.320.7245.1332

[94] Offie P. Soldin, When Thyroidologists Agree to Disagree: Comments on the 2012 Endocrine Society Pregnancy and Thyroid Disease Clinical Practice Guideline, The Journal of Clinical Endocrinology & Metabolism, Volume 97, Issue 8, 1 August 2012, Pages 2632–2635, https://doi.org/10.1210/jc.2012-2529

[95] https://www.ncbi.nlm.nih.gov/pmc/articles/PMC6726361/pdf/dic-8-212597.pdf

[96] Hoermann R, Midgley JEM, Larisch R, Dietrich JW. Recent Advances in Thyroid Hormone Regulation: Toward a New Paradigm for Optimal Diagnosis and Treatment. Front Endocrinol (Lausanne). 2017;8:364. Published 2017 Dec 22. doi:10.3389/fendo.2017.00364

[97] Villar HC, Saconato H, Valente O, Atallah AN. Thyroid hormone replacement for subclinical hypothyroidism. Cochrane Database Syst Rev. 2007;2007(3):CD003419. Published 2007 Jul 18. doi:10.1002/14651858.CD003419.pub2

[98] Bekkering G E, Agoritsas T, Lytvyn L, Heen A F, Feller M, Moutzouri E et al. Thyroid hormones treatment for subclinical hypothyroidism: a clinical practice guideline BMJ 2019; 365 :l2006

[99] https://www.liebertpub.com/doi/10.1089/ct.2019%3B31.285-287

CHAPTER 8

[100] Calvo RM, Garcia L, Vesperinas G, Corripio R, Rubio MA, et al. (2017) Deiodinases in Human Adipose Tissue from Obese Patients. Differences by Gender and Anatomical Depot. JSM Thyroid Disord Manag 2(1): 1009

101 Antonio C. Bianco and Brian W. Kim, "Deiodinases: Implications of the Local Control of Thyroid Hormone Action," Journal of Clinical Investigation 116, no. 10 (2006): 2571–9, doi:10.1172/JCI29812

102 Ibid

103 Robin P. Peeters, MD, PhD, and Theo J Visser, PhD, "Metabolism of Thyroid Hormone," iIn: K. R. Feingold, B. Anawalt, A. Boyce, et al., editors. Endotext [Internet]. South Darmouth, MA: MDText.com, Inc.; 2000–. Available from www.ncbi.nlm.nih.gov/books/NBK285545/

104 Antonio Mancini, Chantal Di Segni, Sebastiano Raimondo, Guilio Olivieri, Andrea Silvestrini, Elisabetta Meucci, and Diego Currò, "Thyroid Hormones, Oxidative Stress, and Inflammation," Mediators of Inflammation (2016): 6757154, doi:10.1155/2016/6757154

105 Antonio C. Bianco and Brian W. Kim, "Deiodinases: Implications of the Local Control of Thyroid Hormone Action," Journal of Clinical Investigation 116, no. 10 (2006): 2571–9, doi:10.1172/JCI29812

106 Antonio Mancini, Chantal Di Segni, Sebastiano Raimondo, Guilio Olivieri, Andrea Silvestrini, Elisabetta Meucci, and Diego Currò, "Thyroid Hormones, Oxidative Stress, and Inflammation," Mediators of Inflammation (2016): 6757154, doi:10.1155/2016/6757154

107 Antonio C. Bianco and Brian W. Kim, "Deiodinases: Implications of the Local Control of Thyroid Hormone Action," Journal of Clinical Investigation 116, no. 10 (2006): 2571–9, doi:10.1172/JCI29812

108 Ibid

109 Sherine M. Abdalla and Antonio C. Bianco,. "Defending Plasma T3 Is a Biological Priority,." Clinical Endocrinology 81, no. 5 (2014): 633–41, doi:10.1111/cen.12538

110 Sanya Kalra and Sachin Kumar Khandelwal, "Why Are Our Hypothyroid Patients Unhappy? Is Tissue Hypothyroidism the Answer?," Indian Journal of Endocrinology and Metabolism 15, Suppl 2 (2011): S95–8, doi:10.4103/2230-8210.83333

111 Apostolos Chatzitomaris, Rudolf Hoermann, John E. Midgley, Steffen Hering, Aline Urban, Barbara Dietrich, Assjana Abood, et al., "Thyroid Allostasis–Adaptive Responses of Thyrotropic Feedback Control to Conditions of Strain, Stress, and Developmental Programming," Frontiers in Endocrinology 8 (2017): 163, doi:10.3389/fendo.2017.00163

112 Ibid

113 Antonio Mancini, Chantal Di Segni, Sebastiano Raimondo, Guilio Olivieri, Andrea Silvestrini, Elisabetta Meucci, and Diego Currò, "Thyroid Hormones, Oxidative Stress, and Inflammation," Mediators of Inflammation (2016): 6757154, doi:10.1155/2016/6757154

114 Apostolos Chatzitomaris, Rudolf Hoermann, John E. Midgley, Steffen Hering, Aline Urban, Barbara Dietrich, Assjana Abood, et al., "Thyroid Allostasis–Adaptive Responses of Thyrotropic Feedback Control to Conditions of Strain, Stress, and Developmental Programming," Frontiers in Endocrinology 8 (2017): 163, doi:10.3389/fendo.2017.00163

115 Sanya Kalra and Sachin Kumar Khandelwal, "Why Are Our Hypothyroid Patients Unhappy? Is Tissue Hypothyroidism the Answer?," Indian Journal of Endocrinology and Metabolism 15, Suppl 2 (2011): S95–8, doi:10.4103/2230-8210.83333

[116] Antonio C. Bianco and Brian W. Kim, "Deiodinases: Implications of the Local Control of Thyroid Hormone Action," Journal of Clinical Investigation 116, no. 10 (2006): 2571–9, doi:10.1172/JCI29812

[117] Hennemann G, Docter R, Friesema EC, de Jong M, Krenning EP, Visser TJ. Plasma membrane transport of thyroid hormones and its role in thyroid hormone metabolism and bioavailability. Endocr Rev. 2001 Aug;22(4):451-76. doi: 10.1210/edrv.22.4.0435. PMID: 11493579.

[118] Cicatiello AG, Di Girolamo D, Dentice M. Metabolic Effects of the Intracellular Regulation of Thyroid Hormone: Old Players, New Concepts. Front Endocrinol (Lausanne). 2018 Sep 11;9:474. doi: 10.3389/fendo.2018.00474. PMID: 30254607; PMCID: PMC6141630.

[119] Antonio C. Bianco, "Cracking the Code For Thyroid Hormone Signaling," Transactions of the American Clinical and Climatological Association 124 (2013): 26–35.

[120] Rashmi Mullur, Yan-Yun Liu, and Gregory A. Brent, "Thyroid Hormone Regulation of Metabolism," Physiological Reviews 94, no. 2 (2014): 355–82, doi:10.1152/physrev.00030.2013

[121] Giuseppe Ferrandino, Rachel R. Kaspari, Olga Spadaro, Andrea Reyna-Neyra, Rachel J. Perry, Rebecca Cardone, Richard G. Kibby, et al., "Pathogenesis of Hypothyroidism-Induced NAFLD Is Driven by Intra- and Extrahepatic Mechanisms," Proceedings of the National Academy of Sciences of the United States of America 114, no. 43 (2017): E9172–80, doi:10.1073/pnas.1707797114

[122] Sinha R, Yen PM. Cellular Action of Thyroid Hormone. [Updated 2018 Jun 20]. In: Feingold KR, Anawalt B, Boyce A, et al., editors. Endotext [Internet]. South Dartmouth (MA): MDText.com, Inc.; 2000-. Available from: https://www.ncbi.nlm.nih.gov/books/NBK285568/

[123] McAninch EA, Bianco AC. Thyroid hormone signaling in energy homeostasis and energy metabolism. Ann N Y Acad Sci. 2014;1311:77-87. doi:10.1111/nyas.12374

[124] Groeneweg S, van Geest FS, Peeters RP, Heuer H, Visser WE. Thyroid Hormone Transporters. Endocr Rev. 2020 Apr 1;41(2):bnz008. doi: 10.1210/endrev/bnz008. PMID: 31754699.

[125] Steve R. Pieczenik and John Neustadt, "Mitochondrial Dysfunction and Molecular Pathways of Disease," Experimental and Molecular Pathology 83, no. 1 (2007): 84–92, doi:10.1016/j.yexmp.2006.09.008

[126] Douglas C. Wallace, "A Mitochondrial Paradigm of Metabolic and Degenerative Diseases, Aging, and Cancer: A Dawn for Evolutionary Medicine," Annual Reviews of Genetics 39, no. 1 (2005): 359–407, doi:10.1146/annurev.genet.39.110304.095751

[127] Steve R. Pieczenik and John Neustadt, "Mitochondrial Dysfunction and Molecular Pathways of Disease," Experimental and Molecular Pathology 83, no. 1 (2007): 84–92, doi:10.1016/j.yexmp.2006.09.008

[128] Haim Einat, Peixiong Yuan, and Husseini K. Manji, "Increased Anxiety-Like Behaviors and Mitochondrial Dysfunction in Mice with Targeted Mutation of the Bcl-2 Gene: Further Support for the Involvement of Mitochondrial Function in Anxiety Disorders," Behavioural Brain Research 165, no. 2 (2005): 172–80, doi:10.1016/j.bbr.2005.06.012

129. Steve R. Pieczenik and John Neustadt, "Mitochondrial Dysfunction and Molecular Pathways of Disease," Experimental and Molecular Pathology 83, no. 1 (2007): 84–92, doi:10.1016/j.yexmp.2006.09.008
130. M. Corral-Debrinski, J. M. Shoffner, M. T. Lott, and D. C. Wallace, "Association of Mitochondrial DNA Damage with Aging and Coronary Atherosclerotic Heart Disease," Mutation Research/DNAging 275, no. 3–6 (1992): 169–80, doi:10.1016/0921-8734(92)90021-g
131. Suzanne Nelso Steen, Robert A. Opplieger, and Kelly D. Brownell, "Metabolic Effects of Repeated Weight and Regain in Adolescent Wrestlers," JAMA 260, no. 1 (1988): 47–50, doi:10.1001/jama.1988.03410010055034
132. D. L. Elliot, L. Goldberg, K. S Kuehl, and W. M. Bennett, "Sustained Depression of the Resting Metabolic Rate After Massive Weight Loss," American Journal of Clinical Nutrition 49, no. 1 (1989): 93–6, doi:10.1093/ajcn/49.1.93
133. Steve R. Pieczenik and John Neustadt, "Mitochondrial Dysfunction and Molecular Pathways of Disease," Experimental and Molecular Pathology 83, no. 1 (2007): 84–92, doi:10.1016/j.yexmp.2006.09.008
134. Stefaina Fulle, Patrizia Mecocci, Giorgio Fanó, Iacopo Vecchiet, Alba Veccini, Delia Racciotti, Antonio Cherebini, et al., "Specific Oxidative Alterations in Vastus Lateralis Muscle of Patients with the Diagnosis of Chronic Fatigue Syndrome," Free Radical Biology and Medicine 29, no. 12 (2000): 1252–59, doi:10.1016/S0891-5849(00)00419-6
135. Robert Buist, "Elevated Xenobiotics, Lactate and Pyruvate in C.F.S. Patient s," Journal of Orthomolecular Medicine 4, no. 3 (1989): 170–2.
136. Steve R. Pieczenik and John Neustadt, "Mitochondrial Dysfunction and Molecular Pathways of Disease," Experimental and Molecular Pathology 83, no. 1 (2007): 84–92, doi:10.1016/j.yexmp.2006.09.008
137. Josephine S. Modica-Napolitano and Perry F. Renshaw, "Ethanolamine and Phosphoethanolamine Inhibit Mitochondrial Function in Vitro: Implications for Mitochondrial Dysfunction Hypothesis in Depression and Bipolar Disorder," Biological Psychiatry 55, no. 3 (2004): 273–7, doi:10.1016/S0006-3223(03)00784-4
138. A. Gardner and R. G. Boles, "Mitochondrial Energy Depletion in Depression with Somatization," Psychotherapy and Psychosomatics 77, no. 2 (2008): 127–29, doi:10.1159/000112891
139. Stephanie Burroughs and Denise French, "Depression and Anxiety: Role of Mitochondria," Current Anesthesia & Critical Care 18, no. 1 (2007): 34–41, doi:10.1016/j.cacc.2007.01.007
140. Steve R. Pieczenik and John Neustadt, "Mitochondrial Dysfunction and Molecular Pathways of Disease," Experimental and Molecular Pathology 83, no. 1 (2007): 84–92, doi:10.1016/j.yexmp.2006.09.008
141. Jane H. Park, Kenneth J. Niermann, and Nancy Olsen, "Evidence for Metabolic Abnormalities in the Muscles of Patients with Fibromyalgia," Current Rheumatology Reports 2, no. 2 (2000): 131–40, doi:10.1007/s11926-000-0053-3
142. M. B. Yunus, U. P. Kalyan-Raman, and K. Kalyan-Raman, "Primary Fibromyalgia Syndrome and Myofascial Pain Syndrome: Clinical Features and Muscle Pathology," Archives of Physical Medicine Rehabilitation 69, no. 6 (1988): 451–4.

[143] M. E. Everts, C. F. Lim, E. P. Moerings, R. Docter, T. J. Visser, M. De Jong, E. P. Krenning, and G. Hennemann, "Effects of a Furan Fatty Acid and Indoxyl Sulfate on Thyroid Hormone Uptake in Cultured Anterior Pituitary Cells," American Journal of Physiology 268, 5 Pt 1 (1995): E974–9, doi:0.1152/ajpendo.1995.268.5.E974

[144] Nancy M. DeMarco, Donald C. Beitz, and Gernett B. Whitehurst, "Effect of Fasting on Free Fatty Acid, Glycerol and Cholesterol Concentrations in Blood Plasma and Lipoprotein Lipase Activity in Adipose Tissue of Cattle," Journal of Animal Science 52 (1981): 75–82, doi:10.2527/jas1981.52175x

[145] Steve R. Pieczenik and John Neustadt, "Mitochondrial Dysfunction and Molecular Pathways of Disease," Experimental and Molecular Pathology 83, no. 1 (2007): 84–92, doi:10.1016/j.yexmp.2006.09.008

[146] Elaine M. Kaptein, Eben I. Feinstein, John T. Nicoloff, and Shaul G. Massry, "Serum Reverse Triiodothyronine and Thyroxine Kinetics in Patients with Chronic Renal Failure" Journal of Clinical Endocrinology & Metabolism 57, no. 1 (1983): 181–9, doi:10.1210/jcem-57-1-181

[147] Elaine M. Kaptein, "Clinical Relevance of Thyroid Hormone Alterations in Nonthyroidal Illness," Thyroid Int 4 (1997): 22–5.

[148] Gabriela Brenta, "Why Can Insulin Resistance Be a Natural Consequence of Thyroid Dysfunction?," Journal of Thyroid Research (2011): 152850, https://doi.org/10.4061/2011/152850.

[149] Jula Szendroedi, Albrecht Ingo Schmid, Martin Meyerspeer, Camilla Cervin, Michaela Kacerovsky, Gerhard Smekal, Sabine Gräser-Lang, et al., "Impaired Mitochondrial Function and Insulin Resistance of Skeletal Muscle in Mitochondrial Diabetes," Diabetes Care 32, no. 4 (2009): 677–9, doi:10.2337/dc08-2078

[150] Kitt F. Petersen, Sylvie Dufour, and Gerald I. Shulman, "Decreased Insulin-Stimulated ATP Synthesis and Phosphate Transport in Muscle of Insulin-Resistant Offspring of Type 2 Diabetic Parents," PLoS Medicine 2, no. 9 (2005): e233, doi:10.1371/journal.pmed.0020233

[151] M. A. Abdul-Ghani, R. Jani, A. Chavez, M. Molina-Carrion, D. Tripathy, and R. A. DeFronzo, "Mitochondrial Reactive Oxygen Species Generation in Obese Non-Diabetic and Type 2 Diabetic Participants," Diabetologia 52, no. 4 (2009): 574–82, https://doi.org/10.1007/s00125-009-1264-4

[152] Steve R. Pieczenik and John Neustadt, "Mitochondrial Dysfunction and Molecular Pathways of Disease," Experimental and Molecular Pathology 83, no. 1 (2007): 84–92, doi:10.1016/j.yexmp.2006.09.008

[153] Carmen Gomez, Manuel J. Bandez, and Ana Navarro, "Pesticides and Impairment of Mitochondrial Function in Relation with the Parkinsonian Syndrome," Frontiers in Bioscience 12 (2007): 1079–93, doi:10.2741/2128

[154] T. Hutchin and G. Cortopassi, "A Mitochondrial DNA Clone Is Associated with Increased Risk for Alzheimer's Disease," Proceedings of the National Academy of Sciences of the United States of America 92, no. 15 (1995): 6892–5, doi:10.1073/pnas.92.15.6892

[155] Kitt F. Petersen, Sylvie Dufour, and Gerald I. Shulman, "Decreased Insulin-Stimulated ATP Synthesis and Phosphate Transport in Muscle of Insulin-Resistant Offspring of Type 2 Diabetic Parents," PLoS Medicine 2, no. 9 (2005): e233, doi:10.1371/journal.pmed.0020233

156 M. A. Abdul-Ghani, R. Jani, A. Chavez, M. Molina-Carrion, D. Tripathy, and R. A. DeFronzo, "Mitochondrial Reactive Oxygen Species Generation in Obese Non-Diabetic and Type 2 Diabetic Participants," Diabetologia 52, no. 4 (2009): 574–82, https://doi.org/10.1007/s00125-009-1264-4

157 Robin P. Peeters, MD, PhD, and Theo J Visser, PhD, "Metabolism of Thyroid Hormone," iIn: K. R. Feingold, B. Anawalt, A. Boyce, et al., editors. Endotext [Internet]. South Darmouth, MA: MDText.com, Inc.; 2000–. Available from www.ncbi.nlm.nih.gov/books/NBK285545/

158 Stephanie Burroughs and Denise French, "Depression and Anxiety: Role of Mitochondria," Current Anesthesia & Critical Care 18, no. 1 (2007): 34–41, doi:10.1016/j.cacc.2007.01.007

159 Munira Baqui, Diego Botero, Balazs Gereben, Cyntia Curcio, John W. Harney, Domenico Salvatore, Kenji Sorimachi, et al., "Human Type 3 Iodothyronine Selenodeiodinase Is Located in the Plasma Membrane and Undergoes Rapid Internalization to Endosomes." Journal of Biological Chemistry 278, no. 2 (2003): 1206–11, doi:10.1074/jbc.M210266200

160 Sinha R, Yen PM. Cellular Action of Thyroid Hormone. [Updated 2018 Jun 20]. In: Feingold KR, Anawalt B, Boyce A, et al., editors. Endotext [Internet]. South Dartmouth (MA): MDText.com, Inc.; 2000-. Available from: https://www.ncbi.nlm.nih.gov/books/NBK285568/

161 Antonio C. Bianco and Brian W. Kim, "Deiodinases: Implications of the Local Control of Thyroid Hormone Action," Journal of Clinical Investigation 116, no. 10 (2006): 2571–9, doi:10.1172/JCI29812

162 van der Spek AH, Fliers E, Boelen A. The classic pathways of thyroid hormone metabolism. Mol Cell Endocrinol. 2017 Dec 15;458:29-38. doi: 10.1016/j.mce.2017.01.025. Epub 2017 Jan 18. PMID: 28109953.

163 Ibid

164 E. A. McAninch and A. C. Bianco, "Thyroid Hormone Signaling in Energy Homeostasis and Energy Metabolism," *Ann N Y Acad Sci* 1311 (2014), 77–87, doi:10.1111/nyas.12374.

165 Fröhlich E, Wahl R. Thyroid Autoimmunity: Role of Anti-thyroid Antibodies in Thyroid and Extra-Thyroidal Diseases. Front Immunol. 2017;8:521. Published 2017 May 9. doi:10.3389/fimmu.2017.00521

166 Mancini A, Di Segni C, Raimondo S, et al. Thyroid Hormones, Oxidative Stress, and Inflammation. Mediators Inflamm. 2016;2016:6757154. doi:10.1155/2016/6757154

167 Paul J. Davis, "How Thyroid Hormone Works Depends on Cell Type, Receptor Type and Hormone Analogue: Implications in Cancer Growth," Discovery Medicine, accessed December 3, 2019, www.discoverymedicine.com/Paul-J-Davis/index.php

168 Meng-Ti Hsieh, Le-Ming Wang, Chun A. Changou, Yu-Tang Chin, Yu-Chen S. H Yang, Hsuan-Yu Lai, Shen-Yang Lee, et al., "Crosstalk Between Integrin αvβ3 and ERα Contributes to Thyroid Hormone-Induced Proliferation of Ovarian Cancer Cells," Oncotarget 8, no. 15 (2017): 24237–49, doi:10.18632/oncotarget.10757

169 Elena Shinderman-Maman, Keren Cohen, Dotan Moskovich, Aleck Hercbergs, Haim Werner, Paul J. Davis, Martin Ellis, and Osnat Ashur-Fabian, "Thyroid Hormones

Derivatives Reduce Proliferation and Induce Cell Death and DNA Damage in Ovarian Cancer," Scientific Reports 7, no. 16475 (2017), doi:10.1038/s41598-017-16593-x

CHAPTER 9

[170] Naviaux RK. Metabolic features of the cell danger response. Mitochondrion. 2014 May;16:7-17. doi: 10.1016/j.mito.2013.08.006. Epub 2013 Aug 24. PMID: 23981537.

[171] "5 Roles Mitochondria Play in Cells," Immunology & Microbiology, dated June 6, 2017. www.technologynetworks.com/immunology/lists/5-roles-mitochondria-play-in-cells-289354

[172] Martin Picard, Bruce S. McEwen, Elissa S. Epel, and Carmen Sandi, "An Energetic View of Stress: Focus on Mitochondria," Frontiers in Neuroendocrinology 49 (2018): 72–85, doi:10.1016/j.yfrne.2018.01.001

[173] Elizabeth A. McAninch and Antonio C. Bianco, "Thyroid Hormone Signaling in Energy Homeostasis and Energy Metabolism," Annals of the New York Academy of Sciences 1311 (2014): 77–87, doi:10.1111/nyas.12374

[174] Daolin Tang, Rui Kang, Carolyn B. Coyne, Herbert J. Zeh, and Michael T. Lotze, "PAMPs and DAMPs: Signal 0s That Spur Autophagy and Immunity," Immunological Reviews 249, no. 1(2012): 158–75, doi:10.1111/j.1600-065X.2012.01146.x

[175] Guo Q, Wu Y, Hou Y, et al. Cytokine Secretion and Pyroptosis of Thyroid Follicular Cells Mediated by Enhanced NLRP3, NLRP1, NLRC4, and AIM2 Inflammasomes Are Associated With Autoimmune Thyroiditis. Front Immunol. 2018;9:1197. Published 2018 Jun 4. doi:10.3389/fimmu.2018.01197

[176] Kawashima A, Yamazaki K, Hara T, Akama T, Yoshihara A, Sue M, Tanigawa K, Wu H, Ishido Y, Takeshita F, Ishii N, Sato K, Suzuki K. Demonstration of innate immune responses in the thyroid gland: potential to sense danger and a possible trigger for autoimmune reactions. Thyroid. 2013 Apr;23(4):477-87. doi: 10.1089/thy.2011.0480. Epub 2013 Mar 18. PMID: 23234343; PMCID: PMC3610444.

[177] Chen Y, McMillan-Ward E, Kong J, Israels SJ, Gibson SB. Oxidative stress induces autophagic cell death independent of apoptosis in transformed and cancer cells. Cell Death Differ. 2008 Jan;15(1):171-82. doi: 10.1038/sj.cdd.4402233. Epub 2007 Oct 5. PMID: 17917680.

[178] Daolin Tang, Rui Kang, Carolyn B. Coyne, Herbert J. Zeh, and Michael T. Lotze, "PAMPs and DAMPs: Signal 0s That Spur Autophagy and Immunity," Immunological Reviews 249, no. 1(2012): 158–75, doi:10.1111/j.1600-065X.2012.01146.x

[179] Kawashima A, Yamazaki K, Hara T, Akama T, Yoshihara A, Sue M, Tanigawa K, Wu H, Ishido Y, Takeshita F, Ishii N, Sato K, Suzuki K. Demonstration of innate immune responses in the thyroid gland: potential to sense danger and a possible trigger for autoimmune reactions. Thyroid. 2013 Apr;23(4):477-87. doi: 10.1089/thy.2011.0480. Epub 2013 Mar 18. PMID: 23234343; PMCID: PMC3610444.

[180] Ibid

[181] Kawashima A, Tanigawa K, Akama T, Yoshihara A, Ishii N, Suzuki K. Innate immune activation and thyroid autoimmunity. J Clin Endocrinol Metab. 2011 Dec;96(12):3661-71. doi: 10.1210/jc.2011-1568. Epub 2011 Sep 28. PMID: 21956420.

[182] Giuliani C, Verrocchio S, Verginelli F, Bucci I, Grassadonia A, Napolitano G. Hormonal Regulation of the MHC Class I Gene in Thyroid Cells: Role of the Promoter "Tissue-Specific" Region. Front Endocrinol (Lausanne). 2021 Dec 6;12:749609. doi: 10.3389/fendo.2021.749609. PMID: 34938270; PMCID: PMC8685237.

[183] Norikazu Harii, Christopher J. Lewis, Vasilly Vasko, Kelly McCall, Uruguaysito Benavides-Peralta, Xiaolu Sun, Matthew D. Ringel, et al., "Thyrocytes Express a Functional Toll-Like Receptor 3: Overexpression Can Be Induced by Viral Infection and Reversed by Phenylmethimazole and Is Associated with Hashimoto's Autoimmune Thyroiditis," Molecular Endocrinology 19, no. 5 (2005): 1231–50, doi:10.1210/me.2004-0100

CHAPTER 10

[184] Sun X, Liu W, Zhang B, Shen X, Hu C, Chen X, Jin S, Jiang Y, Liu H, Cao Z, Xia W, Xu S, Li Y. Maternal Heavy Metal Exposure, Thyroid Hormones, and Birth Outcomes: A Prospective Cohort Study. J Clin Endocrinol Metab. 2019 Nov 1;104(11):5043-5052. doi: 10.1210/jc.2018-02492. PMID: 30994896.

[185] Lourbopoulos AI, Mourouzis IS, Trikas AG, Tseti IK, Pantos CI. Effects of Thyroid Hormone on Tissue Hypoxia: Relevance to Sepsis Therapy. J Clin Med. 2021;10(24):5855. Published 2021 Dec 14. doi:10.3390/jcm10245855

[186] Mancini A, Di Segni C, Raimondo S, et al. Thyroid Hormones, Oxidative Stress, and Inflammation. Mediators Inflamm. 2016;2016:6757154. doi:10.1155/2016/6757154

[187] Davies PH, Franklyn JA. The effects of drugs on tests of thyroid function. Eur J Clin Pharmacol. 1991;40(5):439-51. doi: 10.1007/BF00315221. PMID: 1884719.

[188] Ruiz-Núñez B, Tarasse R, Vogelaar EF, Janneke Dijck-Brouwer DA, Muskiet FAJ. Higher Prevalence of "Low T3 Syndrome" in Patients With Chronic Fatigue Syndrome: A Case-Control Study. Front Endocrinol (Lausanne). 2018;9:97. Published 2018 Mar 20. doi:10.3389/fendo.2018.00097

[189] Kobayashi R, Hasegawa M, Kawaguchi C, et al. Thyroid function in patients with selenium deficiency exhibits high free T4 to T3 ratio. Clin Pediatr Endocrinol. 2021;30(1):19-26. doi:10.1297/cpe.30.19

[190] Gilbert ME, O'Shaughnessy KL, Axelstad M. Regulation of Thyroid-disrupting Chemicals to Protect the Developing Brain. Endocrinology. 2020;161(10):bqaa106. doi:10.1210/endocr/bqaa106

[191] Mancini A, Di Segni C, Raimondo S, et al. Thyroid Hormones, Oxidative Stress, and Inflammation. Mediators Inflamm. 2016;2016:6757154. doi:10.1155/2016/6757154

[192] Roberts SC, Bianco AC, Stapleton HM. Disruption of type 2 iodothyronine deiodinase activity in cultured human glial cells by polybrominated diphenyl ethers. Chemical Research in Toxicology. 2015 Jun;28(6):1265-1274. DOI: 10.1021/acs.chemrestox.5b00072. PMID: 26004626; PMCID: PMC4827872.

[193] Guo Q, Wu Y, Hou Y, et al. Cytokine Secretion and Pyroptosis of Thyroid Follicular Cells Mediated by Enhanced NLRP3, NLRP1, NLRC4, and AIM2 Inflammasomes Are Associated With Autoimmune Thyroiditis. Front Immunol. 2018;9:1197. Published 2018 Jun 4. doi:10.3389/fimmu.2018.01197

194 Kawashima A, Yamazaki K, Hara T, Akama T, Yoshihara A, Sue M, Tanigawa K, Wu H, Ishido Y, Takeshita F, Ishii N, Sato K, Suzuki K. Demonstration of innate immune responses in the thyroid gland: potential to sense danger and a possible trigger for autoimmune reactions. Thyroid. 2013 Apr;23(4):477-87. doi: 10.1089/thy.2011.0480. Epub 2013 Mar 18. PMID: 23234343; PMCID: PMC3610444.

195 Fröhlich E, Wahl R. Thyroid Autoimmunity: Role of Anti-thyroid Antibodies in Thyroid and Extra-Thyroidal Diseases. Front Immunol. 2017;8:521. Published 2017 May 9. doi:10.3389/fimmu.2017.00521

CHAPTER 11

196 Pustorino S, Foti M, Calipari G, Pustorino E, Ferraro R, Guerrisi O, Germanotta G. Interazioni funzionali tra tiroide e motilità gastrointestinale [Thyroid-intestinal motility interactions summary]. Minerva Gastroenterol Dietol. 2004 Dec;50(4):305-15. Italian. PMID: 15788986.

197 J. Jung, C. H. Lee, S. H. Son, et al., "High Prevalence of Thyroid Disease and Role of Salivary Gland Scintigraphy in Patients with Xerostomia," *Nuclear Medicine and Molecular Imaging* 51, no. 2 (2017), 169–77, doi:10.1007/s13139-016-0455-4.

198 X. Sun, L. Lu, Y. Li, R. Yang, L. Shan, and Y. Wang, "Increased risk of thyroid disease in patients with Sjogren's syndrome: a systematic review and meta-analysis," *PeerJ*. 7, no. 6737 (March 19, 2019), doi:10.7717/peerj.6737.

199 Agha-Hosseini F, Shirzad N, Moosavi MS. Evaluation of Xerostomia and salivary flow rate in Hashimoto's Thyroiditis. Med Oral Patol Oral Cir Bucal. 2016;21(1):e1-e5. Published 2016 Jan 1. doi:10.4317/medoral.20559

200 R. Daher, T. Yazbeck, J. B. Jaoude, and B. Abboud, "Consequences of Dysthyroidism on the Digestive Tract and Viscera," World Journal of Gastroenterology 15, no. 23 (2009): 2834–8, doi:10.3748/wjg.15.2834

201 Olga Yaylali, Suna Kirac, Mustafa Yilmaz, et al., "Does Hypothyroidism Affect Gastrointestinal Motility?," Gastroenterology Research and Practice, vol. 2009, Article ID 529802, 7 pages, (2009), https://doi.org/10.1155/2009/529802

202 Ibid

203 A. D. Patil, "Link between Hypothyroidism and Small Intestinal Bacterial Overgrowth," Indian Journal of Endocrinology Metabolism 18, no. 3 (2014): 307–9, doi:10.4103/2230-8210.131155

204 Olga Yaylali, Suna Kirac, Mustafa Yilmaz, et al., "Does Hypothyroidism Affect Gastrointestinal Motility?," Gastroenterology Research and Practice, vol. 2009, Article ID 529802, 7 pages, (2009), https://doi.org/10.1155/2009/529802

205 A. D. Patil, "Link between Hypothyroidism and Small Intestinal Bacterial Overgrowth," Indian Journal of Endocrinology Metabolism 18, no. 3 (2014): 307–9, doi:10.4103/2230-8210.131155

206 Ernesto Cristiano Lauritano, Anna Lisa Bilotta, Maurizio Gabrielli, Emidio Scarpellini, Andrea Lupascu, Antonio Laginestra, Marialuisa Novi, et al., "Association Between Hypothyroidism and Small Intestinal Bacterial Overgrowth," Journal of Clinical Endocrinology & Metabolism 92, no. 11 (2007): 4180–4, https://doi.org/10.1210/jc.2007-0606

207 Rastgooye Haghi A, Solhjoo M, Tavakoli MH. Correlation Between Subclinical Hypothyroidism and Dyslipidemia. Iran J Pathol. 2017 Spring;12(2):106-111. Epub 2017 Apr 1. PMID: 29515631; PMCID: PMC5831065.

208 Rizos CV, Elisaf MS, Liberopoulos EN. Effects of thyroid dysfunction on lipid profile. Open Cardiovasc Med J. 2011;5:76-84. doi:10.2174/1874192401105010076

209 Duntas LH, Brenta G. A Renewed Focus on the Association Between Thyroid Hormones and Lipid Metabolism. Front Endocrinol (Lausanne). 2018 Sep 3;9:511. doi: 10.3389/fendo.2018.00511. PMID: 30233497; PMCID: PMC6129606.

210 Ibid

211 Afghani E, Lo SK, Covington PS, Cash BD, Pandol SJ. Sphincter of Oddi Function and Risk Factors for Dysfunction. Front Nutr. 2017;4:1. Published 2017 Jan 30. doi:10.3389/fnut.2017.00001

212 Hagit Shapiro, Aleksandra A. Kolodziejczyk, Daniel Halstuch, and Eran Elinav, "Bile Acids in Glucose Metabolism in Health and Disease," Journal of Experimental Medicine 215, no. 2 (2018): 383–96, doi:10.1084/jem.20171965

213 A. Eshraghian and A. Hamidian Jahromi, "Non-Alcoholic Fatty Liver Disease and Thyroid Dysfunction: a Systematic Review," World Journal of Gastroenterology 20, no. 25 (2014): 8102–9, doi:10.3748/wjg.v20.i25.8102

214 S. M. Abdalla and A. C. Bianco, "Defending Plasma T3 Is a Biological Priority," Clinical Endocrinology (Oxf). 81, no. 5 (2014): 633–41, doi:10.1111/cen.12538

215 https://www.niddk.nih.gov/health-information/endocrine-diseases/hypothyroidism

216 Rastgooye Haghi A, Solhjoo M, Tavakoli MH. Correlation Between Subclinical Hypothyroidism and Dyslipidemia. Iran J Pathol. 2017 Spring;12(2):106-111. Epub 2017 Apr 1. PMID: 29515631; PMCID: PMC5831065.
Rizos CV, Elisaf MS, Liberopoulos EN. Effects of thyroid dysfunction on lipid profile. Open Cardiovasc Med J. 2011;5:76-84. doi:10.2174/1874192401105010076

217 Duntas LH, Brenta G. A Renewed Focus on the Association Between Thyroid Hormones and Lipid Metabolism. Front Endocrinol (Lausanne). 2018 Sep 3;9:511. doi: 10.3389/fendo.2018.00511. PMID: 30233497; PMCID: PMC6129606.

218 Klein JR. The immune system as a regulator of thyroid hormone activity. Exp Biol Med (Maywood). 2006;231(3):229-236. doi:10.1177/153537020623100301

219 Kell DB, Pretorius E. No effects without causes: the Iron Dysregulation and Dormant Microbes hypothesis for chronic, inflammatory diseases. Biol Rev Camb Philos Soc. 2018;93(3):1518–1557. doi:10.1111/brv.12407

220 J. R. Klein, "The Immune System as a Regulator of Thyroid Hormone Activity," Experimental Biology and Medicine (Maywood) 231, no. 3 (2006): 229–36, doi:10.1177/153537020623100301

221 A. Kawashima, K. Yamazaki, T. Hara, et al., "Demonstration of Innate Immune Responses in the Thyroid Gland: Potential to Sense Danger and a Possible Trigger for Autoimmune Reactions," Thyroid 23, no. 4 (2013): 477–87, doi:10.1089/thy.2011.0480

222 L. Pesce and P. Kopp, "Iodide Transport: Implications for Health and Disease," International Journal of Pediatric Endocrinology 2014, no. 1 (2014): 8, doi:10.1186/1687-9856-2014-8

CHAPTER 12

[223] Saran S, Gupta BS, Philip R, et al. Effect of hypothyroidism on female reproductive hormones. Indian J Endocrinol Metab. 2016;20(1):108–113. doi:10.4103/2230-8210.172245

CHAPTER 15

[224] Koutras DA. Disturbances of menstruation in thyroid disease. Ann N Y Acad Sci. 1997;816:280–284. doi:10.1111/j.1749-6632.1997.tb52152.x
[225] Singla R, Gupta Y, Khemani M, Aggarwal S. Thyroid disorders and polycystic ovary syndrome: An emerging relationship. Indian J Endocrinol Metab. 2015;19(1):25–29. doi:10.4103/2230-8210.146860

CHAPTER 16

[226] Verma I, Sood R, Juneja S, Kaur S. Prevalence of hypothyroidism in infertile women and evaluation of response of treatment for hypothyroidism on infertility. Int J Appl Basic Med Res. 2012;2(1):17–19. doi:10.4103/2229-516X.96795
[227] Sarkar D. Recurrent pregnancy loss in patients with thyroid dysfunction. Indian J Endocrinol Metab. 2012;16(Suppl 2):S350–S351. doi:10.4103/2230-8210.104088
[228] Lee JH, Park YW, Lee SW. The Relationships between Thyroid Hormone Levels and Lower Urinary Tract Symptoms/Benign Prostatic Hyperplasia. World J Mens Health. 2019;37(3):364–371. doi:10.5534/wjmh.180084
[229] Chen D, Yan Y, Huang H, Dong Q, Tian H. The association between subclinical hypothyroidism and erectile dysfunction. Pak J Med Sci. 2018;34(3):621–625. doi:10.12669/pjms.343.14330
[230] Gabrielson AT, Sartor RA, Hellstrom WJG. The Impact of Thyroid Disease on Sexual Dysfunction in Men and Women. Sex Med Rev. 2019;7(1):57–70. doi:10.1016/j.sxmr.2018.05.002
[231] Bauer M, Heinz A, Whybrow PC. Thyroid hormones, serotonin and mood: of synergy and significance in the adult brain. Mol Psychiatry. 2002;7(2):140–156. doi:10.1038/sj.mp.4000963
[232] Sze M. Ng, Gabriella Watson, Mark A. Turner, Paul Newland, and A. Michael Weindling, "Is Dopamine an Iatrogenic Disruptor of Thyroid and Cortisol Function in the Extremely Premature Infant?," Advances in Endocrinology 2014, Article ID 973184 (2014), 4 pages, https://doi.org/10.1155/2014/973184
[233] E. Fröhlich and R. Wahl, "Thyroid Autoimmunity: Role of Anti-Thyroid Antibodies in Thyroid and Extra-Thyroidal Diseases," Frontiers in Immunology 8 (2017): 521, doi:10.3389/fimmu.2017.00521
[234] Shokri-Kojori E, Wang GJ, Wiers CE, Demiral SB, Guo M, Kim SW, Lindgren E, Ramirez V, Zehra A, Freeman C, Miller G, Manza P, Srivastava T, De Santi S, Tomasi

D, Benveniste H, Volkow ND. β-Amyloid accumulation in the human brain after one night of sleep deprivation. Proc Natl Acad Sci U S A. 2018 Apr 24;115(17):4483-4488. doi: 10.1073/pnas.1721694115. Epub 2018 Apr 9. PMID: 29632177; PMCID: PMC5924922.
235 Green ME, Bernet V, Cheung J. Thyroid Dysfunction and Sleep Disorders. Front Endocrinol (Lausanne). 2021 Aug 24;12:725829. doi: 10.3389/fendo.2021.725829. PMID: 34504473; PMCID: PMC8423342.
236 Cleveland Clinic, "Vital Signs," retrieved from https://my.clevelandclinic.org/health/articles/10881-vital-signs.
237 Robson A. Dyspnoea, hyperventilation and functional cough: a guide to which tests help sort them out. Breathe (Sheff). 2017 Mar;13(1):45-50. doi: 10.1183/20734735.019716. PMID: 28289450; PMCID: PMC5343732.
238 Steffen PR, Austin T, DeBarros A, Brown T. The Impact of Resonance Frequency Breathing on Measures of Heart Rate Variability, Blood Pressure, and Mood. Front Public Health. 2017;5:222. Published 2017 Aug 25. doi:10.3389/fpubh.2017.00222
239 Bernardi L, Sleight P, Bandinelli G, et al. Effect of rosary prayer and yoga mantras on autonomic cardiovascular rhythms: comparative study. BMJ. 2001;323(7327):1446-1449. doi:10.1136/bmj.323.7327.1446
240 M. A. Russo, D. M. Santarelli, and D. O'Rourke, the physiological effects of slow breathing in the healthy human. *Breathe* 12, no. 4 (2017), 298–309, doi: 10.1183/20734735.009817.

CHAPTER 17

241 Raymond St. Marie, and Kellie S. Talebkhah, "Neurological Evidence of a Mind-Body Connection: Mindfulness and Pain Control," American Journal of Psychiatry 13, no. 4 (2018): 2–3, doi:10.1176/appi.ajp-rj.2018.130401; Tarani Chandola, Eric Brunner, and Michael Marmot, "Chronic Stress at Work and the Metabolic Syndrome: Prospective Study," BMJ 332, no. 7540 (2006): 521–25, doi:10.1136/bmj.38693.435301.80
242 Ronald Glaser, and Janice K. Kiecolt-Glaser, "Stress-Induced Immune Dysfunction: Implications for Health," Nature Reviews Immunology 5, no. 3 (2005): 243–51, doi: 10.1038/nri1571; Leigh A. Rozlog, Janice Kiecolt-Glaser, Phillip T. Marucha, John F. Sheridan, and Ronald Glaser, "Stress and Immunity: Implications for Viral Disease and Wound Healing," Journal of Periodontology 70, no. 7 (1999): 786–92, doi:10.1902/jop.1999.70.7.786
243 Dan Malm, Bengt Fridlund, Helena Ekblad, Patric Karlström, Emma Hag, and Amir H. Pakpour, "Effects of Brief Mindfulness-Based Cognitive Behavioural Therapy on Health-Related Quality of Life and Sense of Coherence in Atrial Fibrillation Patients," European Journal of Cardiovascular Nursing 17, no. 7 (2018): 589–97, doi:10.1177/1474515118762796; Sonya Kim, Vance Zemon, Marie M. Cavallo, Joseph F. Rath, Rollin McCraty, and Frederick W. Foley, "Heart Rate Variability Biofeedback, Executive Functioning and Chronic Brain Injury," Brain Injury 27, no. 2 (2013): 209–22, doi:10.3109/02699052.2012.729292
244 Samereh Abdoli, Kobra Rahzani, Marjan Safaie, and Amin Sattari, "A Randomized Control Trial: The Effect of Guided Imagery with Tape and Perceived Happy Memory

on Chronic Tension Type Headache," Scandinavian Journal of Caring Sciences 26, no. 2 (2011): 254–61, doi: 10.1111/j.1471-6712.2011.00926.x; Victoria Kress, Nicole Adamson, Carrie Demarco, Matthew J. Paylo, and Chelsey A. Zoldan, "The Use of Guided Imagery as an Intervention in Addressing Non-Suicidal Self-Injury," Journal of Creativity in Mental Health 8, no. 1 (2013): 35–47, doi:10.1080/15401383.2013.763683

[245] Francine Shapiro, "The Role of Eye Movement Desensitization and Reprocessing (EMDR) Therapy in Medicine: Addressing the Psychological and Physical Symptoms Stemming from Adverse Life Experiences." Permanente Journal 18, no. 1 (2014): 71–7, doi:10.7812/TPP/13-098

[246] D. Church, A. De Asis, and A. J. Brooks, "Brief Group Intervention Using EFT (Emotional Freedom Techniques) for Depression in College Students: A Randomized Controlled Trial," *Depression Res Treat.* 57172 (2012), doi:10.1155/2012/257172.

CHAPTER 18

[247] Hart PD, Buck DJ. The effect of resistance training on health-related quality of life in older adults: Systematic review and meta-analysis. Health Promot Perspect. 2019;9(1):1–12. Published 2019 Jan 23. doi:10.15171/hpp.2019.01

[248] Tofas T, Draganidis D, Deli CK, Georgakouli K, Fatouros IG, Jamurtas AZ. Exercise-Induced Regulation of Redox Status in Cardiovascular Diseases: The Role of Exercise Training and Detraining. Antioxidants (Basel). 2019;9(1):13. Published 2019 Dec 23. doi:10.3390/antiox9010013

[249] Mcleod JC, Stokes T, Phillips SM. Resistance Exercise Training as a Primary Countermeasure to Age-Related Chronic Disease. Front Physiol. 2019;10:645. Published 2019 Jun 6. doi:10.3389/fphys.2019.00645

[250] Westcott WL. Resistance training is medicine: effects of strength training on health. Curr Sports Med Rep. 2012;11(4):209–216. doi:10.1249/JSR.0b013e31825dabb8

CHAPTER 20

[251] https://www.epa.gov/newsreleases/epa-releases-first-major-update-chemicals-list-40-years

[252] Krimsky S (2017) The unsteady state and inertia of chemical regulation under the US Toxic Substances Control Act. PLoS Biol 15(12): e2002404. https://doi.org/10.1371/journal.pbio.2002404

[253] Miller AB, Sears ME, Morgan LL, et al. Risks to Health and Well-Being From Radio-Frequency Radiation Emitted by Cell Phones and Other Wireless Devices. Front Public Health. 2019;7:223. Published 2019 Aug 13. doi:10.3389/fpubh.2019.00223

[254] Baby NM, Koshy G, Mathew A. The Effect of Electromagnetic Radiation due to Mobile Phone Use on Thyroid Function in Medical Students Studying in a Medical College in South India. Indian J Endocrinol Metab. 2017;21(6):797–802. doi:10.4103/ijem.IJEM_12_17

255. Mortavazi S, Habib A, Ganj-Karami A, Samimi-Doost R, Pour-Abedi A, Babaie A. Alterations in TSH and Thyroid Hormones following Mobile Phone Use. Oman Med J. 2009;24(4):274–278. doi:10.5001/omj.2009.56
256. Asl JF, Larijani B, Zakerkish M, Rahim F, Shirbandi K, Akbari R. The possible global hazard of cell phone radiation on thyroid cells and hormones: a systematic review of evidences. Environ Sci Pollut Res Int. 2019;26(18):18017–18031. doi:10.1007/s11356-019-05096-z
257. Alexx Stuart, personal communication.
258. Ghassabian A, Pierotti L, Basterrechea M, et al. Association of Exposure to Ambient Air Pollution With Thyroid Function During Pregnancy. JAMA Netw Open. 2019;2(10):e1912902. doi:10.1001/jamanetworkopen.2019.12902
259. Caitlin G. Howe, Sandrah P. Eckel, Rima Habre, et al. (2018) "Association of Prenatal Exposure to Ambient and Traffic-Related Air Pollution With Newborn Thyroid Function. Findings From the Children's Health Study" JAMA Network Open 1(5):e182172 doi: 10.1001/jamanetworkopen.2018.2172
260. Gawda A, Majka G, Nowak B, Marcinkiewicz J. Air pollution, oxidative stress, and exacerbation of autoimmune diseases. Cent Eur J Immunol. 2017;42(3):305–312. doi:10.5114/ceji.2017.70975
261. Fiore M, Oliveri Conti G, Caltabiano R, et al. Role of Emerging Environmental Risk Factors in Thyroid Cancer: A Brief Review. Int J Environ Res Public Health. 2019;16(7):1185. Published 2019 Apr 2. doi:10.3390/ijerph16071185
262. https://www.epa.gov/report-environment/indoor-air-quality
263. https://www.ewg.org/release/meets-all-government-standards-ewg-s-2019-tap-water-database-details-unsafe-contamination
264. Kim MJ, Moon S, Oh BC, et al. Association between perfluoroalkyl substances exposure and thyroid function in adults: A meta-analysis. PLoS One. 2018;13(5):e0197244. Published 2018 May 10. doi:10.1371/journal.pone.0197244
265. https://www.epa.gov/pfas/basic-information-pfas
266. Ghassabian A, Trasande L. Disruption in Thyroid Signaling Pathway: A Mechanism for the Effect of Endocrine-Disrupting Chemicals on Child Neurodevelopment. Front Endocrinol (Lausanne). 2018;9:204. Published 2018 Apr 30. doi:10.3389/fendo.2018.00204
267. https://money.howstuffworks.com/personal-finance/budgeting/10-marked-up-items-in-the-grocery-store.htm
268. https://www.rd.com/advice/saving-money/10-outrageous-markups-youd-never-guess-you-were-paying/
269. https://davidsuzuki.org/queen-of-green/dirty-dozen-cosmetic-chemicals-avoid/
270. Xu X, Liu A, Hu S, Ares I, Martínez-Larrañaga MR, Wang X, Martínez M, Anadón A, Martínez MA. Synthetic phenolic antioxidants: Metabolism, hazards and mechanism of action. Food Chem. 2021 Aug 15;353:129488. doi: 10.1016/j.foodchem.2021.129488. Epub 2021 Mar 5. PMID: 33714793.
271. Chung KT, Murdock CA, Stevens SE Jr, Li YS, Wei CI, Huang TS, Chou MW. Mutagenicity and toxicity studies of p-phenylenediamine and its derivatives. Toxicol Lett. 1995 Nov;81(1):23-32. doi: 10.1016/0378-4274(95)03404-8. PMID: 8525495.

272 Melnick RL, Mahler J, Bucher JR, Hejtmancik M, Singer A, Persing RL. Toxicity of diethanolamine. 2. Drinking water and topical application exposures in B6C3F1 mice. J Appl Toxicol. 1994 Jan-Feb;14(1):11-9. doi: 10.1002/jat.2550140104. PMID: 8157864.

273 Panchal, Sneha & Verma, Ramtej. (2016). Effect of diethanolamine on testicular steroidogenesis and its amelioration by curcumin. Asian Pacific Journal of Reproduction. 5. 10.1016/j.apjr.2016.01.008.

274 Estill M, Hauser R, Nassan FL, Moss A, Krawetz SA. The effects of di-butyl phthalate exposure from medications on human sperm RNA among men. Sci Rep. 2019 Aug 27;9(1):12397. doi: 10.1038/s41598-019-48441-5. PMID: 31455814; PMCID: PMC6711971.

275 National Research Council (US) Committee on Toxicology. Formaldehyde - An Assessment of Its Health Effects. Washington (DC): National Academies Press (US); 1980. EFFECTS ON HUMANS. Available from: https://www.ncbi.nlm.nih.gov/books/NBK217652/

276 Crinnion WJ. Toxic effects of the easily avoidable phthalates and parabens. Altern Med Rev. 2010 Sep;15(3):190-6. PMID: 21155623.

277 https://www.scientificamerican.com/article/toxic-perfumes-and-colognes/

278 Jang HJ, Shin CY, Kim KB. Safety Evaluation of Polyethylene Glycol (PEG) Compounds for Cosmetic Use. Toxicol Res. 2015;31(2):105-136. doi:10.5487/TR.2015.31.2.105

279 Dann AB, Hontela A. Triclosan: environmental exposure, toxicity and mechanisms of action. J Appl Toxicol. 2011 May;31(4):285-311. doi: 10.1002/jat.1660. PMID: 21462230.

CHAPTER 23

280 https://www.pharmacist.com/article/national-rx-drug-abuse-summit-pharmacists-role-responsibility

www.ingramcontent.com/pod-product-compliance
Lightning Source LLC
Chambersburg PA
CBHW020624220526
45464CB00001B/11